D0811346

NUTRITION, STRESS, AND TOXIC CHEMICALS

NUTRITION, STRESS, AND TOXIC CHEMICALS

An Approach to
Environment-Health
Controversies

Arthur J. Vander, M.D.

Ann Arbor   The University of Michigan Press

Library of Congress Cataloging in Publication Data

Vander, Arthur J   1933–
   Nutrition, stress, and toxic chemicals.

   Bibliography: p.
   Includes index.
   1.   Diseases—Causes and theories of causation.
2.   Environmentally induced diseases.   3.   Nutrition.
4.   Health.   I.   Title. [DNLM: 1. Diet—Adverse effects—
Popular works.   2.   Disease—Etiology—Popular works.
3.   Stress, Psychological—Popular works.   4.   Environ-
mental pollutants—Adverse effects—Popular works.
QZ 40 V228q]
RB151.V33   616.07′1   80-28078
ISBN 0-472-09329-0
ISBN 0-472-06329-4 (pbk.)

To Betsy, Eugene, and Jessica

Preface

States of health or disease are the expression of the success or failure experienced by the organism in its efforts to respond adaptively to environmental challenges.

René Dubos, *Man Adapting*

The skeptics in medicine have a hard time of it. It is much more difficult to be convincing about ignorance concerning disease mechanisms than when you are making claims for full comprehension, especially when the comprehension leads, logically or not, to some sort of action. When it comes to serious illness, the public tends, understandably, to be more skeptical about the skeptics, more willing to believe the true believers. It is medicine's oldest dilemma, not to be settled by candor or by any kind of rhetoric; what it needs is a lot of time and patience, waiting for science to come in, as it has in the past, with the solid facts.

Lewis Thomas, "On Magic in Medicine," *New England Journal of Medicine*

I know of no safe depository of the ultimate powers of society but the people themselves; and if we think them not enlightened enough to exercise their control with a wholesome discretion, the remedy is not to take it from them but to inform their discretion.

Thomas Jefferson

This book deals with the influence of certain environmental factors, broadly defined, on human health. It treats questions like: Do high-fat foods increase the risk of heart attacks? Does saccharin, when ingested in moderate amounts, cause cancer? Is "stress" a major cause of physical disease? Scientists have made enormous progress during the past few decades in their attempts at solving the causal mysteries of diseases such as cancer and heart disease, and one of my goals is to describe the present state of our knowledge in these areas. However, we clearly have a long way to go, and so I must emphasize immediately what the book does *not* do. It does not provide conclusive answers to any of the three questions raised above (or to many of the others which prey on our minds). The simple truth is that more often than not, the environmental causes of our modern scourges, including cancer and heart disease, remain uncertain. (There are exceptions: Despite the prattle of the tobacco industry, the evidence that cigarette smoking is the major cause of lung cancer is incontrovertible). Indeed, were answers available, my belief that there is a need for this book would be greatly diminished, for I am not concerned here with resolving any particular environment-health question but rather with the methods and information required to approach all such questions.

We are bombarded almost daily with conflicting pronouncements on the health consequences of environmental factors, many delivered with the utmost certainty and with ringing calls to action. The public is bewildered as to why scientists cannot agree among themselves, and many persons turn away altogether from scientifically based medicine and public health. Some of the blame for this situation lies with scientists themselves, for we have often made pronouncements unjustified by the strength of our evidence and have raised expectations out of proportion to what our state of knowledge permitted us to deliver. At least an equal fraction of blame must fall on popular writers who have churned out how-to-live-to-one-hundred books and articles based on poorly documented or nonexistent scientific data. The medical fields most subject to this kind of popular treatment are those which deal with the role of food, stress, and potentially harmful nonnutritive man-made environmental chemicals.

But the major reason for so much of our confusion and uncertainty in these areas is simply that the research required to answer questions such as those raised above is extremely difficult to perform. As Lewis Thomas, a prominent medical researcher and administrator (and author of *Lives of a Cell*), comments, we need "a lot of time and patience," and, I would add, a good deal of public understanding, interest, and support. The major aim of this book is to enhance understanding, with the hope that interest and support will follow.

I have been guided in this endeavor by one overriding principle: There are no shortcuts to an understanding of both our present state of knowledge and the research techniques used to obtain this knowledge. A major problem in most science writing for the public or for college students is that the reader is simply told what the writer believes to be the truth but is rarely shown, except in a very superficial way, the basic information and research which underlie the final conclusion. For example, that saccharin causes bladder cancer in mice is the "truth," and that this has been observed only when extremely large doses of saccharin are used is the superficial description of the research underlying this truth. I believe it is not very convincing to the lay public to add either that "these high doses are absurd and have no relevance for people" or that "use of these high doses is the standard procedure in cancer tests and they are quite relevant to people." There is no substitute here for fighting one's way through several pages of theory and calculations in order really to see which of these statements should be given credence.

Let me hasten to add that mastery of the level of scientific knowledge required to understand the bases of most environment-health controversies is well within the capabilities of any intelligent layperson with no previous scientific background. In some circles, it has become fashionable to deny this, to argue that the scientific bases of these controversies are so complex that even scientists often can't understand them. I firmly believe this to be the exception rather than the rule; it is your health and life which is at stake, and I'll take my stand with Thomas Jefferson that it is the responsibility of those who possess the knowledge to try to "inform [the public's] discretion."

The first chapter of this book is really the most important one. It briefly describes the scientific methodology used to approach any environment-health controversy, emphasizing particularly the potential weaknesses and sources of misinterpretation in each method. The second chapter takes off from the quote by René Dubos cited at the beginning of this preface. Our bodies are not passively acted upon by environmental factors, but attempt to respond adaptively to them, and these responses must be taken into account in any attempt to understand how disease might arise.

Thus, these first two chapters provide our "first principles." Each subsequent chapter then presents either the additional general concepts germane to the field under discussion (nutrition, for example) or a detailed analysis of a specific controversy in that field. My choice in this latter regard, although to a large degree arbitrary, has been guided by considerations of contemporary interest, importance, and how well the controversy illustrates potential scientific errors and sources of confusion. In particular, I have chosen several controversies which deal with our two major killers—cancer and heart disease—and have included detailed analyses of the basic processes involved in these diseases, irrespective of cause.

Again, I wish to emphasize that my aim has not been to "settle" these controversies. Accordingly, I have not multiplied examples unnecessarily simply because there are so many interesting ones. So it is almost certain you will not find some of the questions you may find most pressing (the effects of radiation, physical inactivity or exercise, salt, sugar, oral contraceptives, etc.). My hope is that, having completed this book, you will be able not only to follow future developments in the specific controversies I have chosen to cover, but also to apply what you have learned to those controversies I have not described. You should at least know the right questions to ask and be able to tell when you are being sold a bill of goods.

Also, I have not restricted myself to environmental "hazards" but have tried to emphasize that the approach one uses to evaluate hazard is really the same as that which must be applied to the positive goal of defining an optimal environment. The questions, How much dietary iron is harmful? and How much dietary iron is ideal? require similar approaches and types of information for their answers.

Finally, a word about documentation and references. I have in no way attempted to deal with my subject material in the comprehensive systematic manner scholars use when writing for their peers; for this reason I have chosen not to burden the pages with voluminous footnotes and references. I have, of course, provided (in the notes) citations for any quotations used and have also cited research studies which I deal with in detail or which are particularly critical for the controversy in question. The suggested readings at the back of the book are a very small sampling of the works I have used in preparing this book; they are, for the most part, review articles (rather than original research papers) which should permit the reader to go into any given subject in more detail. The extensive bibliographies in many of them also provide to an interested reader an efficient entry to the original scientific literature.

Contents

Part I | First Principles

Chapter 1 | Methods for Detecting Environmental Factors in Disease

Disease Patterns

There is no better illustration of the impact of a changing environment than the profound alteration of disease patterns which has occurred in the United States (and all other Westernized or "developed" nations) during the past 100 years (Table 1–1). Infectious diseases such as influenza, pneumonia, and tuberculosis were the major killers a century ago, but their place has now been taken by the so-called chronic degenerative diseases, notably cardiovascular diseases (those involving the heart and blood vessels), and cancer. No one doubts that the decrease in the infectious diseases was due to environmental alteration—modern sanitation, better nutrition, vaccines, and (to a much lesser extent) specific medical therapies. The assumption is often made that, with the "conquest" of the serious infectious diseases, people are simply living to be old enough to succumb eventually to the chronic degenerative diseases. There is certainly a good deal of truth to this view for in most societies the incidence of cardiovascular diseases and cancer do increase with age.* But this view ignores several striking facts. First, these diseases do not strike only the aged—cancer is the second leading cause

---

*Disease rates are usually given in terms either of incidence—the number of new cases per year in a particular population (usually per 100,000 persons)—or of mortality rate—the number of people in the population who die of the disease over a given time period (also per 100,000 population).

TABLE 1–1   The Ten Leading Causes of Death in the United States in 1900 and 1975

Rank	Cause of Death	Crude Death Rate per 100,000 Population	Percentage of Total Deaths
	1900		
	All causes	1,719.1	100.0
1	Influenza and pneumonia	202.2	11.8
2	Tuberculosis	194.4	11.3
3	Gastroenteritis	142.7	8.3
4	Diseases of heart	137.4	8.0
5	Cerebral hemorrhage	106.9	6.2
6	Chronic nephritis (kidney disease)	81.0	4.7
7	Accidents	72.3	4.2
8	Cancer	64.0	3.7
9	Certain diseases of infancy	62.6	3.6
10	Diphtheria	40.3	2.3
	1975		
	All causes	888.9	100.0
1	Diseases of heart	336.2	37.8
2	Cancer	171.7	19.3
3	Stroke	91.1	10.3
4	Accidents	48.4	5.4
5	Influenza and pneumonia	26.1	2.9
6	Diabetes mellitus (sugar diabetes)	16.5	1.9
7	Cirrhosis of liver	14.8	1.7
8	Arteriosclerosis	13.6	1.5
9	Suicide	12.7	1.4
10	Diseases of infancy	12.5	1.4

Source: From S. S. Epstein, *The Politics of Cancer*, (San Francisco: Sierra Club Books, 1978), p. 16.
1900 data: "Facts of Life and Death," National Center for Health Statistics, Public Health Service Publication no. 600,
1970, table 12; 1975 data: American Cancer Society, "1978 Cancer Facts and Figures" (New York, 1977).

of deaths in males for all age-groups except 15 to 34 years and in females for all ages up to 75 years, except 35 to 54 years, when it is the leading disease! Second, these diseases are not inexorable concomitants of aging, as evidenced by their profoundly different incidences in any given age-group from society to society; in some, the entire relationship between age and cardiovascular diseases is shifted upward twenty to thirty years (for example, 70-to-80-year-old Japanese, until recently at least, manifested the same mortality rate from heart attacks as did 50-to-60-year-old Americans).

Evidence from a comparison of different societies is, of course, always subject to the criticism that differences in disease incidences simply reflect genes, not environment. While this is certainly true with regard to some diseases, genetic variability among populations does not seem to make a major contribution to the interpopulation differences in cardiovascular and cancer rates. We know this because, in the great majority of cases, people emigrating from one place to another take on most of the disease incidence characteristics of their new homeland within a few generations, even when the emigrants and their children tend to marry exclusively within their own group. For example, Japanese-American men in the San Francisco Bay area who have taken on an American life-style have essentially the same incidence of coronary heart disease as white native Americans, five times higher than the rate for age-matched native Japanese or Japanese-Americans in the same area who live a traditional Japanese life-style. That more than one generation is often required to achieve the pattern typical of the new country reflects not only the time required for culturally determined patterns such as diet to shift but also the fact that the offspring are subjected to the new environment for an entire lifetime, including the *in utero* period. The role of environmental exposure during these early periods is further illustrated by at least one striking exception to the generalizations just stated. The incidences of a few forms of cancer change in the first generation of immigrants only if the change of country occurs before the age of 10; beyond that age, the incidence typical of the original country persists in the first generation, but not in their offspring. It appears that the environmental factors mainly responsible for the ultimate development of these particular cancers later in life have already done their dirty work during the early years of life.

One need not look only at differences between countries, for changes of incidences over time within a single country may be just as striking (as I'll describe in detail later, such comparisons must take into account the relative numbers of older persons in the country at different times). In our own country, this is the case for a large number of diseases, not just the major killers; in the past seventy-five years the incidence of gallstones has increased many hundred-fold, small benign tumors of the large intestine at least one hundredfold, appendicitis fiftyfold, and varicose veins twentyfold.

Similar types of evidence come from a speeding up of the time machine within a single country—the changes that occur when a group of people remain in their own country but move rapidly toward Westernization. The changes that occur in disease are quite similar to those which characterize immigrants to Westernized countries. Thus, the incidence of hypertension (high blood pressure) has skyrocketed in urbanizing blacks in the United States and in Zulus in South Africa.

Taken altogether, the evidence strongly favors the view that the diseases characteristic of industrialized Westernized societies reflect, in large part, the environmental factors present there (diet, degree of stress, environmental chemicals, noise, etc.). These diseases are distinct from what we now recognize as the "aging process"—the progressive loss of cells and malfunction of those cells which remain—but they interact with this process in a vicious cycle, each accelerating the other.

There is little doubt, therefore, that the new killers depend, like the infectious diseases before them, on environmental factors for their emergence. We have come to recognize that it may be more meaningful to speak of "risk factors" rather than of *specific* causes in describing the etiology of many diseases. Unfortunately, the term risk factor is used in several ways by different scientists. It was coined by epidemiologists who, as described later in this chapter, study the association of various factors—diet, cigarette smoking, exposure to noise, industrial and environmental chemicals, etc.— with disease frequency. When a particular factor is found to be associated with a higher incidence of a specific disease, it is termed a risk factor for that disease. This definition, then, does not require that a risk factor actually play a causal role in the disease but rather that it simply have value in predicting the likelihood of the disease developing. Many scientists, however, use the term risk factor only when there is good reason to believe that the factor really plays a causal role in the disease. Atherosclerosis (the occlusive disease of arteries which leads to heart attacks and strokes) is a classic example; it does not have a simple "cause," but instead results from many interplaying environmental factors (diet, smoking, physical inactivity, psychosocial stress, to name just a few of the suspected culprits). The degree of influence of each factor differs to some degree from person to person because of genetic differences. In some diseases, a single factor may be so all-important that it really rates the term "specific cause" (the chemicals in cigarette smoke and lung cancer, for example) but even here, other factors almost always contribute. This is not really a new concept in medicine, for we have recognized for years that environmental factors, malnutrition for example, could greatly enhance the ability of microbes (the "specific cause") to induce disease.

To reemphasize these generalizations, let us look at the situation for cancer, for which exists some of the most convincing evidence relating environmental factors to differences in worldwide incidence rates. Comparisons of these incidences have led to the informed consensus that in approximately 80 to 90 percent of all cancers, environmental factors play important causal roles. The logic is as follows: Cancer incidence and mortality are measured in as many countries as possible. Those countries with the lowest rate for a particular type of cancer are assumed to establish the so-called background rate for that type, i.e., these populations are affected minimally, if at all, by the dominant (unidentified) environmental factor for that type of cancer. The higher cancer rates for all other countries are then attributed to environmental factors (again, unidentified) peculiar to them. Some of the differences between countries probably reflect differences in detection mechanisms and reporting procedures, but these potential sources of inaccuracy are dwarfed by the often huge differences in rates, sometimes as much as 2,000 percent (a twentyfold difference) between the highest and lowest countries.

Genetic differences seem to play a relatively small role in these population differences, as evidenced by the types of emigrant studies mentioned earlier. For example, cancer of the stomach is much commoner in Japan than in America, but cancer of the large intestine, breast, and prostate is much less common. When Japanese migrate to America they take on the American cancer rates for these organs within two generations. Moreover, studies comparing cancer incidences in identical and nonidentical twins (of the same sex) have generally provided little evidence for a strong contribution of genetic constitution.

This is not to deny that genetic differences play some role in susceptibility to cancer. At least one rare genetic abnormality, characterized by loss of the usual repair mechanisms for DNA (see chap. 8), is associated with an extremely high rate of skin cancer. Some cancers also tend to run in families (cancer of the breast, for example, is twice as common in close relatives of patients with breast cancer than in the general population), but, of course, close relatives tend to share the same environment. Finally, as we shall see in chapter 8, there are, in fact, strong theoretical reasons, relating to the body's handling of carcinogenic substances, for believing that genetic differences between individuals (though probably not between entire populations) do play some role in determining just which people, exposed to an environmental carcinogen, will actually develop cancer.

Notice that the logic used in this type of interpopulation analysis does not require any information whatever as to what the relevant environmental factors are, but once a high-risk country for a particular cancer type has been identified, the search is then on for the "peculiar" factor. In many cases it has been identified (for example, the almost fiftyfold higher incidence of mouth cancer in Asia than in America is due to the habit of chewing betel nuts and tobacco leaves), and this, of course, lends further support to the correctness of the logic behind the inference.

The same logic has been used to evaluate the role of environmental changes in a single country over time in disease causation (table 1–1). For example, in 1900 the death rate per 100,000 population in the United States from all forms of cancer was 64.0 and in 1975 it was 171.7, almost a threefold increase. Such numbers are often cited to argue that changes in our environment during the past seventy-five years have caused an epidemic of cancers to emerge. This statement is an exaggeration because it fails to take the aging of our population into account. Since we know that the chances of cancer developing definitely increase with age, then even had all environmental risk factors for cancer remained absolutely constant during the past seventy-five years, the cancer rate would have increased, approximately in proportion to the increased fraction of aged persons in our population. (Notice that I am not saying that aging, per se, causes cancer, only that whatever does cause it is more likely to do so with increased age.) Fortunately statisticians can take this into account either by calculating rates for specific age groups (say 50-to-60-year-olds) or by use of a more complex process which gives a single age-adjusted incidence or mortality rate for the entire population. When this is done, a much less catastrophic picture emerges; taking age into account, the death rate from all cancers has increased only 11 percent in the past forty years.

However, before allowing this number to lull you into the secure feeling that maybe our environment hasn't changed too badly vis-à-vis carcinogens after all, recognize that cancer has a very long latent period and the rates of today reflect exposures of twenty to forty years ago; if the major increase in environmental carcinogens has occurred during the past thirty years, we may be only beginning to see the results now. Disturbingly, the overall age-adjusted cancer rate seems to be rising presently at 1 to 2 percent per year for white Americans. For black Americans the situation is far worse; from 1949 to 1967, while the age-adjusted cancer mortality for whites rose 3 percent, that for blacks rose 32 percent, a true epidemic! This has been ascribed to the increasing affluence of blacks, with its accompanying changes in diet and personal habits, or to their mass migration to the North and into cities with the resultant increased exposure to environmental pollutants, but the real factors are not yet known.

The discussion of the previous two paragraphs focused only on total cancer rates. A truer picture of the contribution of changing environmental factors in the United States emerges when one looks at age-standardized cancer incidence rates for individual body sites (table 1–2); for example, from 1937 to 1969, lung cancer in white males increased 133 percent, whereas stomach cancer in the same group decreased 59 percent. Thus the 11 percent change in total cancer incidence masks the fact that environmental factors for specific cancers really are changing markedly, some down and some up.

The fact that the incidence rates of a large number of specific cancers are decreasing is a reminder that not all environmental changes in the century have favored the growth of cancer, but should also serve as reinforcement for the view that cancer is, in

TABLE 1–2   Changes in Age-Standardized Cancer Incidence from 1937 to 1969.

Cancer Site	Group[a]	Percent Changes 1937–47	Percent Changes 1947–69	Net Change 1937–69
Esophagus	WM	6	−28	Down
	WF	19	−18	Down
	BM	62	101	Up[b]
	BF	57	89	Up[b]
Stomach	WM	−23	−59	Down
	WF	−30	−67	Down
	BM	3	−48	Down
	BF	3	−56	Down
Colon	WM	17	26	Up
	WF	16	−1	Up
	BM	5	90	Up[b]
	BF	37	129	Up[b]
Rectum	WM	16	−22	Down
	WF	25	−29	Down
	BM	59	3	Up
	BF	62	−27	Up
Pancreas	WM	33	22	Up
	WF	12	21	Up
	BM	132	30	Up[b]
	BF	88	127	Up[b]
Lung	WM	115	133	Up[b]
	WF	63	108	Up[b]
	BM	202	234	Up[b]
	BF	71	213	Up[b]
Breast	WF	10	4	Up
	BF	9	25	Up
Uterus	WF	−6	−37	Down
	BF	−12	−49	Down
Ovary	WF	16	−10	Up
	BF	80	16	Up
Prostate	WM	17	23	Up
	BM	63	55	Up[b]
Bladder	WM	22	21	Up
	WF	8	−26	Down
	BM	25	118	Up[b]
	BF	44	−43	Down

Source: From S. S. Epstein, *The Politics of Cancer* (San Francisco: Sierra Club Books, 1978), pp. 18–19. Data from S. J. Cutler and S. S. Devesa, "Trends in Cancer Incidence and Mortality in the USA," in *Host Environment Interactions in the Etiology of Cancer in Man,* ed. R. Doll and I. Vodopija (Lyon, France: International Agency for Research on Cancer, 1973), pp. 15–34.
[a]*WM* = white male; *WF* = white female; *BM* = black male; *BF* = black female.
[b]Total increase exceeds 75 percent.

large part, environmentally induced and can, therefore, be prevented, at least in theory. The "in theory" qualification denotes the fact that, even though an environmental factor is known, it may be impossible to avoid it completely. Sunlight, for example, is probably the major causal environmental factor for the development of skin cancer.

Investigation of Suspected Causal Factors

How do scientists determine just which environmental influences are causal factors for cardiovascular diseases, cancer, liver disease, and other illnesses? Similarly, in a more positive vein, how do they identify what we might call "antirisk factors," influences which optimize health and oppose the development of disease? (Because it would be cumbersome in the remainder of this chapter to add constantly the phrase "antirisk factors" each time it is relevant, the reader should simply assume that the investigatory methods to be described apply equally to the determination of beneficial influences even though reference is made only to disease-producing factors.) One must acquire at least a passing acquaintance with the major types of experiments since much of our present state of uncertainty concerning the scientific facts of any particular controversy stems from problems and limitations in these methods. This chapter will describe mainly the basic principles of such methods, and other chapters will go into the details of specific tests, for example, those used to detect a chemical's likelihood of producing cancer in experimental animals.

One approach to identifying causal factors is to try to discover the biologic mechanisms of the disease, for example, how an atherosclerotic plaque forms in an arterial wall, and then to reason backward from the mechanism to the cause. For example, when researchers found that the dominant component of atherosclerotic plaques is cholesterol, it was logical to hypothesize that a high dietary cholesterol intake might be an important causal factor in the genesis of the plaque. Such a hypothesis can then be subjected to experimental verification. Deductions such as these can be extremely useful in pointing experimental directions to be taken but one must never be seduced by their plausibility into believing that they, in themselves, constitute proof. For the latter, we must depend upon two broad types of research—epidemiology and controlled experiments with human subjects and laboratory animals.

Epidemiology

A discipline which has served medicine well since earliest times, epidemiology is the search for causes of a disease by an attempt to identify the characteristics, both personal and environmental, common to those contracting it. Epidemiologists generally do not manipulate either the environment or the subjects of their studies, but rather make use of the "natural experiments" that people perform on themselves (by smoking or not smoking, consuming different foods, etc.) or that society inflicts on them (by releasing industrial chemicals into the environment, raising the noise level, etc.). Because of the justifiable constraints on human experimentation in the realm of deliberate exposure to potentially toxic environmental factors, epidemiological studies are often the only form of human studies possible. Virtually all the data cited in the first part of this chapter were epidemiological data.

The successes of epidemiology in providing crucial clues to the causal factors in a host of infectious diseases—cholera, yellow fever, and malaria, to name a few—are well known, but epidemiology has had a rougher time with our modern killers because of the complexity of their causes and the long time delays in their development. Nevertheless, epidemiological evidence is often the first clue that a problem exists, as was true for lung cancer and smoking, and sometimes the only one as to cause and prevention (the case for skin cancer and workers' exposure to arsenic).

The basic epidemiological approach is to compare several groups of people that are similar except for some particular factor—the suspected risk factor. The questions take the form: Do workers in plants manufacturing DDT have a higher incidence of bladder cancer than workers of similar age, race, and socioeconomic status who work in automobile factories? Do people drinking fluoridated water have fewer dental caries than those in similar communities having nonfluoridated water? Are the offspring of mothers who smoke smaller than those of similar nonsmoking mothers? Do people who eat large quantities of animal fat suffer more heart attacks than those who do not?

The two basic types of epidemiological studies are retrospective and prospective. In a retrospective (or case-control) study, patients with a particular disease are located and are asked a variety of questions concerning their personal habits, both past and present, and their home and work environments, with emphasis, of course, upon those characteristics suspected of being causal factors in their disease. Their characteristics are then compared, using appropriate statistical methods, to those of a control group of persons who are either healthy or suffering from some unrelated disease. In this way, certain personal habits, environmental exposures, and bodily changes (if physical and chemical measurements of the subjects are a part of the study) can be associated with increased (or decreased) frequency of a particular disease. The best-known example of such a relationship is, of course, smoking and lung cancer.

One important potential defect in retrospective studies is that the presence of the disease being investigated may, itself, have important effects on the individual. For example, a retrospective study of patients with stomach cancer would be likely to reveal that affected persons are more depressed, eat less food, and get less sleep than do healthy control persons. It would be absurd to conclude, on this basis, that risk factors for stomach cancer include depression, poor nutrition, and inadequate sleep, since the causal sequence is much more likely in the opposite direction. In addition, persons who already have a disease are usually aware of suspected risk factors in their disease and are much more likely to recall (or exaggerate) that particular habit or environmental exposure than is a person in the control group.

Because the long-term prospective study avoids, to a large extent, these particular problems, it is usually considered to be more conclusive than a retrospective study, but it is expensive and time-consuming. Prospective studies begin with the selection of a presumably healthy group of subjects, and gather as much information as possible about them at the outset. Then they are followed closely over a period of years to determine which of them contract or die from a specific disease. Such a study for lung cancer was begun in 1959 by the American Cancer Society, and involved approximately one million subjects for a dozen years.

A third type of epidemiological approach is really a variant of the retrospective study, one which ignores individuals and simply correlates the overall rates of various diseases with geographical location. For example, such studies have revealed that urban areas of the United States, particularly those in which petrochemical industries are located, have much higher per capita rates of many cancers than do rural areas. Many examples of such types of study were presented in the first part of this chapter.

These descriptions make it all sound very simple, but in fact, epidemiological studies of chronic diseases, whether retrospective or prospective, are subject to many problems, some inherent in the methodology, some due to poor design of the specific study. First of all, a very large number of subjects is usually required in order for statistical analysis of the data to be meaningful (just what is meant by "statistical analysis" will be described later). For example, one American out of approximately 2,500 will develop lung cancer this year. Clearly if you were doing a prospective study on risk factors for lung cancer, you would have to include a huge number of people in your study (as the 1959 project cited earlier did) in order to insure that enough cases of the disease would develop to work with. This is particularly true when the disease in question has a high background incidence due to risk factors other than the one being studied. For example, because skin cancer is a relatively common form of cancer, its major cause being solar radiation, trying to detect a further increase in skin cancer, due say to a particular cosmetic, is a very difficult task. The problem of numbers applies equally to retrospective studies, and one aid in the identification of a sufficient number of cases of the disease to be studied has been the establishment of state or national registries in which are recorded all new cases of that disease.

A second problem which can prevent the epidemiological discovery of relevant risk factors is the long period of time it takes for chronic disease to develop. Cancer, for example, may have a latency period of many years between exposure to the risk factor and disease manifestation (twenty to forty years, for example, for smoking and lung cancer). It is an incredibly difficult task to follow huge numbers of people for these periods of time. For this reason, some of our best epidemiological data comes from two entire towns—Framingham, Massachusetts, and Tecumseh, Michigan—which have been studied intensively and continuously by epidemiologists for many years.

Retrospective studies are also plagued by such long latencies because it is extremely difficult for people to recall accurately just what they used to eat, how much they smoked, how much they weighed, and so on, for the past twenty years. Similarly, it is equally difficult for the epidemiologist to ascertain just what chemicals, radiation, noise levels, etc., may have been present in the persons' homes or job locations so many years ago.

The longer a prospective study goes on, the more likely it is that a third problem becomes dominant—subjects dropping out or being lost track of. If these occurrences were random, it would not be so bad, but they are often related to the disease itself, or to one of the potential risk factors being studied. For example, suppose a study were being conducted in a town concerning the possible role of job stress in the development of heart disease; if all those with the greatest job stress left the town (because of the stress) and were lost to the study, the results would clearly be useless. To take another example, cited by Dr. Samuel S. Epstein (professor of occupational and environmental medicine, University of Illinois), who believes that inadequate follow-up is the most common error in conducting prospective studies[1]: Industry studies on retirees often find living retirees in a far greater percentage than they find the death certificates of retirees who have died; this, of course, causes a serious underestimate of the death rate for people in that industry.

A fourth problem is that of using the wrong control population. If you wished to study the effect of smoking on death rate, it would be absurd to compare 30-year-old smokers to 60-year-old nonsmokers; the nonsensical conclusion from such a study would almost certainly be that smokers have a lower death rate than do nonsmokers. Age, health status unrelated to the disease being studied, socioeconomic class, sex, genetic background, and many other variables must be matched as closely as possible (unless, of course, one of these variables is the very one being evaluated in the epidemiological study) or else taken into account in the data analysis.

The example I just presented is, of course, ludicrous, but unfortunately there are many others which are much more subtle. Dr. Epstein points out that industrial epidemiological studies often compare a particular disease's rate in the company's workers to that of the general population; this is not acceptable, since the general population includes disabled and chronically ill persons, whereas the industrial population is healthy enough to work.[2] In other words, an increment in disease rate caused by some factor in the working place may be masked by a larger incidence rate in the general population due to other risk factors. As Dr. Epstein concludes, "the only meaningful comparison group for any given work force under investigation is a control group of workers from other industries where there is no exposure to the suspected [risk factors]."[3]

There are still more pitfalls in epidemiological methodology, but the ones I have described should suffice to emphasize this critical generalization: Failure to obtain in any given epidemiological study a significant correlation between the incidence of a disease and a suspected risk factor for that disease proves nothing. What credence should we give the conclusion from a company's epidemiological survey of its workers that a particular industrial chemical does *not* cause cancer when the survey used very few workers, failed to provide adequate follow-up, used an unacceptable control group, and looked at workers exposed for only three years? But even when a study has been carried out properly with large numbers, adequate follow-up, and so on, the difficulties inherent in epidemiological studies are so great that the results of a single negative study usually cannot be taken as conclusive.

Suppose that, despite all these difficulties, a significant association *is* revealed in an epidemiological study. We now have to face not a problem of methodology but one of inference, the crucial inference at the heart of epidemiological research: Is the association simply fortuitous or is it causal? The tobacco companies have never denied that cigarette smoking is associated with an increased incidence of lung cancer, but they do deny that one causes the other. There is something about cigarette smokers, they argue, that causes some people not only to smoke but to develop lung cancer; perhaps they are genetically different or perhaps they do something in association with their smoking, and that "something" is the real culprit.

This argument capitalizes on a truth recognized by all epidemiologists: Association can never absolutely prove causality. Remember that epidemiological studies are not controlled studies, in the sense of all variables, except the one being evaluated, maintained constant (as we'll see is the goal in the next category of experiments to be described). People who smoke are very likely, as a group, to be different from nonsmokers in ways other than smoking, which accounts for their choosing to become smokers in the first place. They were not placed into the smoking or nonsmoking group by experimenters, they chose their group by their previous actions. All the epidemiologist can do is to try to think of all the other ways they might be different (socioeconomic class, religion, coffee drinking, etc.) and match them to the nonsmoking group as best he can, but he well knows that a complete match is impossible. Indeed, where really important "other" variables cannot be matched, the study may simply not be worth doing.

A classic example is the one dealing with London busmen. A comparison of drivers, who of course were sedentary throughout their shift, with ticket-takers, who were constantly walking up and down the stairs of the double-deck buses, revealed that the drivers had a significantly higher incidence of heart attacks. This finding was hailed widely as strong evidence for a protective effect of exercise; the truth is that exercise *might* account for the differences, but so might other variables. For one thing, the men had not been arbitrarily assigned by the bus company to one or the other of the two jobs, but had chosen, themselves, to be drivers or ticket-collectors. As you might predict, those choosing to be drivers had quite different characteristics than did those opting for ticket-collector; they ate more, were significantly heavier, and had very different personalities, just to name a few. A second problem in this study is that the drivers and ticket-takers were exposed on the job not just to different levels of physical activity but to different degrees of stress as well, and no attempt was made to evaluate this other suspected risk factor. All in all, the busmen study really should never have been done, for there were simply too many confounding variables for it to serve as a meaningful test of exercise.

So we must agree with the tobacco industry that epidemiological studies alone never absolutely prove causality, but in the next breath we must emphasize that 100 percent proof is a rarity in any type of science, and that epidemiology alone *can* provide very convincing, if not absolute, evidence. Sir Arthur Bradford Hill, professor emeritus of medical statistics, University of London, has provided a clear-headed approach to the problem:

> We have this situation. Our [epidemiological] observations reveal an association between two variables, perfectly clear-cut and beyond what we would care to attribute to the play of chance. What aspects of that association should we especially consider before deciding that the most likely interpretation of it is causation?[4]

He then provides his list of attributes, including, among others, strength of the association, consistency, specificity, biological gradient, plausibility, and temporality. Let us look at each of these.

His reasons for assigning prime importance to the strength of the association is illustrated by smoking, lung cancer, and coronary thrombosis (heart attacks).

Prospective inquiries into smoking have shown that the death rate from cancer of the lung in cigarette smokers is nine to ten times the rate in nonsmokers and the rate in heavy cigarette smokers is twenty to thirty times as great. On the other hand, the death rate from coronary thrombosis in smokers is no more than twice, possibly less, the death rate in nonsmokers. Though there is good evidence to support causation [vis-à-vis heart attacks] it is surely much easier in this case to think of some features of life that may go hand-in-hand with smoking, features that might conceivably be the real underlying cause or, at the least, an important contributor, whether it be lack of exercise, nature of diet, or other factors. But to explain the pronounced excess in cancer of the lung in any other environmental [and, I would add, genetic] terms requires some feature of life so intimately linked with cigarette smoking and with the amount of smoking that such a feature should be easily detectable. If we cannot detect it or reasonably infer a specific one, then in such circumstances I think we are reasonably entitled to reject the vague contention of the armchair critic "you can't prove it, there may be such a feature."[5]

Moreover, one must not push the demand for strength of association to absurd lengths, as the tobacco industry does when, ignoring the certainty that multiple risk factors and differences in genetic susceptibility always exist for any disease, it argues nonsensically that the association between smoking and lung cancer can't be causal because lots of people smoke yet don't get cancer. Not all people who are exposed to the tubercle bacillus get tuberculosis, either, but that is because other factors are involved in resistance to the tubercle bacillus, not because this bacterium doesn't really cause tuberculosis. Similarly, a few people (very few indeed!) don't smoke, yet get lung cancer anyway, and different populations with the same degree of smoking manifest different rates of lung cancer (but within every population studied, there is an internal correlation between smoking and lung cancer).

Consistency of the association is the second most important characteristic for implicating causality. Has the relationship been repeatedly observed by different persons, in different places, circumstances, and times? By 1964 the association of smoking with lung cancer had been found in twenty-nine retrospective and seven prospective studies, with none finding a lack of association.

By specificity, Sir Hill means that the observed epidemiological association is limited to particular persons and to particular sites and types of diseases, and there is no association between the suspected risk factor and other illnesses. He cautions, however, that absolute specificity is really quite uncommon, for diseases usually have more than one risk factor and any given risk factor may be causal for several diseases.

> In short, if specificity exists we may be able to draw conclusions without hesitation; if it is not apparent, we are not thereby necessarily left sitting irresolutely on the fence.[6]

Biological gradient simply means "dose-response." An epidemiological correlation is much more likely to indicate causality when there is a "more-of-one, more-of-the-other" relationship. The fact that the incidence of lung cancer rises in direct proportion with the number of cigarettes smoked daily, length of time the individual has smoked, and degree of inhalation, adds immensely to the evidence in favor of causation.

Plausibility is another very important influence on our viewing an epidemiological association as causal or merely fortuitous. Let us take a rather absurd example: There is no question that a worldwide epidemiological survey would reveal a very strong association between the per capita number of telephones in a country and its incidence of heart attacks. Does this mean that telephones are a major cause of heart attacks (or vice versa!)? Of course not, and it is extremely unlikely that any scientist would follow up the clue because it is implausible. It is far more likely that telephones themselves don't cause heart attacks (except, perhaps on the occasion of a person with a weak heart being told some unsettling news via the phone) but rather that the number of telephones tends to be high in those countries in which factors truly causal for heart attacks also exist. In this case it is easy to see that the number of telephones in a country is really a marker of the degree of industrialization or Westernization of that country, and that factors to really suspect of being causal are the diet, activity pattern, pollution, and psychosocial environment characteristic of such countries.

Yet, though plausibility is an important attribute, we should avoid rejecting an association just because it seems implausible, for what is biologically plausible depends on the science of the day. For example, until recently, what we knew about the physics of microwaves—a type of radiation emitted by radar, TV transmitters, and many other electronic devices—convinced the government that microwaves could not possibly cause damage to the general public, and so observed correlations between disease and microwave exposure were simply rejected as noncausal; we still don't know whether they are causal but we certainly know that the biological effects of microwaves are much more complex than had been thought at the time the judgment was passed.

On the other hand, the fact that a causal relationship seems quite plausible should not blindly lead us to accept it as true (recall the busmen example). Several epidemiological studies have shown a definite association between coffee drinking and mortality from heart attack. A causal relationship is very plausible since caffeine is know to have powerful effects on the nervous and cardiovascular systems, effects which could easily be seen as tending to produce the conditions required for a heart attack. Yet, further studies revealed that those persons who consumed a good deal of coffee also were the heaviest smokers, so it is probable that the correlation with coffee intake is a "red herring," that the real causal relationship is between cigarette smoking and mortality from heart disease. For this particular example, the issue still remains hotly contested, but it nicely illustrates the great need in any given study for looking simultaneously at as many potential risk factors as possible so as to be able to sort out such interrelations.

By temporality is meant, Which is the cart and which is the horse? I made reference to this problem earlier in this chapter in reference to whether a poor diet, lack of sleep, and depression leads to cancer or vice versa. This problem is particularly relevant with diseases of slow development; indeed, if the onset is extremely insidious, even prospective studies may be influenced, i.e., a significant fraction of the presumably healthy beginning population may, unawares, be affected enough for some of their habits to be altered at the very outset of the study.

To summarize, epidemiological studies provide an important tool for establishing the association of suspected risk factors with specific diseases and for inferring that such an association is causal. When such an association is not observed in any single study, this does not exonerate the risk factor, for given the difficulties inherent in epidemiological research there are many reasons for failing to observe a relationship even when one truly exists. Of course, when failure to establish an association occurs consistently and in studies that are clearly well-designed, exoneration becomes quite likely. On the other hand, demonstration of an association does not, of itself, establish causality, but certainly should start one thinking in that direction. The stronger the association is and the more frequently it can be observed under a variety of conditions and in both retrospective and prospective studies, the stronger becomes the likelihood that the association may be causal. Finding a high degree of specificity, a good dose-response, and proper temporality, and being able to hypothesize a plausible connection also add to the likelihood.

Using these criteria, any objective person would have to conclude, on the basis of the epidemiological evidence alone, that cigarette smoking is the major risk factor for lung cancer, that occupational exposure to arsenic causes skin cancer, that asbestos is the major risk factor for an unusual form of lung cancer, that thalidomide causes birth defects in the offspring of exposed mothers. It is simply incorrect to argue that epidemiological studies never really prove anything, unless one demands a level of certainty from them beyond that expected from any other scientific approach to disease. However, most associations are not nearly as convincing as in the examples just cited, and other types of evidence must be sought from controlled experiments with human subjects and laboratory animals. Moreover, these additional types of evidence should also be sought even when the epidemiological case against a suspected risk factor seems very strong.

Before turning to these other types of investigation, I would like to correct any impression I may have given that the only major misuse of epidemiological data is to demand too much of it, as does the tobacco industry. Our present problem is often in precisely the opposite direction, to fail to apply criteria like Sir Hill's with enough vigor and to foist claims upon the public much too strong for the epidemiological data upon which they are based. This was certainly the case in the busmen and the coffee-heart attack questions described earlier. The outstanding recent example, cited by Lewis Thomas, is the advice on how to add eleven years to your life which has appeared in a recurring Blue Cross advertisement, and has been cited not only in many popular magazines but in many professional journals as well: Eat breakfast, exercise regularly, maintain normal weight (neither too skinny nor too fat), don't smoke cigarettes, don't drink excessively, sleep eight hours each night, and don't eat between meals. This battery of rules is based on a single prospective epidemiological study carried out on 7,000 people, 45 years of age or older, who were followed for five years, at which point the causes of the 371 deaths which had occurred in the interim were analyzed and correlated with the questionnaire answers given at the outset of the study. What do you think about the likelihood that the inferences drawn from this study are correct?

Controlled Human and Animal Experiments

Animal experiments provide the means for a direct, controlled evaluation of suspected relationships between environmental factors and specific diseases. If dietary cholesterol is suspected of causing atherosclerosis, then feed laboratory animals a diet rich in cholesterol and see if they develop more atherosclerosis than a control group of animals (of the same species, age, sex, and background—preferably litter mates of the animals given the high-cholesterol diet) fed exactly the same diet minus the cholesterol (the total calories would be kept constant by substituting for the cholesterol an innocuous nutrient with the same caloric value). Even in such a straightforward experiment, there are potential pitfalls. For example, if the cholesterol changes the palatability of the food, the "high-cholesterol" rats might eat more or less total food than the controls so that any observed difference in their incidence of atherosclerosis could be due to differences in total food intake rather than cholesterol intake (this problem can be circumvented by pair-feeding the animals, i.e., not allowing them free access to food but administering equal amounts to both groups). The point of this example is that, to be meaningful, the two groups of animals must be subjected to exactly the same environments except for the factor being studied.

The other point of the example is to emphasize that experiments with laboratory animals are much more difficult to perform than the public generally realizes.

> The day-to-day practical difficulties of managing animal experiments almost have to be endured personally to be appreciated: feeding uniformly and on schedule, keeping the cages, tanks, or stalls clean, controlling the ambient temperature, protecting the animals from disease and vermin, keeping records, collecting specimens, arranging matings, performing deliveries, shielding the young from harm, conducting autopsies [and I would add behavioral studies], and in general taking every possible measure to ensure that whatever unusual effects are observed will not be due to uncontrolled or unnoticed variation in experimental conditions but will be solely and compellingly attributable to the hazard under suspicion. And this perhaps with many hundreds or thousands of smelly, squealing, squirming, defecating, biting animals.[7]

All these difficulties are greatly increased in long-term, multigeneration studies, now the rule in much animal testing, particularly in the field of toxicology. Such studies are, however, essential, since short-term (acute) animal experiments bear little relevance to the human predicament—long-term low-level exposures and slowly progressing diseases which may have very long latent periods.

The greatest advantage of animal experimentation, of course, is that experiments can be performed that would be unacceptably hazardous to human subjects. Unhappily, the other side of the coin is that any results determined using experimental animals might not be applicable to human beings. If the great problem of inference in epidemiological studies is distinguishing causality from mere association, then that for animal experiments is extrapolating the results from animals to people. Man is a unique species, and no other animal, not even other closely related primates, duplicates precisely his responses to environmental factors. There are many examples of this fact. Thalidomide, for example, is 10 times less toxic in baboons than in man, 100 times less in rats, and 700 times less in cats.

Yet, just as I argued in the case of epidemiological evidence, this knowledge that extrapolation of animal data to human beings is not perfectly reliable does not detract from the tremendous importance of such experiments and should not paralyze us in their use. It does mean that we should try to minimize the problem through certain features of experimental design. Whenever economically feasible, several species should be used, including the one which previous studies of the organ system likely to be affected indicate is most like man's. The route of exposure should be, whenever possible, the same as that experienced by people. Where appropriate, the tests should be for very long periods of time to mimic the chronicity of environmental exposures. A variety of doses should be tried, including the level to which the human population at risk is exposed. However, in the absence of an observable effect, much higher doses should also be tried, both because human sensitivity may be much greater than any of the species tried (as in the thalidomide case) and because of problems inherent in trying to find subtle or delayed effects in manageable numbers of animals. This last feature is typical of chemical carcinogens, and I'll go into detail about its implications in chapter 9.

There is yet another reason for using large doses where appropriate. We now recognize that combinations of risk factors can be synergistic, i.e., can exert effects far greater than the sum of their individual effects. In other words, their effects don't merely add, they reinforce each other. Laboratory research is difficult enough when only one factor is being evaluated, and it is quite impossible to test for more than a few synergistic effects at a time. We will simply never be able to work out, in the laboratory, all the potential possible synergistic effects in air pollution, for example, in which there exist, to mention just a few, carbon monoxide, nitrogen oxide, ozone, peroxides, sulfur oxides, viruses, bacteria, and pollen. For this reason, the toxic action of these substances may be far greater in the actual environment than our laboratory tests of individual substances at the usual exposure level suggest. (On the other hand [there always seems to be an "other hand"], various agents may interact in antagonistic rather than synergistic ways, so that the effective dose in the lab may overestimate the effective dose in the environment.)

In conclusion, the single most important generalization relevant to animal testing is that the great majority of physiological differences between human beings and experimental animals are quantitative not qualitative. Therefore, even though there are no hard and fast rules which can be used to sanction extrapolation, common sense dictates that a strong effect, consistent among species studied, plausible with regard to present knowledge of the field, and, very importantly, confirmatory of clues provided by human epidemiological studies, all make it very likely that at least a qualitative extrapolation to human beings is warranted. For example, this description nicely characterizes the results of experiments showing that several of the chemicals found in cigarette smoke are able to cause cancer in experimental animals. This example raises another obvious but crucial point; animal studies cannot find a particular kind of response unless it is looked for! Tests for mutagenesis (the production of mutations in reproductive cells), teratogenesis (birth defects), carcinogenesis (production of cancer), and behavioral alteration (often without observable changes in the brain), have only come into being in the past ten to fifteen years and still are in a primitive state of development.

Finally, animal experiments have yet another major advantage over epidemiological studies. Animal testing of new chemicals not yet introduced into the environment, or of new types of radiation-emitting equipment, allows for evaluation of toxicity prior to exposure of the entire population to the agent.

Let us now take a brief look at controlled human experimentation, perhaps the most difficult of all scientific approaches to environmental risk factors. The major feature which distinguishes controlled human experimentation from the pure epidemiological approach is that, as in controlled animal experiments, the scientist deliberately introduces changes into the environment or the subjects' lifestyle, occupation, etc. For example, instead of asking whether people who spontaneously eat different amounts of cholesterol differ in their incidences of heart attacks, the researcher deliberately sets the cholesterol intakes of his subjects and then observes the consequences. Comparison between groups is usually required, so that in our cholesterol experiment two or more groups of subjects would be placed on deficient intakes.

The crucial point is that this type of experiment avoids (at least at the outset) the problems of self-selection that plague epidemiological studies. Recall that the London busmen chose to be either ticket-takers or drivers; in a controlled experiment, newly hired men would be randomly assigned to one or the other of the two positions. People choose to be sedentary in their spare time or to jog; in a controlled experiment, a group of people similar to each other in as many respects as possible would be randomly placed into groups, one nonjoggers and the other jogging a specified number of miles per week (better yet would be several groups of joggers doing different distances so that a dose-response could be constructed for the effects of jogging on the disease in question—heart attacks, strokes, colds, or whatever).

The phrase in parentheses in the last paragraph—"at least at the outset"—denotes a fact of life which is the dismay of experimenters and a major pitfall of this kind of research. It is one thing to assign a person to a nonjogging group or a jogging one, but it is another matter altogether to keep him there. As the study progresses, many of the subjects simply stop complying. Some of the nonjoggers can't stand being sedentary and begin to jog, while some of the joggers just simply refuse to jog because they don't like it. You might think this problem could be solved easily by just dropping noncompliers from the study, or transferring them to the group they vote for with their feet, but such is not the case. Whether you drop them altogether or transfer them, the result is the same—soon you have a self-selection epidemiological study rather than a controlled experiment! The remaining joggers clearly are different from the nonjoggers, otherwise they would not have continued to jog (or chosen to transfer to a jogging group). When noncompliance becomes great enough, therefore, the study becomes worthless as a controlled experiment.

But noncompliance is not the only problem in back of "at least at the outset." Again, let's look at joggers, this time assuming, miraculously, perfect compliance. To the researcher's chagrin, at the first year's follow-up he finds that, because of their exercising, almost all of the joggers have lost about fifteen pounds and are therefore lighter than the nonjoggers (the weights were carefully matched at the beginning of the study). Therefore, any difference observed between joggers and nonjoggers in, let's say, heart attack rate, might be due to their differences in body weight rather than to the jogging per se. But that isn't all; many of the joggers, feeling healthier, have decided to alter some of their other habits—they have given up smoking, spend more time with their children, enjoy sex more with their wives, have cut down on their beef intake, and so on. All these habits had been carefully matched across groups at the outset and all are now different; jogging is no longer the unique factor distinguishing the groups.

I have taken a somewhat extreme example to make the point, and the moral is not to ignore such studies, but to recognize that confounding variables may occur in even the best-designed study. Again, we must use our common sense and look for strength of association, consistency between studies, plausibility, and coherence with regard to the epidemiological studies and animal experiments evaluating the same risk factor.

There are many other important methodological problems inherent in human experimentation. As with epidemiological studies, extremely large numbers of subjects may be required, and the follow-up may be for many years, all of which is extremely costly in terms of both scientific manpower and money. Beyond these constraints of practicality exist profound ethical problems inherent in the exposure of human beings to suspected risks. Much has been written of late concerning this immensely important issue, and I will not deal with it here except to emphasize the obvious: The decision as to whether a particular experiment is acceptable is not a scientific question (once the soundness of the experimental design is assured) but a value judgment to be determined not by scientists alone but by society.

Fortunately, the experiment can sometimes be done in a way which eliminates risk to the subjects rather than increasing it. If a particular chemical is suspected of causing disease in workers manufacturing it, then the results of installing in the factory a new protective system can be evaluated by measuring disease incidences before and after installation. The influence of maternal malnutrition on fetal death rate can be evaluated not by deliberately starving mothers but by giving supplements to malnourished mothers. (Yet this last example hides a less obvious but nevertheless potent ethical problem— is it ethical to withhold supplements from another group of matched malnourished mothers so their offspring can serve as controls? How important is it for society to know whether maternal malnutrition is bad for the offspring's development? Should we just assume that it is on the basis of inconclusive epidemiological evidence and animal studies possibly not meaningful for human beings?)

If people are often too skeptical about extrapolation from animal studies to human beings, they are usually not skeptical enough about the interpretation of controlled studies performed on human subjects. From descriptions of research results appearing in the mass media one often cannot tell whether the experimenters themselves have overinterpreted their data or whether the science writer or journalist has butchered the description of a well-performed experiment or added unwarranted interpretations of his own. Here is a reasonable facsimile of some mass-media science news:

> In a recent study done at a famous teaching hospital, schizophrenic patients were given vitamin Z and showed substantial improvement. One who had been hospitalized for five years was ultimately able to return to his family. It is clear from this study and many others like it that vitamin Z deficiency is presently exacting a terrible toll in this country. Think of the huge number of people whose headaches, irritability, and depression could be eliminated by a diet rich in vitamin Z.*

---

*If you think this item represents a gross caricature of popular science writing, just thumb through any of the nutrition books by the late Adelle Davis. Here is an example taken at random from *Lets Get Well* (New York: Harcourt, Brace & World, 1965, p. 225): "I have seen a number of persons who have recovered completely from multiple sclerosis [a neuromuscular disease usually characterized by striking waxing and waning of symptoms!] when dietary improvement was made soon after the disease had been diagnosed. These individuals have stayed on the antistress program, and a highly adequate diet. In some cases, 600 units of vitamin E taken with each meal . . . have brought spectacular success. Recently I was talking to a young woman who told me that for several years she had been an invalid because of this disease but that after following an excellent diet she had no signs of the illness except occasional foot cramps which disappeared when she increased her magnesium intake." There is absolutely no evidence from controlled experiments that vitamin E or magnesium influences the course of multiple sclerosis.

Let's analyze this little item for its classical flaws. In so doing, we will really be establishing a checklist to go over mentally when reading such articles. First of all, be wary of the appeal to authority in the first line—even if it is a "famous teaching hospital" (and one can't tell since it is not named), there is no law forbidding famous scientists (even Nobel laureates) from losing their objectivity on certain issues.

Second, we are not told whether the experiment was done in a double-blind manner. One of the major pitfalls of human experimentation is failure to take the "placebo effect" into account. We know with absolute certainty that a person's perception of disease can be influenced by his expectations. Moreover, I believe with equal certainty (not shared by all scientists) that not just the perception but the disease process itself is responsive to psychological factors. The term, placebo effect, simply denotes the fact that many persons improve when they are given a medication, diet, or physical therapy they believe in. For this reason, it is desirable that the control group in any experiment be subject to the same expectation of success (or toxicity, in the case of the testing of a suspected risk factor) as is the group actually exposed to (or removed from contact with) the factor being studied. In studies of medication, the field in which the placebo effect was first recognized, this is routinely accomplished by use of the double-blind study—neither the subject nor the experimenter knows who is receiving the placebo (a nonactive medication) or the drug. Of course, it is often impossible to apply these methods to the evaluation of environmental risk factors (a person clearly knows when he is being exposed to no noise or loud noise, workers know whenever safety systems are being installed, people know the difference between granola and a beefsteak).

The particular study described by our newspaper article is not really difficult to do as a double-blind. It requires first of all that the subjects not know whether they are getting vitamin Z or a placebo. But this "single-blind" is not enough—the personnel performing all phases of the study (selecting the subjects, handing out the pills, checking for signs and symptoms, performing lab tests, carrying out statistical analyses of the data) also must be kept ignorant of which subjects are receiving which pill. The need for double-blind studies in the evaluation of therapeutic efficacy (or degree of toxicity) does not mean that scientists are deliberately dishonest but only that they are human beings, like the rest of us, and cannot avoid either unconsciously acting differently toward subjects known to be receiving their favored medication or making judgments prejudiced in favor of their enthusiasms. The latter is particularly true when the data being collected require subjective evaluations (just how "runny" must a nose be before its owner is said to have a cold) but is still a problem even when the data collected are objective (the patient's white blood cell count, for example); most scientists will admit how much more critically they treat lab tests which disagree with their prejudices and how easy it is to find a reason for throwing out or ignoring that test.

After the study is deemed completed, the code (set up by persons others than the persons doing the research) is "broken" to permit the analysis of the data, i.e., the comparison between the control group of schizophrenics (who receive no vitamin Z) and the group receiving the vitamin. Also, in advance, the researchers must carefully specify the criteria to be used to evaluate "improvement" (we haven't any idea from the article what they were).

Even if there were something about the study that precluded use of a double-blind plan, a control group must still be used. This is an absolute requirement, not just an important one, for the natural history of schizophrenia is often characterized by remissions; without an untreated group for comparison, it would be impossible to know what fraction of the "improvement" could be ascribed not to vitamin Z but to spontaneous remission or some other aspect of therapy correlated with the vitamin administration.

The next problem in our example is the total lack of quantitation of both the dose of vitamin Z and the response to it. Exactly how much did each criterion of improvement change? If the major criterion was "returned home," what percentage of the control and treated groups went home? Was the difference significant using appropriate statistics (I'll describe what I mean by appropriate statistics in a subsequent section)? The anecdote about the single patient is gratuitous and, in the absence of information on how many untreated patients also improved enough to go home, is also meaningless.

Let us assume, for the moment, that the study really was done properly, that in a double-blind procedure, when a group of schizophrenic patients were given a specified dose of vitamin Z (let us say, ten times the amount usually recommended as minimal for the general population), significantly more of them than of those patients in the control group were able to return home and resume their jobs.

These are the facts of the study, and they warrant the inference that very large doses of vitamin Z, under the conditions used in this study, are useful in the treatment of schizophrenia. The facts do not warrant any of the other inferences cited in the article. The fact that one illness attributable to brain malfunction—schizophrenia—is responsive to very large amounts of vitamin Z says nothing of the possible responsiveness of other disorders—headaches, irritability, and depression. Moreover, extrapolation from studies of one type of population (in this case, schizophrenic people) to others or to the general population is not warranted. This is an extremely common mistake in much popular writing about nutrition. For example, persons with the disease "functional hypoglycemia" have many disturbing symptoms several hours after eating a pure carbohydrate breakfast, but this does not warrant the inference that normal people will also suffer these symptoms, though to a lesser degree, after a pure carbohydrate breakfast. On a more sophisticated plane, patients with one of the diseases causing profound elevation of plasma cholesterol concentration live longer if their dietary cholesterol is reduced but, as we shall see, this doesn't necessarily mean that the general population, with its lower level of plasma cholesterol, will also live longer on low-cholesterol diets.

Similarly, extrapolation from one level of medication, nutrient, or environmental exposure to another level is not warranted. The fact that very large doses of vitamin Z might help schizophrenics does not mean that half the dose will help these patients half as much, or twice the dose twice as much. In subsequent chapters I shall describe in detail some of the implications of this dose-response problem.

To reiterate, interpretation of facts gained from controlled human experimentation can be extrapolated only with great caution beyond the type of population tested, the doses these people were exposed to, and the other environmental factors in existence during the experiment. Of course, such extrapolations can, and should be, set forth as hypotheses and then tested for specifically. If vitamin Z, in large doses, helps schizophrenics, it is logical to test it on depressed persons; if patients with unusually high concentrations of plasma cholesterol suffer from fewer heart attacks when eating low-cholesterol diets, it is logical to test the effects of such a diet on the general population.

There is another major question to ask when reading or listening to the latest science report, regardless of whether the experiment was performed on animals or people: Has the information been published in a scientific journal? After a manuscript has been submitted to a scientific journal for consideration, it is reviewed for the journal by at least two experts in the field who then advise the journal editor as to disposition. Sometimes the manuscript is simply rejected on the grounds of scientific problems, but often it is returned to the original scientist with comments and suggestions concerning data analysis, the need for additional experiments, alternate interpretations, and so on. There follows an often spirited and prolonged interaction between the scientist and reviewers (the journal editor acting as middleman, since in most cases, the reviewers remain unknown to the scientist), resulting ultimately in a report acceptable to all. Now, this process is by no means foolproof in spotting errors or problems, and it also sometimes results in the rejection of important contributions because of prejudice on the part of the reviewers (controversy and disagreement are the rule in science, not the exception). Nevertheless, peer review is the best present means we have for avoiding the publication of unsound experimental data and interpretations. Unfortunately, most newspapers, magazines, and television programs do not inform the audience of the source of their information, and do not state whether it appeared in a scientific journal. Moreover, more and more science news comes "hot off the podium," that is, from coverage of meetings at which scientists present their most recent findings; these presentations have generally not been subjected to peer review and its winnowing effect.

Statistical Evaluation of Data

I have frequently made reference to "statistical evaluation" and the term "significant" without defining them. Although statistical methods constitute the single most pervasive tool in making inferences from data, I have saved them for last, partly because they apply equally to epidemiology and controlled lab animal and human experiments, and partly because they seem to turn people off. The tobacco industry repeats over and over again, "mere statistics, no real proof," and this somehow mesmerizes people; the fact is that "mere statistics" is not to be contrasted with "real proof" but underlies our inferences concerning the latter.

I have neither the knowledge nor the desire to present a crash course in statistics and so I promise to define and explain only four terms: arithmetic mean, standard deviation, *P* value, and correlation coefficient.

Statistical analysis of the data generated by epidemiological studies or controlled experiments is required for the simple reason that the population actually studied is almost always relatively small compared to the entire relevant population. If you wished to know whether there exists a difference in the arithmetic mean (average) of the height of students in two adjacent classrooms it would be a relatively easy matter to take all the students in each room, measure their heights, and calculate the arithmetic mean (by adding all the heights and dividing by the number of students). If the means for the two rooms differ, even by a small amount, you are completely justified in saying so; no inference is involved (except that your measuring devices are good and you know how to use them).

Let's make the task more difficult: Are the mean heights of all children in two particular schools different? Again, if you have the time and energy, all students could be measured, and an absolutely certain answer given. Now for a large jump in difficulty: Are the mean heights of all 10-year-old children in Detroit and Chicago different (or in the United States versus Canada or North America versus South America)? The problem here is that we simply cannot measure all the children, and so we must resort to measuring a sample of the whole population.

How many children do we need for our sample? That depends largely on how much variation there is in the population. For example, if all 10-year-olds in the school were exactly the same height, a nonsensical possibility, one child would do! In contrast, if heights varied enormously, then we woud need a very large sample for it to be reasonably representative of the entire population of 10-year-olds in that city. The way we select our sample is just as important as the total number selected. For example, we can't take all our sample from one ethnic group in the city, since ethnic groups differ considerably in their mean heights. The actual amount of variability in whatever sample we do finally use is quantified for us by a single calculation (based on how much *each* individual value in the sample differs from the arithmetic mean of *all* the samples) and is known as the standard deviation.

Let's assume we have a fairly good sized sample and we have been careful in the way we chose it; nevertheless, it is a virtual certainty that the mean we calculate for our sample will only rarely be exactly the same as the true mean for the entire population, unless we take such a large sample that you might as well have done the entire population. Knowing this, we have a problem when we try to answer the original question about the mean heights of 10-year-olds in Detroit and Chicago. The mean of our sample from Chicago turns out to be 5'2" and that from Detroit 5'3". A skeptic would rightly say: "Your data don't convince me that Detroit children are really taller; 1 inch certainly isn't much, and if you did the study over again, using a new sample, I'll bet the difference observed would disappear."

Here is where statistical analysis is helpful. It allows you to predict just what the odds are that the 1-inch difference seen between your population samples really represents a true difference between total-population means and not a spurious one reflecting solely the factor of chance in your sample selection. Exactly how these tests work and how they are performed need not concern us here; suffice it to say that their use requires only a knowledge of the different sample means, how much variation there is within each of the samples (given by the value of the standard deviation), and how many individuals there are in each sample. The value that comes out of the computer in most of these tests is termed a P (for probability) value. Its limits are zero and 1.0 and it states simply what the likelihood is that the difference observed between our sample means could have occurred by chance even though the total-population means are identical. For example, if the P value in our study turns out to be 0.20, this means that, were we to do the test 100 times, using 100 different samples, a difference of 1 inch (Detroit greater than Chicago) would have been found in twenty of these studies even though the true total-population means were identical. In other words, there is a 20 percent probability that chance alone, not a true difference in populations, explains the results of our study. The lower the P value, then, the less the probability that chance explains the data and the greater the likelihood that a true population difference exists.

I said that the lower limit of P is zero, but such values never really are obtained although they can certainly get very low indeed (a P value of 0.001 signifies, for example, that in only 1 out of 10,000 times would the observed difference between sample means have occurred by chance, i.e., the odds are 10,000 to 1 that the populations really differ).

Since a zero P value is unattainable, then statistical analysis can never establish the presence of a true difference with 100 percent certainty. Once more we see that all inferences concerning "truth" from experiments are relative. Given such relativity, scientists have established cutoff points for themselves; most accept a P value of 0.05 or less as convincing enough to accept any difference generated by their experiments as representing a true difference. They are saying that twenty-to-1 odds are pretty reasonable. So when you read that a difference is statistically significant (the adjective is often omitted), you know that the P value is no greater than 0.05 (and may be much less).

Let us take an example of why it is so important to have statistics presented and not just be guided by statements concerning the magnitude of the difference observed in an experiment. Company A claims that people using its cold remedy had, in well-controlled studies, 25 percent fewer colds than did a control group of people; those using a competitor's remedy had only 10 percent fewer colds. When you write, asking for the statistical evaluation of the data, they hem and haw, but finally send it to you. You find that the P value for their product's 25 percent difference is 0.2, whereas that for their competitor's product is 0.01. Now you see why they were reluctant to send the data. The P value of 0.2 means that all scientists would reject the claim that their product has been proven to have an effect on the incidence of colds, even though the number, 25 percent, seems so large! On the other hand, although the competitor's 10 percent reduction is small, the odds are 100 to 1 that it represents a real effect. How is it that the 25 percent number turns out not to be significant whereas 10 percent is? Remember that the calculation of the P value for any particular difference between the means depends only on the number of subjects (or animals) used in the study and the amount of variability, expressed as the standard deviation, in the results. The company's records show that equal numbers of persons were used in both studies so the only remaining possibility is that there was much greater variability in the group using the company's product.*

---

*How variability can give a large mean difference but a high P value can be illustrated by the following data. Suppose each of the 10 subjects in a drug-treated group has 2 colds per year, so that the mean per capitum colds is also 2. Suppose 9 of the 10 control subjects have 2 colds per year but the tenth person has 10 colds! The mean for this control group is therefore $29/10 = 2.8$ colds per year. This is 40 percent higher than the mean for the drug-treated group, so the company might report that its drug reduces colds by 40 percent. This would, however, be a statistically unjustified statement, for the P value for this comparison would be much higher than 0.05. In this gross example, the statistical analysis only corroborates your common sense recognition that the company's claim, while numerally true, is due to a fluke.

There are a variety of tests for determining the significance of a difference between groups (or a difference in the same persons of a single group before and after a single manipulation, say, reducing the group's dietary cholesterol), but they all end up expressing the likelihood of the difference being significant in terms of a P value or its equivalent. It cannot be stressed too strongly that such statistical tests never indicate how *important* the difference is, only how likely it is to represent a true difference. Thus, in our example, you can be highly confident that the cold remedy with the P value of 0.01 truly exerts an anticold effect, but you may decide that the actual decrease in colds it produces—only 10 percent—is simply too unimportant for you to bother taking the drug.

Now for our last statistical concept, one crucial for epidemiological research, which is concerned with possible quantitative interrelationships between variables. Such a relationship is called a correlation. A correlation is basically a statistical tool which tells you how useful knowing the value of one characteristic is in predicting the value of the second. Returning to our example of 10-year-olds, if you were given the heights of all the people in the class, you would be able to make reasonable estimates of their weights. In a few cases, those of the very skinny or very fat, you would be way off, but for most of the students you would be fairly close, especially if we started you off with a few representative values.

A calculator or computer usually performs the calculations, but you can visualize a correlation this way (fig. 1–1): On a piece of graph paper, one characteristic such as weight is plotted on the horizontal axis, with the subjects' corresponding second characteristic (height) plotted on the vertical axis. This yields one point for each of the subjects. In the simplest type of correlation, a linear correlation, the points will seem to lie along a straight line if the linear correlation is a good one. Mathematically, there is a single line which comes as close as possible to all the points, and this is the line which the calculator or computer yields for you. It will then compute for you a number, termed r or the correlation coefficient, which states how nicely the points really fit the line, i.e., how strongly one characteristic serves as a prediction of the other. The maximum value of r is 1.0 which means that all the points are smack on the line and one characteristic perfectly predicts the other. An r of zero means that the points scatter randomly and that one characteristic is utterly useless as a prediction of the other.

The *r* value can also be less than zero, having negative values up to −1. A value of −1 also means perfect predictability except that instead of the two variables getting larger together, the second variable gets smaller as the first gets larger. The two variables are said to be negatively correlated. Such a relationship occurs, for example, in a correlation in adults of age and ability to perform endurance exercise; the older the persons, the fewer miles they are able to jog (of course, there would be a good deal of variability in such a response, well-trained older persons being able to jog further than completely untrained young adults). Thus, the closer *r* is to 1 or to −1, the better the correlation.

So far, I have been careful to emphasize that the correlation coefficient is a measure of how well one characteristic's magnitude predicts another. Of course, what epidemiologists have in mind when they do their experiments is the likelihood that predictability may signify causality, but no matter how strong the correlation, it remains just that—a correlation. As I have described in the section on epidemiology, the strength of the correlation (or association, as I referred to it there) is one important factor in the inference of causality, but there is nothing magical about the statistic which

Fig. 1–1.   Correlation between height and weight in a group of women.
The line gives the "best fit" of the data. It is a linear correlation because it is a straight line.

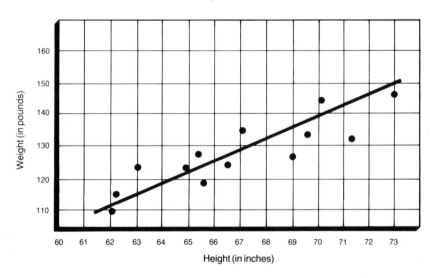

can mathematically transform correlation (a fact) into causality (an inference).*

The correlation coefficient is particularly useful in epidemiological studies of diseases for which multiple causes exist, since it is rarely possible to match populations for all these factors. For example, remember I mentioned the study which found an association between coffee intake and coronary heart disease; the interpretation was confounded by the fact that those with high coffee intake also tended to be heavier smokers than those in the control group. The correlation coefficients from many other studies correlating cigarette smoking and coronary artery disease were used to estimate how much of the increased coronary artery disease suffered by those with high coffee intake could really be ascribed to their smoking, and it turned out that most of it could be. Thus, after "factoring out" smoking, the association between coffee intake and coronary artery disease became much less striking.

---

*In graphic representations of correlations (such as fig. 1–1), you can usually tell the investigator's assumptions about the direction of causality by what gets placed on the horizontal (x) and vertical (y) axes. The "causing" variable is generally on the former and the "caused" on the latter. Thus, we would plot number of cigarettes per day on the x axis and cancer incidence on the y.

Chapter **2** | Biological Responses to Environmental Challenges

The body rarely, if ever, submits passively to environmental perturbations. Any significant change in the physicochemical or psychosocial environment calls forth a variety of responses, both physiological and behavioral, most of which constitute the body's attempt to adapt to the perturbation. When external temperature rises or falls, responses tend to minimize any change in internal temperature; when the oxygen concentration in the air is low, responses maintain oxygen supply to the cells; when a foreign chemical is present in the environment, responses minimize its accumulation in the body. In all these cases, the overall effect of the body's responses is to minimize the displacement of some physiological variable (body temperature, oxygen supply to cells, body concentrations of foreign chemicals) from its preperturbation value.

The purpose of this chapter is to lay a foundation of basic principles upon which the specific details of the body's multitude of responses can be laid.

Homeostasis

All those responses mentioned in the preceding paragraph fit nicely into the central paradigm of physiology, the science which deals with bodily function. The fluids within a person's body constitute an internal environment, which is maintained relatively constant in the face of changes in the external environment, i.e., the environment surrounding the person. This stability, known as homeostasis, is achieved by regulation and integration of the cells, tissues, and organs of the body.

Consider regulation of internal body temperature. Our subject is a resting, lightly clad man in a room having a 70°F temperature and moderate humidity. His internal body temperature is 98.6°F and he is losing heat to the external environment—the air surrounding him and the walls of the room. But the chemical reactions occurring within the cells of his body are producing heat at a rate precisely equal to the rate of total heat loss, so that his body undergoes no net gain or loss of heat, and his internal temperature remains constant. Here is the first crucial generalization about homeostasis: Stability of an internal environmental variable is achieved by balancing input and outputs. In this case, the variable—internal temperature—remains constant because heat production (input) equals heat loss from the body (output).

Now we lower the temperature of the room rapidly to 45°F and keep it there. This, of course, immediately increases the loss of heat from his warm skin, upsetting the dynamic balance between heat gain and loss; internal body temperature, therefore, starts to fall. But very rapidly, a variety of physiological responses occurs which limit the fall (fig. 2–1). First, the blood vessels to the skin narrow, reducing the amount of warm blood brought to the skin, and reducing heat loss. However, at a room temperature of 45°, the degree of blood vessel constriction undergone by our subject is not able to eliminate completely the extra heat loss from the skin. He curls up so as to reduce the surface area of skin available for heat loss, and this helps a bit, but excessive heat loss still continues. He has a strong desire to put on more clothing ("voluntary" behavioral responses are often crucial components in homeostasis), but none is available. Clearly, then, if excessive heat loss (output) cannot be prevented then the only way of restoring the balance between heat input and output is to increase input, and this is precisely what occurs. He begins to shiver, and the chemical reactions responsible for the rhythmic muscular contractions which constitute shivering produce large quantities of heat. The end result of all these responses is that heat loss from the body and heat production by the body are both high, but are once again equal, so that body temperature stops falling. Indeed, heat production may transiently exceed heat loss so that body temperature may begin to go back to the value originally existing before the room temperature was lowered. It will stabilize at some value a bit below this original value. Here is a second crucial generalization about homeostasis: Stability of an internal environmental variable depends not upon the absolute magnitudes of opposing inputs and outputs, but only upon the balance between them.

This entire sequence of events is, of course, familiar to everyone, since the ultimate responses—blanching of the skin, curling up, and shivering—are visible, but what about the internal workings which underlie them? The narrowing of the skin blood vessels is the direct consequence of contraction of the small muscles which encircle

Fig. 2–1. **Reflex for maintaining body temperature relatively constant when room temperature decreases.**

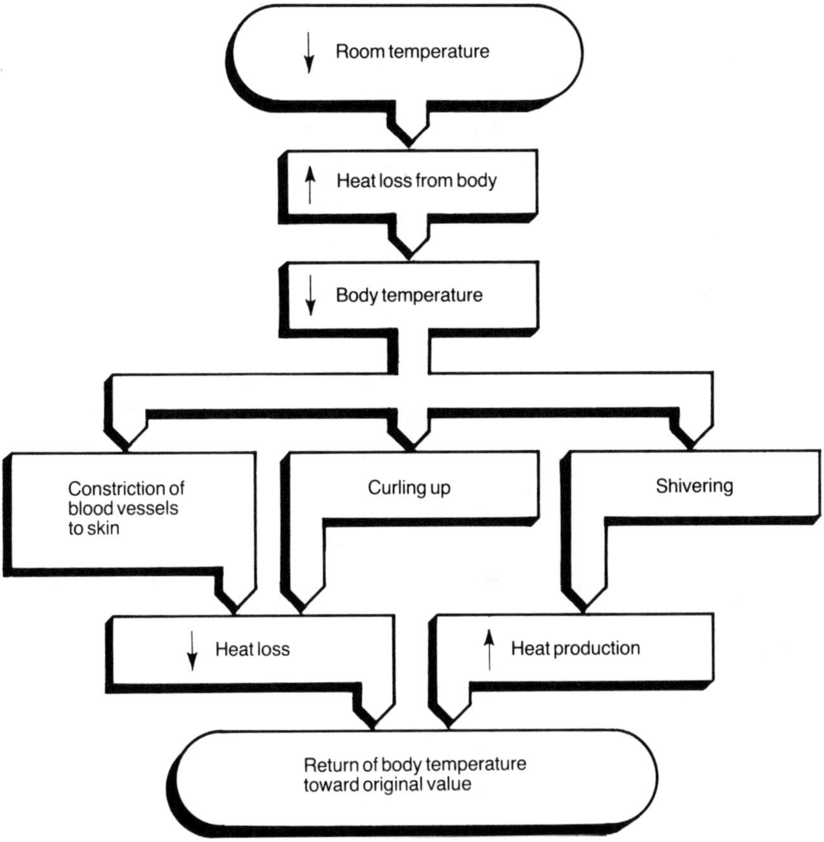

BIOLOGICAL RESPONSES TO ENVIRONMENTAL CHALLENGES

them; these muscles had been receiving only a few signals via the nerves to them to contract when the person was in the 70°F room, but the nerve signal rate was greatly increased in the cold room. Similarly, the nerves supplying the large external muscles of the body markedly increased their rates of signaling during exposure to the cold (of course, not only were the rates increased but the pattern was altered so as to produce shivering, not running or random rapid movements). But this begs the critical question. What stimulated all these nerves to increase their firing? They were being controlled by other nerve centers in the brain which were in turn being controlled by nerve signals coming from small groups of temperature-sensitive nerve cells in various parts of the body. The chain of events can be summarized (fig. 2–1): decreased room temperature → increased heat loss from body → decreased internal body temperature → increased activity of temperature-sensitive nerve cells in the brain → increased activity of a series of nerve cells, the last of which stimulate the skin blood vessel muscles and the skeletal muscles.

To generalize from this example: A homeostatic control system usually contains an internal component capable of detecting changes in the variable (temperature, in our example) being regulated, and there is a continuous flow of information from this "detector" via more or less complex chains of interconnecting components to the apparatus (skeletal muscles, for example), which alters its rate of output (heat, in our example).

I should emphasize that not all homeostatic responses involve systems as complex as the classic reflex just described. In some cases, the entire response occurs locally with no participation of nerves, hormones, or any other part of the body. For example, if you cut yourself, prevention of blood loss—a homeostatic response—is achieved by purely local changes, in this case contraction of the small muscle fibers surrounding the blood vessels followed by blood clotting. Sometimes the trigger to a response acts directly on the relevant cells. DDT, for example, acts directly on liver cells to stimulate the formation of proteins which then permit the cells to break down the DDT.

There remains one more component of the homeostatic system which we have described but not named: feedback. The ultimate effects of the change in output by the system must somehow be made known ("fed back") to the detectors which initiated the sequence of events. Look again at the sequence of events in our example. When the body temperature originally began to fall, this was "detected" by thermodetectors which alter their signal output and initiate the reflexes leading to decreased heat loss via the skin and increased heat production by skeletal muscles. These latter processes not only prevent the body temperature from falling further but tend to raise it back toward its original value. The thermodetectors immediately "detect" this alteration and decrease their output toward the original value, thereby reducing the signals to the skin blood vessels and skeletal muscles. This type of feedback, in which an increase in the activity of the final components (vessel muscles and skeletal muscles, in our example) results in a decrease in the original signal to the entire system, is known as negative feedback. It leads to stability of the system and is crucial to the operation of homeostatic mechanisms.

A third generalization about homeostatic control systems follows from this description of their components and the nature of negative feedback: They cannot maintain *complete* constancy of the internal environment, but can only *minimize changes.* Imagine for the moment that the reflex responses to persistent cold really did return body temperature completely to normal; what would happen to the output of the first component, the thermodetectors? Recall that it was the drop in body temperature that elicited the change in output from these detectors in the first place. If the body temperature were to return completely to its original value, so would the output of the thermodetectors, and the entire reflex would be abolished; the blood vessels would stop constricting, shivering would cease, and body temperature would once again fall since the compensations would no longer be present. In other words, as long as the exposure to cold continues, some decrease in body temperature must persist to serve as a signal maintaining the reflex. (Of course, whenever the person is able to extricate himself from the cold environment, then his body temperature will return completely to the precold value). Just how big this so-called error-signal is depends on the magnitude of the stress as well as on the sensitivity of the detectors, the efficiency of the component interconnections and the responsiveness of the final apparatus in the control system. The temperature-regulating systems of the body are extremely sensitive so that body temperature normally varies by only 1 to 2°F even in the face of marked changes in the external environment.

Inherent in the last sentence is a fourth generalization about homeostasis: Even in reference to a single person (so as to ignore interperson variation), any regulated variable in the body (temperature, plasma sugar, etc.) cannot be assigned a single "normal" value, but will span a more or less narrow range of values, depending on the external environmental conditions. The more precise the homeostatic mechanisms are for regulating this variable, the narrower will be the range.

Does it really matter for the health of the body where along its normal range a particular variable sits? Let us take another example, this time from nutrition. Sodium is an essential nutrient for the body, and the control systems which regulate total body sodium are remarkably precise. These control systems have as their targets the kidneys, and they operate by inducing the kidneys to excrete daily into the urine an amount of sodium approximately equal to the amount ingested. Imagine now a person with a daily intake and output of 7 g, and a stable amount of sodium in his body. Tomorrow the person changes his diet so that his daily consumption rises to 15 g and remains there indefinitely. On this same day, the kidneys excrete into the urine somewhat more than 7 g but certainly not all of the ingested 15 g. The result is that some excess sodium is retained in the body on that day. The kidneys do somewhat better on day two but it is probably not until day three or four that they are excreting 15 g. From this point on, output from the body once again equals input, and sodium balance is stable. But, and this is the important point, the person has perhaps 2 to 3 percent more sodium in his body than when he was eating the lesser amount of sodium. It is this 2 to 3 percent extra sodium which constitutes the signal for the reflexes driving the kidneys to excrete 15 g/day rather than 7 g/day. An increase of 2 to 3 percent doesn't seem like much but it is possible that over many years, this little extra might facilitate the development of certain diseases, notably high blood pressure.

The moral to be drawn from this last discussion is that the concept of homeostasis is an ideal, for total constancy of the internal environment can never be achieved. No matter how good the body's control systems are, all regulated variables will manifest a range of values ("operating points") dependent on the degree of environmental stress. Knowledge of these facts makes mandatory a consideration of the overall significance for the individual's health or disease of where along the range the variable rests.

One more disclaimer: Homeostatic control mechanisms are not the exclusive adaptive machinery of the body, nor is it possible (or desirable) for everything to be maintained relatively constant. Indeed, one often finds adaptive responses which seem to fly in the face of homeostasis. For example, the aborigines of Australia sleep unclothed on the ground despite winter night temperatures below freezing; during the night, their body temperature may fall by 2 to 3°F, yet they never shiver! This "failure of homeostasis" actually has important survival value for the aborigines. Shivering uses a great deal of energy, which must be supplied by food, a very scarce commodity in the outback of Australia. Instead of using their own energy to maintain body temperature at night the aborigines simply allow themselves to cool down and then warm up the next morning at the expense of the sun. Of course, addicts to homeostasis simply point out that we had our eyes on the wrong variable, that total body energy stores, not temperature, were being homeostatically regulated. This is not a trivial point. Adaptive responses frequently represent a trade-off in which one variable (in this case, temperature constancy) is sacrificed in order to regulate a more critical variable (in this case, total body energy content). Of course, we have said nothing about how the aborigines came to be able to perform this trick, and it is time we turned to the entire question of how adaptive responses, homeostatic or not, arise.

Gene-Environment Interactions

Homeostatic control systems such as those described in the previous section are biological adaptations which favor survival in specific environments. The origin of such adaptations, like that of all characteristics of the body—anatomic structure, physiologic activities, and behavior—can be understood only in terms of the individual's genetic endowment and the interactions of the genes with the external environment. Each of us begins as a single cell, the fertilized ovum, which gives rise to the entire body by cell division and differentiation. All the information required to achieve this enormous task is present in the genes of the fertilized ovum and is passed on (with a few exceptions) to each new cell arising from cell division. However, every step in the construction process requires not merely the information present in the genes but appropriate interaction of these genes with the environment.

The information coded into the genes are blueprints for the construction of all the million or more types of proteins present in the body. Proteins are very large molecules, ranging in molecular weight from 10,000 to 1,000,000 or more, but they are all made of sequences of much smaller subunits known as amino acids, each having a molecular weight of approximately 100. Although there are only twenty kinds of amino acids, there is no problem in forming a million unique linear sequences from them, since each sequence contains 100 to 10,000 amino acids.

How is it possible that a code containing only information required for protein synthesis can serve as instructions for construction of the entire body? Why is no code needed for synthesis of all the nonprotein molecules? The answer is that proteins control the production and destruction of all these other molecular types.

Biochemical reactions proceed relatively slowly unless accelerated by certain types of protein molecules collectively called enzymes. There is a remarkable degree of specificity in these enzyme-accelerated reactions such that any given enzyme will speed up only a limited number of reaction types, often only one. For example, the enzyme which accelerates the first step in the synthesis of glycogen (the storage form of carbohydrate) from glucose accelerates no other reaction; similarly, no other enzyme will accelerate this step. The result of all this specificity is that the types of molecules which get made or destroyed in the body depend on the types of enzymes present; for example, if the body makes none of the enzyme molecules needed to accelerate the synthesis of glycogen, then it will contain virtually no glycogen. Thus, the genetic code specifying what proteins the body can make indirectly specifies all the rest of the bodily components and physiological response capabilities as well. As an example of this, consider eye color, which is due to the presence of particular kinds of nonprotein colored molecules (pigments) within cells of the eye. Different sequences of enzyme-accelerated reactions are required to synthesize the various pigments, and the genes for eye color do not code for the pigments, themselves, but rather for the enzymes in the synthetic pathways.

Of course, what I have been describing is a gross oversimplification. For the body to construct itself, it is not enough merely to specify directly (for proteins) or indirectly (for nonprotein molecules) the types of molecules to be built. These molecules must be built (or broken down) at the right times and locations and combined into appropriate units to form cells, tissues, and organs. We are many decades, perhaps centuries, away from understanding how this all occurs.

To reiterate, the genes code for amino acid sequences of all the protein types in the body, but now we must back up and describe just what the genes actually are and how their code is put into action. As every school child must know by now, genes are segments of the DNA molecules packed into each cell's nucleus. Each DNA molecule comprises an intercoiled pair of chains, each chain composed of four kinds of small molecular building blocks called nucleotides. Just as proteins are variable sequences of amino acids, so DNA molecules are variable sequences of nucleotides. If one pictures each type of nucleotide as a letter in an alphabet, then each sequence of three nucleotides "spells" a three-letter word. Sixty-four such words are possible with a four-letter alphabet, more than the twenty needed to code for the twenty different amino acids. Thus, the sequences of nucleotides along a DNA molecule form a code for the sequences of amino acids in proteins. What does the word "gene" really mean in the context of this system? A single DNA molecule contains so many nucleotide sequences that it codes for many different types of proteins. Accordingly, a DNA molecule may be viewed as containing many informational units strung together, and each unit constitutes a single gene. Most genes contain the information (i.e., the nucleotide sequence) needed to code for the synthesis of one type of protein.

The biochemical steps by which the nucleotide-sequence code of DNA is translated into the actual synthesis of proteins is quite complex and need not concern us except for one intermediate step. The cell's DNA is trapped in the nucleus, whereas its protein-synthesizing apparatus is in the cytoplasm. Therefore, each DNA molecule "directs" the synthesis in the nucleus of another type of molecule called messenger RNA (mRNA), which comprises a single chain of nucleotides, analogous to those contained in DNA molecules. In the process, the DNA code is transcribed into an mRNA code, and the mRNA molecules leave the nucleus, enter the cytoplasm, and direct the synthesis of the proteins for which they code. Some of the proteins synthesized under the direction of mRNA are structural elements, but most function as enzymes, accelerating specific chemical reactions which, taken all together, constitute the sum total of your anatomical and physiological traits. The set of genes you possess constitutes your *genotype*, but the expression of the genes via the chain of events summarized in figure 2–2 produces your *phenotype*, the actual "you."

This is where the environment comes into play, for environmental factors can exert profound influences at each of the steps required for gene expression. Given any particular genotype, different environments, by altering gene expression, can produce a spectrum of phenotypes, an incredible variety of "yous." This is *phenotypic plasticity*, the ability to manifest different traits and different magnitudes of any particular trait or physiological response, depending on the environment. In the same breath, I must emphasize that phenotypic plasticity of any given characteristic is not an infinite continuum; one's genes set the possible range of plasticity, and the environment, by influencing the expression of the genes, determines whether (and how much) any given trait or response within this range will be manifested.

There are three major ways in which environmental factors influence expression of any particular gene: They alter the rate of formation of mRNA from DNA; they alter the ability of the enzyme, once formed, to function; they supply the substrates required for the reaction which the enzyme accelerates.

Altered Rate of mRNA Synthesis. It is axiomatic that a cell cannot make an enzyme for which it does not have a gene to code. However, even though the appropriate gene is present, the cell may not make an enzyme at all or may make it at variable rates. That this must be the case becomes obvious when one recollects that almost all cells

Fig. 2–2. **Pathway by which DNA "directs" the production of molecules in the body.**

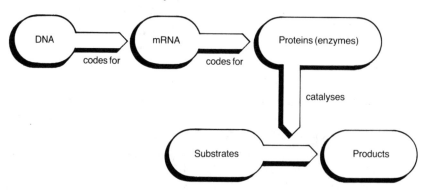

in the body have precisely the same genes, yet each cell type differs from all others, i.e., has a unique set of protein types and/or different amounts of shared protein types. This reflects differential rates of transcription of the various genes. Thus, the genes which code for contractile proteins are extremely busy transcribing mRNA in muscle cells but are completely inactive in nerve cells; the genes which code for the protein hormone, insulin, are very active in certain cells of the pancreas but completely inactive in all other cells of the body, and so on down the list of the body's million types of protein. It is the turning on or off (sometimes irreversibly) of genes which is responsible for differentiation, during embryonic and fetal development, of the totipotential fertilized ovum into the myriad types of body cells. But we are not here concerned with this mind-boggling process of development but rather with the fact that once certain genes of any given cell type have been granted, during development, the potential capacity for transcribing their particular mRNAs, the actual rates at which such transcription occurs can still be greatly influenced by environmental factors throughout that individual's life.

The best studied example of this phenomenon is the enzyme galactosidase in the bacterium Escherichia coli (E. coli). This enzyme catalyzes the splitting of lactose ("milk sugar") into a molecule of glucose and a molecule of galactose:

$$\text{Lactose} \xrightarrow{\text{galactosidase}} \text{glucose} + \text{galactose}$$

When E. coli are grown in a medium devoid of lactose, the bacteria synthesize galactosidase at an extremely slow rate and therefore contain almost none of the enzyme (about three molecules per cell). Within minutes after adding lactose to the medium, the rate of synthesis of galactosidase increases enormously and maintains this pace so that each bacterium contains about 3,000 molecules of galactosidase. This is an example of *enzyme induction*, an induced increase in the rate of mRNA synthesis leading to increased synthesis of the enzyme which that particular mRNA directs. The advantage of such a system is that the cell need not expend energy synthesizing an enzyme unless there is a substrate present for the enzyme to act upon.

Using the same type of logic, one can predict the phenomenon of *enzyme repression*, the other side of the coin, as it were. It makes no sense for the cell to expend energy synthesizing an enzyme when the product of the reaction that enzyme catalyzes is already available in large amounts. To take another example involving bacteria: The synthesis of the amino acid, histidine, requires a series of reactions catalyzed by ten different enzymes; when E. coli are grown in a medium to which histidine has been added, the cells do not synthesize these ten enzymes, but simply use the histidine supplied in the medium. In contrast, when no histidine is added to the medium the cells do synthesize the ten enzymes. Thus, the presence of histidine represses the synthesis of the enzymes required for its own synthesis; it does so by blocking the transcription of the genes which code for the enzymes.*

The impression should not be left that environmental inducers and repressors of gene transcription are always substrates or products of the reactions requiring the enzymes coded for by the affected genes. In many cases, the environmental factor may have no discernable relation to such reactions at all. This is a very important point. Enzyme repression by product should be recognizable to the reader as a completely intracellular homeostatic regulatory mechanism for maintaining product concentration relatively constant; in contrast, if anything but the product of a reaction represses the formation of the enzyme required for the product's formation, the result will be an abnormal reduction in cell concentration of product. Similarly, enzyme induction by an environmental factor other than the substrate for that enzyme will result in depletion of substrate and excessive formation of product. As we shall see, many environmental pollutants do just this.

Alteration of Enzyme Activity. The ability of an enzyme to accelerate a reaction (that is, how "active" an enzyme molecule is) is often subject to considerable variation. Other molecules may combine with it, altering its shape, and so-called cofactors may be needed for its normal function. By providing more or less of these factors which alter enzyme activity, the environment may exert profound effects on the rates at which chemical reactions proceed.

---

*One might imagine that enzyme induction and repression are effected simply by having the environmental factors (lactose and histidine, in our examples) combine with the relevant genes along the DNA chain and somehow stimulate or inhibit their transcription of mRNA, but such is not the case. The process is far more elegant, and descriptions of it can be found in any basic textbook of biology, physiology, or biochemistry.

One example of such influences is the phenomenon called *end-product inhibition*, in which the end product of a series of enzyme-catalyzed reactions decreases the activity of the enzyme in the series (by combining with it and changing its shape). This bears a superficial resemblance to the process of enzyme repression described in the previous section, and it may be worthwhile to emphasize how different the processes really are. In enzyme repression the product inhibits the *synthesis* of the enzyme by blocking DNA transcription; in end-product inhibition, the product does not influence the synthesis of the enzyme but rather decreases the *activity* of the already-formed enzyme. Of course, the significance to the cell is similar, since in both cases the presence of large amounts of product feeds back to decrease any further formation of product. Again, it should be clear that end-product inhibition represents a homeostatic process, whereas environmentally-induced inhibition (or enhancement) or enzyme activity by anything other than products (or substrates) of that enzyme can cause significant nonhomeostatic perturbations of the cell's chemistry.

Alteration of Substrate Supply. This influence on gene expression is simpler to visualize than the preceding categories. A cell may have an enzyme and this enzyme may be highly active, but if no substrate is present, obviously no reaction can occur. (I have stated this as an all-or-nothing proposition, but of course there is really a quantitative gradation of chemical reaction rates, depending upon just how much substrate is present.) Accordingly, the environment, by supplying or withholding substrate, can influence gene expression in this straightforward manner. An example, which we shall go into in detail in a later chapter: We have enzymes capable of converting perfectly harmless substances into cancer-producing molecules; accordingly, we carry within our genes (which code for these enzymes) the potential for producing cancer, but this expression of the genetic potential will occur only if the substrates (the "harmless molecules") are supplied by the environment (in cigarette smoke, for example).

Another example, one of the most striking illustrations I know of how the environment can influence phenotype: The genetic disease known as phenylketonuria (PKU) is due to the inherited absence of a single gene, the one which codes for the enzyme catalyzing the conversion of phenylalanine into tyrosine. A usual diet provides considerable amounts of phenylalanine, most of which is converted, in a normal person, to tyrosine. In children suffering from PKU, this conversion cannot occur, and the phenylalanine builds up in the blood and causes brain damage leading to mental retardation. The treatment? Provide a phenylalanine-free diet and the infant will be normal. Thus, the phenotype of these children spans the range from mental retardation to normal brain function depending on the phenylalanine content of their diets.

I hope that this description of the mechanisms by which the environment influences genetic expression reinforces the fact that human phenotypic plasticity is acted upon all the time, not only intermittently when environmental stresses are very great. The entire development and everyday functioning of the individual is conditioned by the total environment. For example, several profound physical and physiological changes have occurred in the peoples of the Western world during the past 100 years, and these changes must be attributed purely to environmental influences, since 100 years is much too short for genetic change to have played a role. Most visible is people's rate of growth, but even more remarkable has been the change in the rate of sexual maturation; in Norway, the average age at which menstruation begins has dropped from 17 to 13 during the past 110 years. It is quite likely that changes in nutrition have been the major environmental factors responsible for inducing this change, since the age of menarche seems to correlate well with body size, weight, or fat content.

To reiterate, at all times environment shapes our physical functioning and behavior. However, the most profound and lasting—often irreversible—effects occur during prenatal and early postnatal periods. This fact is expressed by the concept of *critical periods*, which states that developing organ systems are most susceptible to environmental influence at certain times, often during their periods of maximal cell division. (Growth of an organ or tissue depends upon increases both in cell number and in the size of individual cells; in most organs, cells stop increasing in number at some point in development, and subsequent growth is due mainly to enlargement of cells.) The critical period differs from organ to organ, in large part because of differences in the timing of maximal cell division; for example, this occurs very early in the development of the brain and very late in the case of the heart. This explains why environmental influences may exert no effect when present at certain times but may be extremely influential at others. For example, thalidomide caused its tragic defects in embryonic limb development only when mothers had taken it during the period when the limb buds of the fetus were appearing (approximately twenty to forty days after conception).

We are just beginning to appreciate how susceptible the developing embryo or fetus is to environmental influences. Altered nutrition, infection, external environmental temperature and humidity, noise, degree of crowding, sensory stimuli, and psychic or physical stress to the pregnant mother are only a few of the influences shown, in experimental animals, to influence the offspring's rate of growth, ultimate size, resistance to stress, capacity to learn, etc. These effects remain all through adult life and, most amazingly, often are manifest in the next generation as well. (This is not genetic inheritance of acquired characteristics, but can be explained by the persisting altered physiology of the first-generation female during her subsequent pregnancy. For example, a female rat whose growth was permanently stunted by nutritionally depriving her mother during pregnancy will in turn bear stunted offspring because of her permanently altered capacity to handle nutrients properly.)

Examples of postnatal critical-period influences are equally common. Single injections into newborn mice of particulate materials from urban air tend to increase frequency of cancer in those mice during adult life. Single injections of male sex hormone into newborn female rats causes the failure of normal sexual function to appear later in life. Permanent blindness is the result of not allowing an animal exposure to light during the first few weeks of life.

I have used examples from experiments on animals because such results are quite clear-cut, but the thalidomide example illustrates that human beings are not immune to such prenatal and postnatal phenomena and there are tragic human analogues of almost all the animal experiments. Diethylstilbestrol (DES), for example, is known to cause uterine cancer, after a delay of many years, in the offspring of mothers given this chemical at a critical period during pregnancy.

Alterations of Adaptive Capacity

We can now apply this information on gene-environment interactions in answering the question: How can adaptive capacity be altered? One way is by alteration of gene structure (genotype) and the other is by environmentally induced changes in gene expression with no change in genotype; the first category is called *genetic adaptation* and the second *acclimatization*.

Genetic Adaptation

Let us again look at thermoregulatory responses, this time taking, simply for variety, response to heat rather than cold. A familiar example of an adaptive response is the sweating which occurs when one is in a hot environment. This homeostatic response, which has survival value in a hot environment because it prevents a potentially dangerous rise in body temperature, requires the presence of sweat glands, nerves to the glands, internal temperature-detection devices, and the appropriate wiring circuits connecting all these components into a completely automatic self-contained control system. All these components exist because we have genes which code for their proteins. They are present more or less in all persons (except for a tiny number of people who, as a consequence, cannot survive for long in hot environments), because the genes which code for them are passed on from generation to generation. The origin of these particular gene types is described by basic evolutionary theory (fig. 2–3). Long ago they arose by mutations from already existing genes and not only persisted but spread widely during subsequent generations until they existed in virtually all individuals, simply because the possession of these genes carried immense survival value and, therefore, greater reproductive capacity, given the requirement for early humans (or their ancestors) to perform considerable physical exertion in the heat. To generalize, a gene which codes for a potential adaptation arises from a mutation, and the environment then selects for it if it is adaptive for that particular environment. For the general biologist the only measure of adaptiveness is the extent to which the individual possessing that gene can reproduce relative to those who do not possess it. Thus the mark of evolution is a change in the gene-frequencies within a population, and *natural selection* may be defined as any environmental force that causes a given gene, once having arisen, to increase or decrease over generations.

Let me reemphasize the phrase "adaptive for that particular environment." One cannot call a gene "good" or "bad" without reference to the environment. Perhaps the most striking illustration of this principle is the gene responsible for sickle-cell anemia. The "sickle-cell gene" codes for an abnormal hemoglobin molecule which causes red blood cells, in the low oxygen environment of capillaries, to be distorted from their normal disk shape into the shape of sickles. These sickled cells clog the vessels, causing damage, and are soon themselves destroyed by the body so that the patient becomes anemic. Most sufferers from this inherited disease die in childhood so that the gene responsible for it should be quite low in the population, at a level maintained only by continued mutations forming the gene. Geneticists were, therefore, amazed to find that in many tropical countries, the gene is present in as much as 40 percent of the population and is stable at this value. The puzzle was solved when two facts were realized. First, the gene usually causes death only when the offspring receives it from each parent, and almost all of the 40 percent of those people with the gene had only one such gene, the other gene coding for hemoglobin being normal. Second, the

Fig. 2–3. Pathway by which mutations lead to evolution.

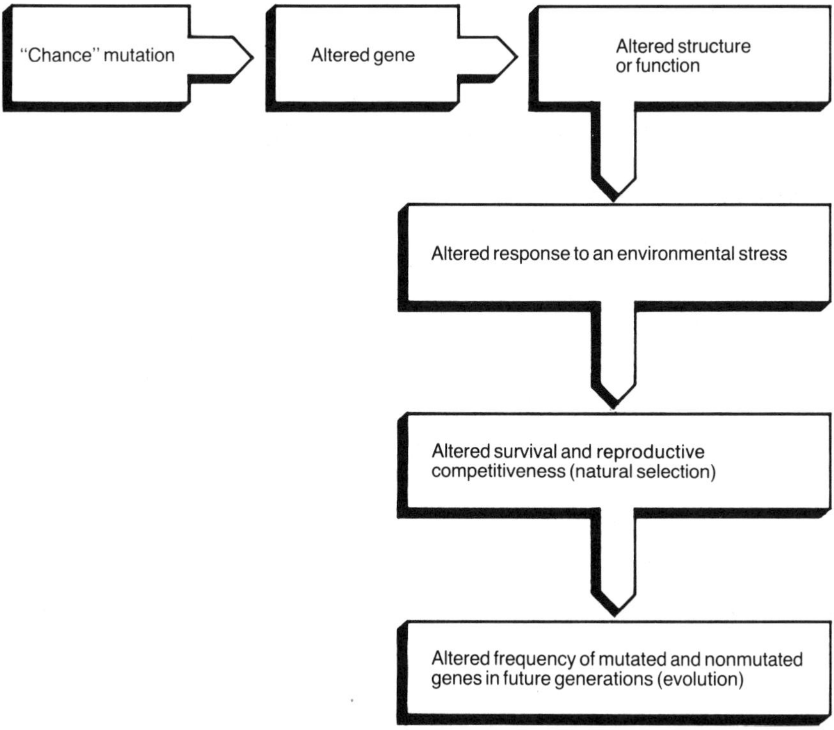

presence of one sickle-cell gene caused the red blood cell to be far more resistant to the parasite causing malaria, a disease endemic to those countries manifesting the high frequency of sickle-cell genes. Thus, the survival advantage conferred on those living in malaria-infested environments by a single sickle-cell gene maintains a high frequency of the gene even though it is deleterious in double dose. The sickle-cell gene is both "good" and "bad" in these countries, depending on whether the person has one or two of them. In contrast, there is absolutely no survival value of the gene in nonmalarial countries such as the United States, and the gene frequency is slowly diminishing here.

To return to our basic theme, what causes gene mutations, i.e., the alteration in gene structure upon which natural selection can then act? Here is a source of potential misunderstanding. We know that most, if not all mutations, are caused by environmental forces (mainly radiation and chemicals), but the crucial point is that any changes in adaptability resulting from the mutation are *not* directed toward that environmental factor responsible for the mutation. In our earlier example, there is absolutely no reason to suspect that exposure of our ancestors to heat was the trigger which caused the genetic mutations favorable for development of sweat glands; rather we presume that these genes were formed as a result of mutations that occurred by chance (in the sense that they were random, indeterminate, and unpredictable), and were then selected for by the hot environment.

Unless this fact is appreciated, it is all too easy to believe complacently but wrongly that environmental hazards are likely ultimately to induce genetic changes which lead specifically to better adaptability against that hazard. Many environmental hazards do increase the rate of mutations in our genes, but there is not the slightest shred of evidence that the resulting changes in structure and function are protective against the mutagenic substance itself. To the contrary, it seems almost certain that the great majority of mutations result in changes that are detrimental to survival. To protect against mutations, living organisms have evolved intracellular mechanisms for repairing damaged DNA. For example, there exist enzymes which "recognize" certain forms of damaged DNA, and catalyze both the excision of these segments from the DNA molecule and the normal resynthesis of the excised region, using the complementary undamaged DNA strand as a template. First discovered in bacteria, DNA repair mechanisms are known also to exist in mammalian cells and play active roles in protecting us against mutations. One present theory of aging, in fact, postulates that a progressive failure of DNA repair accounts for the loss of function characteristic of aging.

There is no question that humankind is still undergoing biological evolution, but it is quite impossible, on the basis of present information, to predict in just what directions or how quickly. The rate of evolutionary change depends on both the mutation rate and the selection pressure (i.e., the degree to which the environment confers relative reproductive success on the bearers of various genes). On the one hand, it is likely, although unproven, that the mutation rate of human genes is increasing because of our increased exposure to ionizing radiation and chemical mutagens (agents which cause mutations). Indeed, the creation of some monitoring system for mutation rate in human beings is considered by most geneticists to be essential so that we may quickly detect the presence of any new potent environmental mutagen. Any such system would require the monitoring of from one to ten million people, as the following analysis shows.

The present spontaneous mutation rate in human beings is estimated at one mutation per 100,000 gene loci per generation. Since the total number of gene loci in each cell of an individual is approximately 100,000, we can expect one mutation per person. How can we detect these? One way is to screen newborns for the fifty or so easily detectable diseases each of which is due to a single dominant mutation. The incidence of all these diseases taken together should be fifty per 100,000 births, and some simple statistics reveal that we would need to monitor at least 127,000 births to convince ourselves that an observed rate of seventy-five per 100,000 (50 percent greater than normal) was really different from the present rate of fifty per 100,000. At a birth rate of 20 per 1,000 population, we have to monitor a total population of six to ten million people.

An easier approach is to look not for diseases (phenotypic sentinels), but for changes in proteins. There are at least twenty blood proteins in which alteration of a single amino acid, due to a mutation in the gene coding for that protein, can be detected with a chemical analysis. Routine analysis of these blood proteins (biochemical sentinels) in only 18,000 births per year (to be expected in a population of one million people) would yield conclusive evidence of a 50 percent increase in mutation rate were such to occur. Neither of these systems nor any others proposed is presently in use despite the immense importance of knowing whether our mutation rate really is increasing.

What about selection pressure, the other factor determining the rate of evolutionary change? One might predict that selection pressure, too, is increasing because our rapidly changing environment puts a greater variety of biological demands on people. However, and this is one of the major themes of this book, we simply do not know to what degree most of our present environmental threats really influence survival and reproductive potential. Moreover, selection pressure has been drastically reduced in the case of persons suffering from diseases treatable with modern medical care, since these persons are now able to live through their reproductive years and reproduce successfully. An example is retinoblastoma, the eye cancer of children, which is almost always fatal if not treated. The gene for retinoblastoma is estimated to arise in approximately one sex cell (sperm or ovum) out of 50,000; previously this gene disappeared with the early death of its bearer, but now treatment permits 70 percent of the gene-bearers to survive, reproduce, and pass the defect on to half their children.

Even taking into account these unknowns, it is almost certain that evolution continues to be an extremely slow process and that our ability to adapt to present environmental problems will not be appreciably enhanced by widespread genetic change for many generations.

This is not something to complain about when one realizes the alternative, for evolution can theoretically be very rapid under one of two conditions—marked increase in either the mutation rate or the selection pressure. In either case, the result would be massive increases in death or misery. In the first case, although some mutations that might be beneficial for our present environment might emerge, it is generally agreed among geneticists that a much larger fraction of such mutations would be detrimental to their bearers. To illustrate the second case—a marked increase in selection pressure—the radiation released during a nuclear holocaust might spare only those persons who bear genes conferring upon them extraordinary resistance to the lethal (and sterility-producing) effects of radiation. Only they would survive and so the frequency of that gene in the population would have greatly increased. This, by definition, is evolution, but at what a price!

It is not very comforting to find natural phenomena which bear at least a superficial resemblance to this latter type of "instant" evolution. One of these is the population crash so typical of certain rodent species. As I shall describe in detail in a later chapter, these species manifest profound swings in population; at the crest of a population rise there is a rather sudden and huge increase in death rate, decrease in birth rate, and a mass migration. The result is a profound drop in population size and the beginning of a new cycle. The important point for our present discussion is that all these events affect mainly the subordinate members of the community, leaving the most dominant individuals relatively unscathed. If (and it is a big "if") the dominance-subordinance hierarchy of these rodent populations were the reflection of genetic differences, then each population crash would be a strong selector for certain genes, i.e., evolution would take a quantum leap with each crash. However, we do not know to what extent the dominance-subordinance hierarchy really does reflect genetic differences among animals.

There is another reason other than its slow pace which precludes evolution from protecting us from the diseases we fear most. Unlike the infectious diseases which, in concert with malnutrition, strike most commonly before the age of five, the present scourges of Westernized countries—heart disease, strokes, and cancer—affect most people beyond their major reproductive years. Since natural selection acts by favoring reproductive success of individuals, there is no reason to assume that evolution will slowly select against any genes which predispose to these diseases. Indeed, some have argued that natural selection may actually be favoring such genes! This concept is intimately associated with the biological "value" or "disvalue" of the aged to those still in their reproductive years. Does having a large number of elderly people in a society hinder or help the other members of that society to survive through their reproductive years and breed successfully?

Acclimatization

In contrast to the altered adaptability occurring as a result of genetic change, acclimatization is an adaptive change induced during the individual's own lifetime by an environmental stress with no alteration in his genetic endowment (fig. 2–4). It follows that an acclimatization is not passed on genetically to one's offspring.

To clarify the distinctions between acclimatization and genetic alteration as the causes of altered adaptability, let us again take sweating as an example and perform a simple experiment. On day one we expose a person for thirty minutes to a temperature of 37°C and ask him to do a standardized exercise test. He soon begins to sweat and the volume of sweat produced is measured (simply by weighing him before and after the test). Then, for one week, he enters the 37°C heat chamber for one or two hours per day and exercises. On day eight, his sweating rate is again measured during the same exercise test performed on day one; the striking finding is that he begins to sweat earlier and much more profusely than on day one; accordingly, his body temperature does not rise nearly to the same degree. He has acclimatized to the heat, that is, he has undergone an adaptive change induced by exposure to the heat, to which he is now specifically better adapted, but with no change in his gene structure. In a sense, acclimatization may be viewed as an environmentally induced improvement in the functioning of an already existing genetically based homeostatic system. Repeated or prolonged exposure to the environmental stress enhances the responsiveness of the system to that particular type of stress.

Let us take another example, one which vividly illustrates the generalization that a homeostatically regulated variable cannot be interpreted without regard to the environmental setting. Approximately 45 percent of a person's blood is composed of red blood cells when he is dwelling at sea level. If he moves to the mountains (let's say at 12,000 ft) and remains there, the relative amount of his blood which is red cells slowly increases. This is an excellent acclimatization to life at high altitude because almost all blood oxygen is carried in the red cells, and the relative increase in red cells increases the oxygen-carrying capacity of the blood and thereby helps to

Fig. 2–4. Pathway for acclimatization.

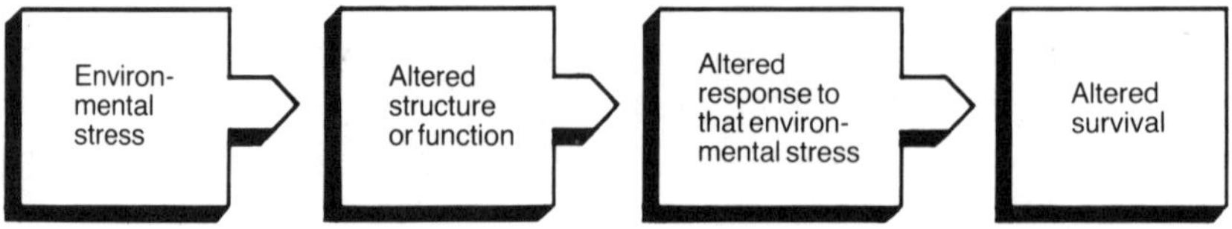

| Environmental stress | Altered structure or function | Altered response to that environmental stress | Altered survival |

maintain the oxygen concentration in the tissues. This is precisely the same type of change that occurs in a sea-level dweller who develops severe enough lung disease to impair oxygen delivery. The point is that a high level of red cells in the blood is a sure sign of disease in a sea-level dweller but a perfectly normal finding in high-altitude dwellers.

It has proven very difficult to determine for any particular acclimatization just which components of the control system the acclimatization has sensitized, but the right questions are easy to phrase on the basis of our earlier description of homeostatic control systems. For our example of sweating we would come up as a start with the following: Is the sensitivity of the thermosensitive elements increased so that they respond to smaller deviations of temperature from normal? Are the nerve-cell wiring connections in the system more responsive to signals? Are the sweat glands enlarged and so more able to respond to a given signal? Are those sweat gland enzymes responsible for the actual production of the sweat more numerous or more active?

For the biochemist, the fun only begins when the control system component affected by the acclimatization has been identified, for then he can go to work on the series of questions predictable from our earlier description of gene expression—just which step(s) from DNA transcription to the actual enzyme-catalyzed reaction has been altered in this component by the repeated exposure of the overall system to the environment stimulus?

In the example above, the heat acclimatization of our subject is completely reversible in that, if the daily exposures are discontinued, then within a relatively short time his sweating rate during future tests will revert to its preacclimatized value. However, not all acclimatization is reversible. If the acclimatization is induced very early in the individual's life, at the "critical period" for development of that structure or response, it may be irreversible. For example, the barrel-shaped chests of Andean natives does not represent a genetic difference between them and their lowland countrymen, but rather an irreversible acclimatization induced during the first few years of their lives by their exposure to the low-oxygen environment of high altitude. It remains even though the individual moves to a lowland environment later in life and stays there. Lowland children who suffered oxygen deprivation from heart or lung disease during their early years show precisely the same chest shape.

These so-called developmental acclimatizations are very common responses to a wide variety of environmental stresses. They take the form not only of anatomical changes, as in the example cited, but of physiological responses as well. For example, because of their developmental acclimatizations, the Andean natives have a greater maximal capacity for exercise at high altitude than do lowlanders who have moved to the mountains beyond childhood and remained there the rest of their lives. The latter never reach the level of acclimatization achieved by those born in the mountains.

Physiological Differences Between People

A question which always captures both the scientific and popular imagination is the extent to which phenotypic differences between people represent differences in genotype. It may be unnecessary to state that we cannot tell whether two persons' genes are different by looking at their DNA molecules; their phenotypes are all we can work with. (In this regard we are in the same predicament as natural selection which does not discriminate against genes directly but rather against the phenotypes of the persons bearing them; thus, retinoblastoma genes cannot be eliminated by themselves but only through the death of their bearers.)

No one denies that most of the obvious physical (anatomical) differences between Chinese and Norwegians reflect differences in the genotypes of these groups. However, it has proven extremely difficult to determine whether physiological (i.e., functional, as opposed to anatomical) differences between peoples represent genetic differences or merely phenotypic differences reflecting the diverse environments. Indeed, it is no exaggeration to say that very few physiological differences between peoples have been shown conclusively to be the result of genetic differences. We were much more confident of genetically-based physiological variation a decade ago because we did not realize how common developmental acclimatizations are and that, therefore, lack of reversibility of a trait is not necessarily proof of genetic differences.

Paul Baker has described the problem very well in terms of an apparently simple example—hand temperature during exposure to cold.[1] In an earlier example in this chapter, I described how blood vessels to the skin constrict as an adaptive response to cold-exposure; the vessels to the hands are no exception (in us and almost all other peoples), and the result is that the hands become very cold, "wooden," and painful. But this does not occur in Eskimos, who can actually immerse their hands in near-freezing water for many minutes; the blood vessels to their hands do not constrict, blood flow remains high, and no pain is reported. Clearly, this is an excellent adaption for the Eskimos, who must work bare-handed at delicate tasks in the cold, and one might assume that it represents a genetic alteration selected for by the environment. However, although the evidence is not yet conclusive, it seems much more likely that this striking response really represents a developmental acclimatization. Interestingly, Gaspé fishermen manifest precisely the same response.

Let us take another example, because it may represent an analogue to the bacterial galactosidase story described earlier in this chapter. Lactose is milk sugar, and the intestinal enzyme lactase (this is a galactosidase with precisely the same function as the bacterial galactosidase described earlier) must break it down into its two component sugars before they can be absorbed from the intestinal tract into the blood. For want of lactase, most adults cannot digest lactose, and this results in diarrhea whenever they drink fairly large quantities of milk. However, in certain populations, adults do have the enzyme so that they manifest no lactose-intolerance. Yet the story is far more complex than this, for lactase is present in all normal infants, otherwise they would be unable to digest the lactose in milk, the major food during infancy. What happens is that the concentration of this enzyme is very high at birth but then, in most people, it decreases and becomes extremely low or absent altogether after eighteen to thirty-six months. The decrease in the enzyme results from repression of the enzyme which codes for its synthesis. In contrast, in lactose-tolerant populations the gene fails to "turn off" after infancy. These are generally populations who possess large numbers of cattle and continue to drink large quantities of milk beyond early childhood. Here is a classic "nature-nurture" problem, for one can pose very different alternate hypotheses for this phenomenon: (1) the continued presence of milk in the diet somehow causes the gene which codes for lactase not to be repressed; (2) Since it is biologically advantageous for these cattle-rich populations to be able to digest milk, then the survival of individuals with a genetic mutation that led to the persistence of high intestinal lactase beyond infancy would have been favored (natural selection). Norman Kretchmer has beautifully described approaches required to distinguish between these two alternatives and the great difficulties involved in coming to any definite conclusions, even though the population difference in this case reflects a single well-defined enzyme![2] It is sheer hubris to conclude that we presently possess the knowledge and techniques to dissect infinitely more complex nature-nurture problems such as differences in performances on IQ tests?

Maladaptive Responses

It is easy enough to understand how a given environmental threat can cause disease or death if there is no adaptive response at all to it, or if the response is simply not up to the task, as for example, in an overwhelming bacterial infection. What is surprising, however, is that the response, itself, may be outright damaging, i.e., maladaptive.

In many cases this maladaptation is an unavoidable consequence of the body's complexity. The response to a stressor automatically alters many other components of body function, sometimes in a harmful way. For example, as will be described in detail later, when the body responds adaptively to a foreign harmful chemical by increasing the rate at which the liver breaks down the chemical, the rate at which certain essential endogenous chemicals is broken down is also enhanced, with potentially harmful results if the endogenous chemical is already in short supply.

On yet another level of complexity, acclimatization to one stressor may influence the ability to respond to a second, different stressor. For example, rats acclimatized to the cold showed a reduced ability to survive when they were acutely exposed to high altitude. (I certainly do not wish to leave the impression that the response to one stressor always impairs that to a second—these same cold-acclimatized rates have a much greater resistance to the lethal effects of radiation.)

Another type of maladaptation occurs when a response which is highly adaptive in the short term turns out to be harmful if continued for long periods. For example, low levels of irritating air pollutants increase mucus production by the airways, an adaptive response which helps prevent entry of these chemicals into the blood. However, over long periods of time, the accumulation of mucus may predispose to infection in the airways and to serious lung disease.

A third type of maladaptive response is characterized by being inappropriate. Allergies such as hay fever fit into this category. The ragweed pollen which triggers the response is quite harmless, and it is the body's response to the pollen which causes the symptoms—runny nose, sneezing, itching eyes, etc.—so familiar to the miserable victim.

In other cases, the response is appropriate, but excessive. For example, the body may launch such an aggressive attack against a microbial invader that its weapons destroy not only the microbes but adjacent normal cells and tissues as well.

There may well be a common denominator to many of these maladaptive responses, namely the fact that most people now live in environments which, because of human intervention, are very different from the environments in which humankind evolved. It should not be surprising, therefore, that physiological activities and responses which were selected by evolution because of their adaptiveness in one environment might prove to be maladaptive when the environment changes. The potential conflict described above between short-term benefits and long-term losses certainly fits nicely into the category. The reflex stimulating mucus secretion in response to inhaled irritants almost certainly evolved as a purely acute response, for there simply were no chronic irritants present in the air at that time.

It is in the realm of learning and behavior that the most vivid examples of this principle are to be found. It is now axiomatic that the most potent unconscious reinforcers of one's actions are their immediate consequences. In Skinnerian terms, we are more likely to repeat an action if the consequences of that action are pleasurable at the time. In contrast, the long-term consequences of an act simply have no automatic effect on our likelihood of repeating that act (I am speaking here only of unconscious learning and certainly do not want to deal here with the mind-body problem, free will, "conscious" future planning, and the like). Therefore, trouble occurs when the long-term and short-term consequences are different. Cigarette smoking offers a tragic example (short-term pleasure versus long-term lung cancer).

There are many other examples of how profound environmental alterations might cause a previously adaptive response to become maladaptive. When food supply is quite precarious it is adaptive to possess a strong "drive" for food; in contrast, when food is relatively plentiful, such a "drive" may cause overeating, obesity, and its attendant negative health consequences.

Even more interesting implications appear when we look at obesity in terms of homeostatic control systems. One gains weight only when total energy expenditure is less than total energy input (supplied as food), and evolution has provided us with precise regulatory mechanisms which cause a person to increase food intake when his general level of activity has increased. But this relationship does not hold at very low levels of physical activity. In a key study, the caloric intakes and body weights of large numbers of workers in the same factory in India were studied after grouping the men according to the physical exertion required for their jobs. Levels of activity below a certain arbitrary minimum were classified as sedentary. Men performing work loads above the sedentary range displayed the expected pattern, in that caloric intake was directly proportional to work load, and body weights for all groups of men were similar. The unexpected finding was that for men performing very little work (the sedentary range), caloric intake varied *inversely* with work load, i.e., the less physical activity the men performed, the more they ate! Accordingly, these men were considerably fatter, on the average, than the other men. Since this kind of study might be confounded by many other variables, a series of experiments was performed on rats forced to remain sedentary or to exercise; the results were completely analogous to those found in the human study. Clearly, very few if any of our ancestors operated in the sedentary range whereas most Westernized peoples presently do. Does this presently maladaptive relationship represent a holdover from our evolutionary past, in which, somehow, it might have been adaptive in the setting of only brief periods of physical inactivity, or does it simply reflect a homeostatic system out of control because it is being called upon to operate at a level of physical activity not encountered during its evolution?

Maladaptive responses are not the only consequence of the fact that our present environment is so different from that in which humankind evolved. Another is the complete absence of any response! Earlier I emphasized that homeostatic control systems, a major common denominator of our adaptive responses, require biological "detectors" which continuously monitor the variable being regulated (temperature, plasma glucose concentration, plasma oxygen concentration, etc.) and trigger the reflexes required to keep the variable relatively constant. We simply have not had time to evolve appropriate detectors for those environmental factors which have only recently emerged as serious threats. Thus, we are completely unaware of the presence of ionizing radiation until it has already done its damage. Carbon monoxide is another example—people may die of carbon monoxide poisoning without ever being aware they are being exposed to it.* In all these cases, the body does not have the ability to rid itself of the threat before damage is done, and so adaptive responses must be limited simply to repairing the damage.

Conclusion

In the way of concluding this chapter, I cannot do better than quote Frederick Sargent:

> Does man possess the adaptive capacity to meet the environmental challenges and hazards that he himself is creating? . . . Human adaptability identifies a capability of man to people a wide range of habitats successfully. This capability arises from diverse configurations of morphological, biochemical, physiological, and behavioral traits. Because of their evolutionary history, these traits function within constraints defined by the environmental conditions and circumstances through which the human species has passed. The mark of these experiences continues in the genotype of the individual and gene pool of the biological population. Although, within the limits set by these constraints, phenotypic plasticity provides considerable latitude for adjustment to environmental change, there is no assurance that the challenges of really novel environments will be dealt with successfully. Natural selection, of course, in the long run serves to test adaptability, but man has now created a situation where events are transpiring so rapidly that it would seem that there is not time enough for selection to act.[3]

Clearly, the question of man's adaptive capacity cannot be answered in general terms, but requires deep knowledge of the specific effects of each environmental challenge on human performance and response. Precisely the same types of considerations apply to the more positive question of what constitutes an "optimal" environment.

---

*Carbon monoxide and ionizing radiation occur normally in the environment, but modern man has created higher local concentrations of them than existed before.

Part II | Nutrition

Chapter 3 | The Task of Nutritional Science

During its golden age earlier in this century, the science of nutrition made profound contributions to preventive medicine. One-by-one the vitamins were discovered and the diseases associated with their deficiencies conquered. The importance of iron and other trace elements, the relationship between malnutrition and infection, these and many other discoveries provided new insights and weapons against specific diseases. Then, for many years, nutrition became the orphan child of the medical sciences. Its mission seemingly accomplished (at least in the view of nonnutritionists), its content dull and old-fashioned in comparison to newly emerging glamour fields like immunology and molecular genetics, nutrition almost ceased to be taught in medical schools. Even when some instruction was given it was generally in the form of dusty tables of dietary requirements, rules that reminded students of their grade-school days ("eat at least one of the major food categories each day"), and with the clear implication that essentially all the information was already "in," that nutrition was pretty much a dead or dying field, and that real nutritional problems occurred only in a very small fraction of our population.

But during the last few years the climate of opinion has been changing rapidly and drastically. On the one hand it is being argued that the amounts of many nutrients traditionally recommended for prevention of deficiency diseases are too small to promote optimal health, well-being, and longevity. On the other, our diet is even more vigorously criticized as supplying too much of other nutrients—cholesterol, fat, sugar, and salt—and the crucial point is that this accusation is leveled against the "normal" diet of the general population.

Even the Congress of the United States has stated:

> Congress hereby finds that there is increasing evidence of a relationship between diet and many of the leading causes of death in the United States; that improved nutrition is an integral component of preventive health care; that there is a serious need for research on the chronic effects of diet on degenerative diseases and related disorders.[1]

To back up its words, Congress has markedly increased the appropriations for research related to human nutrition. In 1977, all agencies of the federal government spent some $50 million in this area; in 1979, the National Institutes of Health (NIH) and the United States Department of Agriculture (USDA) alone were estimated to spend more than $170 million. Clearly, the hope is that this increased funding will usher in a second golden age for nutrition, one which will illuminate the optimal diet for the maintenance of health and longevity.

This is a tall order and some fear that "another War On Cancer is in the works—that the payoff from increases in nutrition research will fall short of what the dollars promise."[2] Associated with this view is the belief that most of the accusations against our general diet are wrong. This may turn out to be the case, but the theme of this chapter and the next three is that such research is needed, that our knowledge of diet-health interrelations is really in its infancy, not its dotage.

This chapter provides the scientific information and approaches basic to pursuing any question in nutrition, ending with an analysis of the vitamin C controversy as a classic case. The next chapters then provide more specific examples of the types of diet-health problems encountered in nutrition and the present status of scientific knowledge concerning them.

History of Nutritional Patterns

There is still much debate among scientists over what constituted the diet of early humankind and its hominid ancestors, particularly with regard to the relative amounts of animal and plant products consumed. One popular conception is that human beings evolved from "killer apes"—aggressive hunters whose dietary staple was meat. This view is now thought to be incorrect and the hominids and early man are now pictured more as herbivores than carnivores. One reason for this shift in view is new archaeological evidence provided by analysis of fossilized human or hominid feces called coprolites. These contain some animal remains (chicken feathers, small bones, deer hairs) but considerably more seeds, pollen, and other plant matter. Moreover, it is now felt that the archaeological sites laden with fossilized bones of large animals really represent butchering sites, rather than living sites, and so led us to exaggerate the amount of prey eaten by prehistoric peoples.

A second type of evidence is anatomical and physiological. The human digestive tract is much longer than the carnivore's and has a larger surface area. The chemical composition of the saliva, too, is more like a herbivore's than a carnivore's.

Perhaps the most important evidence concerning early food habits comes from studies of contemporary hunting-and-gathering tribes who live much as we believe prehistoric humans did. The !Kung San (formerly called Bushmen) of southern Africa, for example, obtain approximately two-thirds of their calories from vegetable matter. Most striking of all is the sheer variety of their diets—no less than fifty-nine species of plants and seventeen of animals.

> Their ability to adapt to and exploit the food resources of their rather harsh environment is remarkable but not atypical of hunters. Although they prefer wild vegetables and the flesh of certain game animals such as the antelope, they will eat anything they can digest—rats, lions, snakes, hyenas, lizards, frogs, insects, scorpions, grubs, and the available seeds, berries, wild plums, wild melons, wild veld cabbage, and many bulbs and roots. They are not particular about the state of their food and are able to eat meat that is putrid or ostrich eggs already old and smelly. They can also endure the rhythm of feast and famine, eating prodigiously whenever food is abundant, surviving on short rations when necessary, or going completely without food for considerable periods. In half a day, two Bushmen are able to consume a whole sheep or comparable amounts of wild game—intestines and all. This voracious and indiscriminate eating is typical of hunting groups.[3]

If we assume that such a diet was typical of our ancestors, then it is likely that the sheer variety as well as the inclusion of at least some animal matter assured that all essential nutrients were consumed when food was available. Because of the precariousness of the hunt and, perhaps even more important, fluctuations in the availability of plants, there were probably relatively long periods when total food supply was inadequate. Accordingly, a major evolutionary development must have been mechanisms for dealing with alternating periods of feasting and fasting.

The agricultural revolution of 10,000 to 12,000 years ago brought about extraordinary changes in human food habits. First, there occurred an even greater dependence on vegetable sources of food, and this pattern remains the norm today for most nonindustrialized countries. For example, as shown in table 3–1, more than 95 percent of the total calories consumed by Asians comes from vegetable sources; the figure for Africans is about 93 percent.

Even more important than the overall dependency on vegetable sources is the fact that most of the calories for any given people come from a single type of cultivated plant—rice, wheat, corn, potatoes, millet, sorghum, or cassava. For example, half the people in the world obtain nearly 50 percent of their total caloric intake from rice alone.

With these dietary changes came a new set of problems. First, the reduction in the variety of food greatly increased the incidence of chronic deficiencies of various essential nutrients (iron and vitamin A, for example) even when total caloric intake was adequate. Second, the seasonal nature of the staple crop's growth often imposed several months of inadequate intake prior to the next harvest; for example, rural Gambians lose 10 percent of their body weights from June to October, and these seasonal bouts of inadequate caloric intake may have had important physiological consequences for body growth and maturation. Third, the expansion of the total food supply made possible by the agricultural revolution ironically ushered in the age of great famines (table 3–2). An almost total dependence on a single cultivated crop means that whenever the production of that crop fails (usually because of weather or blights, but sometimes because of social upheavals) there are no adequate alternate sources. Moreover, the large increases in population brought about by the shift from hunting and gathering to agriculture means that masses of people, not just small groups, are affected when the crops fail. (During more recent years population growth has been further stimulated by modern public health and medical practices.) Thus, the paradox: A major result of the agricultural revolution has been widespread chronic malnutrition, interrupted by periods of acute starvation affecting huge numbers of people.

TABLE 3–1 Percentage Distribution of Total Calorie Supply by Major Food Groups, by Regions

Region	Grain Products, Roots, and Tubers	Fruits, Nuts, and Vegetables	Sugar	Fats and Oils	Livestock Products	Fish	Total
Geographic regions							
North America	24.4%	9.1%	15.8%	19.9%	30.6%	0.2%	100.0%
Oceania	30.0	5.6	16.3	12.3	35.2	0.6	100.0
Western Europe	43.9	6.4	11.2	16.8	20.8	0.9	100.0
Latin America	50.7	12.3	14.0	8.0	14.7	0.3	100.0
E. Europe & USSR	64.9	3.5	8.6	9.2	14.0	0.4	100.0
Africa	70.1	11.5	4.1	7.5	6.3	0.5	100.0
Asia	74.5	11.4	4.1	5.3	3.8	0.9	100.0
World	62.7	9.6	7.3	8.9	10.8	0.7	100.0
Economic regions							
Developed regions	47.3	5.9	11.1	14.5	20.7	0.5	100.0
Less developed regions	71.7	11.5	5.1	5.8	5.1	0.8	100.0

Source: From Lester R. Brown and Gail W. Finsterbusch, *Man and His Environment: Food* (New York: Harper and Row, 1972), p. 39. Data from U. S. Department of Agriculture.

TABLE 3–2   Reasonably Authenticated Major Famines

Date	Place	Comments
B.C.		
436	Rome	Thousands of starving people threw themselves into the Tiber
A.D.		
310	England	40,000 deaths
917–18	India (Kashmir)	Great mortality
c.1051	Mexico	Caused migration of Toltecs; probable origin of human sacrifice
1064–72	Egypt	Failure of Nile flood for 7 years; cannibalism reported
1069	England	Harrying by Normans; cannibalism
1344–45	India	Many thousands of deaths
1347	Italy	Famine followed by plague (the "Black Death") caused great mortality
1594–98	Asia	In India, great mortality, cannibalism, and bodies not disposed of
1600	Russia	500,000 deaths from famine and plague
1630	India (Deccan)	30,000 deaths in Surat alone
1660–61	India	No rain for 2 years
1677	India (Hyderabad)	Due to excessive rain; great mortality
1769	France	5 percent of population said to have died
1769–70	India (Bengal)	Due to drought; 10 million deaths
1770	Eastern Europe	Famine and disease caused 168,000 deaths in Bohemia, 20,000 in Russia and Poland
1775	Cape Verde Islands	16,000 deaths
1790–92	India (Bombay, Hyderabad)	Boji Bara, or skull famine; bodies not disposed of; great mortality
1803–4	Western India	Due to drought, locusts, and war; thousands died
1837–38	Northwestern India	800,000 deaths
1846–47	Ireland	Due to potato blight; 2 to 3 million deaths
1866	India (Bengal, Orissa)	1 million deaths
1869	India (Rajputana)	1.5 million deaths
1874–75	Asia Minor	150,000 deaths
1876–78	India	5 million deaths
1876–79	North China	Almost no rain for 3 years; deaths estimated at 9 to 13 million
1891–92	Russia	Widespread distress; mortality relatively small
1899–1900	India	1 million deaths
1918–19	Uganda	4,400 deaths
1920–21	Northern China	500,000 deaths
1920–21	Russia	Due to drought; millions died
1929	China (Hunan)	2 million deaths
1932–33	Russia	Due to collectivization; excess mortality estimated at 3 to 10 million
1943	Ruanda-Urandi	35,000 to 50,000 deaths
1943–44	India (Bengal)	Excessive rain and wartime difficulty of supply; 2 to 4 million deaths
1969–70	Biafra	Due to civil war; several hundred thousand deaths (minimum)

Source: Lester R. Brown and Gail W. Finsterbusch, *Man and His Environment: Food* (New York: Harper and Row, 1972), p. 6–7. Copyright © 1972 by Lester R. Brown and Gail W. Finsterbusch. Adapted from the original in *Famine* by Geoffrey B. Masefield, published by Oxford University Press, 1963. Reprinted by permission of Harper and Row Publishers, Inc.

The next great change in nutritional patterns has occurred only during the past 100 years or so in those countries which have industrialized. The diets of most of the inhabitants of these so-called Westernized countries differ profoundly from both the diet of hunter-gatherers and that of persons living in nonindustrialized nations. Table 3–3 lists the major differences.

Perhaps the most striking change has been in the shift from vegetable sources to animal sources; North Americans now obtain less than 25 percent of their caloric needs from grains and other vegetable matter, and more than 30 percent from meat, milk, eggs, and fish. Associated with this has been a large increase in protein intake and an even larger increase in fat intake (even though hunter-gatherers consume a moderate amount of meat, it is game meat, which contains only about one-sixth the fat, on a percentage basis, of our domestic cattle, bred and fed specifically for their rich marbled fat). Total calories have increased as has the supply of sugar (North Americans consume four to five times more sugar than do Asians), salt, and food additives, whereas fiber intake ("roughage") has greatly decreased. Our food supply is now continuous so that periods of fasting are no longer compulsory. Finally, much of our

TABLE 3–3   Changes in Diet as Countries Industrialize

Change	Hypothesized Negative Health Consequences
↑ Protein, particularly from animal sources	↑ Rate of aging process and development of cancer
↑ Fat, particularly from animal sources	↑ Heart attacks, strokes, and cancer
↑ Simple sugars	↑ Dental caries, diabetes mellitus, heart attacks ↑ Deficiencies of trace elements and vitamins
↑ Total calories	↑ Obesity, diabetes mellitus, heart attacks, hypertension
↓ Fiber	↑ Cancer, gallstones, appendicitis, etc.
↑ Salt (sodium chloride)	↑ Blood pressure
Continuous intake	↑ Rate of aging process
↑ Food additives	↑ Cancer
↑ Processing of food	↑ Deficiencies of trace elements and vitamins

food has undergone some form of commercial processing (refining, preserving, etc.).

These changes in dietary habits are major suspects as causal factors in the diseases associated with Westernization. This is one reason that there is so much current interest in the likely food habits of our primitive ancestors; the "argument from evolution" hypothesizes that any food habits profoundly different from those characteristic of prehistoric people and their primate ancestors, that is, different from those present during almost our entire period of evolution, are very likely to be harmful. In other words, the genetic basis for our physiological characteristics has not had time to change appreciably, and our profound biological success as a species means that natural selection must have favored the dietary patterns present during our emergence.

This is a logical inference, but by no means a necessary one for several reasons. First, as pointed out in chapter 2, it is not at all clear in what direction natural selection acts on individuals beyond their prime reproductive years, and the elderly are the major targets for our modern "killer diseases." Second, the present nondietary environment is so different today that dietary factors which may have been highly advantageous during our evolution might be maladaptive today. Nutritional status is so important in determining our resistance to microbial diseases and environmental pollutants to name just two categories of environmental factors, and the relationship with these factors are so complex, that predictions based on the "argument from evolution" alone concerning the beneficial or harmful effects of our present diet are tenuous indeed.

Nevertheless, the association, in our culture, of these new dietary habits and the emergence of the new killer diseases demands looking into. And so a large number of epidemiological studies as well as controlled experiments with laboratory animals and people have been performed; the right-hand column of table 3–3 lists the major negative health consequences which have been hypothesized for each. I cannot emphasize too strongly the word "hypothesized," for only in the case of sugar and dental caries are we presently certain beyond a reasonable doubt that the dietary characteristic is truly a causal factor in the disease listed.

Without question, the single most intensively studied of these hypothesized relationships is that connecting a large intake of animal fat to heart attacks, and I will analyze this hypothesis as a prototype in chapter 6. The uncertainty we shall find there should only underscore the even greater uncertainty associated with the others. The reader should consult the back of the book for suggested readings on each association in the list.

The list also underscores the fact that dietary factors other than nutritional content may have health consequences. Undigestible nonnutrient fiber ("roughage"), for example, may well play a protective role against a variety of diseases. Meal frequency may also be important. Nevertheless, the great majority of all nutritional research centers on the individual dietary nutrients, particularly the so-called essential ones, and their possible influences on disease.

Homeostasis of Essential Nutrients

Nutrition is like a chain in which all of the essential items are the separate links. If the chain is weak or is broken at any point, the whole chain fails. If there are 40 items that are essential in the diet, and one of these is missing, nutrition fails just as truly as it would if half the links were missing. The absolute lack of any item (or of several items) results in ill health and eventually in death. An insufficient amount of any one item is enough to bring distress to the cells and tissues which are most vulnerable to this particular lack. . . . The links in the nutrition chain are chemical links. . . . Water is a chemical; salt is a chemical; sugar is a chemical; bread and milk are each highly complex mixtures of chemicals.[4]

The human body contains an extraordinary number of distinct chemicals, over a million types of proteins alone. Ultimately the sources of all these chemicals is the food we eat, but nature has not left us in the predicament of having to seek out and ingest just the right amounts of more than a million different chemical types. Indeed, the number of nutrients which must be ingested is only around fifty.

How is it possible that only fifty different chemicals provide the raw materials for more than a million unique finished products? One reason is that these finished products are often multiunit complexes of a very few building blocks. For example, as I described in chapter 2, the huge number of distinct types of proteins in the body is constituted by only twenty different amino acids; similarly, our DNA molecules contain only six types of building blocks.

The second reason that such diversity results from only a few raw materials is the remarkable capacity of our body's cells to convert one type of chemical into another. Glucose offers an excellent example. Although this simple sugar is the major metabolic fuel consumed by most of our cells (and the only one which the brain can use under most circumstances), there is absolutely no need ever to consume a single molecule of glucose; the required glucose can be made from other chemicals—lactate, glycerol, or amino acids. Look a little deeper and one finds that lactate, glycerol, and many of the amino acids don't have to be ingested either, for they, too, can be made from other molecules.

Take another example—DNA. These giant molecules, our very blueprints, are composed of deoxyribose, four different "bases," and phosphate. Only the phosphate (because it contains the mineral phosphorus) must be ingested for normal DNA synthesis; the other five building blocks can be synthesized within the body from other raw materials. We not only must construct our own genes but, in large part, the basic building blocks to be used for the construction.

But this wonderful capacity for interconverting chemicals is not infinite, and so we are not freed of the requirement to ingest certain chemicals. These comprise the *essential nutrients*, the fifty or so substances which are required for normal or optimal body function, but which the body either cannot synthesize at all or synthesizes in amounts too small to meet its needs; the essential nutrients must therefore be supplied by the diet. It is not necessary that each of them be ingested every day because we always carry some reserves, but sooner or later, failure to ingest adequate amounts will lead to abnormal function and disease.

Leading the list of essential nutrients are the nine amino acids our bodies cannot synthesize. Without one or more of them, there is inadequate synthesis of structural proteins, antibodies, protein hormones, and most important, enzymes. Because enzymes are required for chemical reactions to proceed normally in the body, deficiency of essential amino acids not only plays havoc with protein metabolism but with all the rest of the body's chemistry as well.

At this point, one might well ask why evolution did not supply us with the capacity to synthesize these nine amino acids. The question becomes even more interesting in the light of the present belief by biologists that the earliest forms of simple unicellular organisms were probably capable of making all their own amino acids. It appears, then, that the more proper phrasing of the question should be: Why did natural selection favor mutations which *eliminated* the genetic coding for those enzymes required to synthesize the nine essential amino acids? One hypothesis holds that, during the earliest evolution of animal cells, these nine amino acids were present in the environment in large quantities, and it was therefore adaptive for cells not to waste energy synthesizing genes which would only end up being repressed all the time anyway. I, for one, am rather uncomfortable about this hypothesis, for it may explain early evolutional events but it certainly gives no satisfactory explanation of why, during the evolution of mammals, the process was not reversed in environments lacking given amino acids, unless one assumes that such environments simply did not exist for long periods of time, at least not until the present era. The only honest answer is, of course, that we do not know.

The other essential carbon-containing nutrients are a small group of fatty acids and the vitamins. The former serve as precursors for a family of chemicals which are involved in cell membrane structure and which modulate a host of physiological events. Some of the vitamins (particularly those that are soluble in water) function as coenzymes (molecules which must be present to facilitate an enzyme-mediated reaction), and others exert a wide variety of physiological actions involving vision, blood clotting, bone mineralization, etc. The same questions I raised for the essential amino acids concerning the evolutionary loss of the enzymatic machinery required for synthesis can be raised for the essential fatty acids and vitamins. Vitamin C is a particularly interesting example since the mutation resulting in loss of the key enzyme required for its synthesis seems to have occurred only about 25 million years ago in an ancestor common to human beings and other primates.

The other essential nutrients do not contain carbon and are therefore called inorganic; they are water (the body normally synthesizes quite a bit of water but not enough to supply its total needs), and approximately twenty minerals (calcium, sodium, iron, chromium, zinc, etc.). Many of these minerals are present in the body in very small quantities and are therefore known as "trace elements," but this designation is in no way meant to denigrate their immense importance for normal body function. The list of essential trace elements has slowly grown over the past few decades as methods for detecting their presence in the body and for designing diets completely free of them (which diets can then be used to test for essentiality) have been improved, and most scientists believe that the list is not yet complete. For the minerals, the question of why we have not evolved the ability to synthesize them does not apply, since biological organisms, not being "nuclear reactors," have no ability to form one mineral element from another.

One last criterion in addition to the supply of all essential nutrients must be met by the diet. The body requires an adequate supply of energy, that is, energy-containing molecules whose breakdown within the body's cells can be used to perform work. This energy, measured in calories, can be supplied by a wide variety of carbohydrates, fats, and protein; i.e., unlike the essential nutrients, there is no single essential energy-containing food. It is the total of all the energy-containing foods that counts so far as calories are concerned.

Because the body's cells depend upon being supplied continuously with essential nutrients, a multitude of homeostatic mechanisms has evolved to assure such supplies in the face of changes in dietary intake. We can apply to these mechanisms the generalizations developed in chapter 2 for homeostatic mechanisms in general.

Figure 3–1 is a generalized scheme of the possible pathways involved in the homeostasis of a nutrient (not every pathway shown is applicable to every substance; for example, sodium cannot be synthesized or catabolized within the body). The pool occupies a position of central importance in this scheme; it is the body's readily available

Fig. 3–1. **Potential pathways involved in the homeostasis of nutrients.** (Redrawn from A. J. Vander, J. H. Sherman, and D. S. Luciano, *Human Physiology: The Mechanisms of Body Function*, 3d ed. [New York: McGraw-Hill, 1980].)

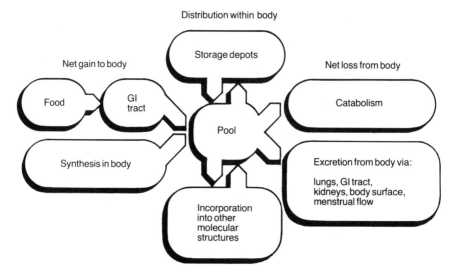

Distribution within body

Net gain to body

Storage depots

Net loss from body

Food

GI tract

Catabolism

Pool

Synthesis in body

Excretion from body via:

lungs, GI tract, kidneys, body surface, menstrual flow

Incorporation into other molecular structures

quantity of the nutrient, and it functions as "middleman," receiving from and contributing to all the other pathways. Those for net gain (input) to the body are to the left of the figure. For essential nutrients, ingestion is, by definition, the really important input route. A few of the essential nutrients, water for example, are synthesized to some extent by the body's cells but not in amounts adequate to maintain normal function. Another potential internal source of a few essential nutrients is the bacteria which inhabit our large intestines and with which we enjoy a symbiotic relationship. These bacteria are capable of synthesizing certain vitamins and perhaps other essential nutrients as well, which are then absorbed into the blood of their human host. Vitamin K is synthesized by these bacteria as are small amounts of vitamin B_{12}. This latter vitamin, required for normal blood formation, is the only nutrient which is completely lacking in purely vegetarian diets, ones which do not include any animal products, and it is quite likely that deficiency of vitamin B_{12} is less common than it ought to be in persons ingesting such a diet, because their gut bacteria contribute some of the vitamin.

The pathways to the right of the figure are sources of net loss (output) from the body. There are two output routes—excretion and catabolism. Excretion means loss from the body by way of the urine, feces, body surface (in sweat, sloughed skin, nails, and hair), menstrual flow, and milk. Excretion is the only output mechanism for the minerals (just as you can't make an atom of zinc, so you can't break it down), but another is available for the carbon-containing (organic) essential nutrients—the amino acids, fatty acids, and vitamins may be broken down (catabolized) within the body.

The central portion of the figure illustrates the distribution of the substance within the body. From the readily available pool, it may be taken up by storage depots; conversely, the nutrient may leave the storage depots to reenter the pool. Finally, the nutrient may be incorporated into some other molecular structure (iodine into the hormone thyroxin, for example); this process is reversible in that the nutrient is liberated again whenever the more complex molecule is broken down. It is distinguished from storage in that the latter has no function other than the passive one of storage, whereas the incorporation of the nutrient into other molecules is done to fulfill an active function of the nutrient (the function of iodine in the body is to provide an essential component of thyroxin).

The orientation of the figure illustrates two important generalizations: (1) as emphasized in chapter 2 for homeostatic control systems in general, total-body balance of the nutrient depends only upon the relative rates of gain and loss; (2) the pool concentration reflects not only total-body gains and losses, but exchanges of the nutrient within the body.

So far as total-body balance is concerned, it should be apparent that there are three possible states for any nutrient: (1) when output (the sum of excretion and catabolism) exceeds input, the amount of that nutrient in the body decreases, a state of negative balance; (2) when input exceeds output, the body content increases, a state of positive balance; (3) when input and output are equal, a stable balance exists. You might assume that the body is much more concerned with preventing negative balances of nutrients than positive because we naturally tend to think of nutrients as "good" chemicals. However, the fact is that many nutrients, although essential ("good" chemicals) when present in normal amounts, are quite toxic to cells when present in unusually high concentration. Remember the brief mention of phenylketonuria in chapter 1—the buildup of phenylalanine (an essential amino acid) in the body due to genetic absence of the enzyme which accelerates its catabolism causes severe brain damage. Iron is another example of an essential nutrient which, in excess amounts, can be highly toxic (in this case, to the liver).

Now we may ask the critical question: When the ingestion of a given nutrient is increased or decreased, which of the pathways involved in its handling is homeostatically controlled so as to maintain or reestablish stable total-body balance? The answer differs from nutrient to nutrient as the examples in the following discussion illustrate.

First, let's look at ingestion as a possible control point. If the dietary availability of a nutrient is low, are we automatically driven to seek out foods containing more of that nutrient? Do we have specific instinctive "hungers" for the various essential nutrients analogous to the one we have for total calories? The answer is a definite "yes" for at least one nutrient—water. Our completely automatic reflex called thirst is a major component of the homeostatic control mechanisms maintaining body water relatively constant. A possible specific hunger for salt (sodium chloride) has also been hypothesized, and there is no question that such a "drive" exists in most experimental animals studied. If a rat is made salt-deficient and then given a choice of pure water or moderately salty water, it will choose the latter and drink large quantities very rapidly, stopping only when the deficiency has been replaced. We simply don't know at present whether salt deficiency induces a similar sort of physiologic salt craving in people. (That people like salt and tend to use it when available is not the question, which is whether they instinctively increase their intake when salt-deficient.)

For substances other than salt and water, the answer is probably "no" if the question insists on a "specific" hunger for the nutrient, but "yes" if one simply asks whether some "nonspecific" factor makes it likely that animals deficient in a particular nutrient will be attracted to foods containing that nutrient. Let me explain. Scientists have shown that rats suffering from a deficiency in thiamine (one of the B-vitamins) prefer thiamine-rich foods when given a choice, niacin-deficient rats prefer niacin-rich foods (but not thiamine-rich ones), and so on. This certainly makes it appear that rats somehow "know" when they are missing a specific nutrient and actively seek out foods containing that nutrient. It turns out that this isn't really the explanation at all, even though the end result is the same as if it were. When rats are vitamin-deficient, they become ill, just as people do; one instinctive response to the illness is to avoid the foods they were eating prior to the onset of the illness and to seek out new foods, one at a time. If the new food contains the missing nutrient, the rat's health improves considerably within a few hours, and this constitutes a strong positive reinforcement (reward) for the rat's continuing to eat the new food. Thus, operant conditioning seems to explain the apparent "instincts" for various essential nutrients* (readers familiar with the basic concepts of operant conditioning will recognize immediately that "a few hours" ought to be much too long a period between behavior and reinforcement, but behaviors associated with eating are the exception to this rule).

Of course, all this work on rats may be interesting, but what is its relevance for human beings? Can we expect some mechanism (whether it be operant conditioning or specific "instinct") automatically to guide us to the ingestion of proper amounts of the various

---

*The reverse of this phenomenon explains "bait-shyness" in animals—their refusal to touch any food which has previously made them ill. This knowledge is presently being used to reduce the killing of lambs by coyotes. Lamb flesh soaked with a mild toxin is placed where coyotes will get at it; the resulting illness causes the coyotes to avoid lambs in the future and actually to retch at the sight of them. Moreover, this avoidance is passed on to the babies because the tastes in the mother's milk and food brought to the den determine the infants' future choice of foods.

essential nutrients? Most scientists believe that any such homeostatic mechanisms, even were they to exist, would be overwhelmed by the cultural factors that operate on human habits. The few studies done on humans to date have used very young children, supposedly less encumbered with cultural dictates; the results are very scanty and quite inconclusive.

Even though a nutrient is ingested, there is no guarantee that it will be absorbed, i.e., transported across the cells lining the digestive tract and into the blood, and so regulation of absorption is a second potential homeostatic control point for maintaining a stable body balance. For the great majority of nutrients—carbohydrates, fats, proteins, water, sodium chloride, and vitamins—absorption is normally close to 100 percent and is not subject to physiological control, but the situation is quite different for many of the minerals. For example, only about 50 percent of ingested calcium is absorbed, the remainder moving through the length of the gut and appearing in the feces. What is much more important, the fraction absorbed is not fixed at 50 percent but is subject to physiological control. When dietary calcium is low and the body becomes calcium-deficient, the resulting low plasma calcium triggers reflexes culminating in increased production of a particular hormone which then stimulates absorption of calcium by the gut; the result is restoration of body calcium toward normal. Iron, zinc, and copper are examples of trace elements whose absorption by the gut is normally incomplete and physiologically regulated; indeed, gut absorption constitutes the main homeostatic control point for these elements.

So far we have looked at the input side for homeostatic control points, but for most essential nutrients, control of output—excretion and catabolism—tend to predominate. The kidneys are the single most important regulatory site for excretion of water, sodium chloride, phosphate, many other minerals, and several of the vitamins. I have already described in chapter 2 how the kidneys can adjust their output of salt so as to maintain stable body sodium balance over a huge range of dietary intakes (0.25 g/day to 30 g/day); this is achieved by means of a variety of reflexes which alter how much salt the kidneys filter out of the blood and how much of this filtered salt is returned to the blood as the filtered fluid moves along the several million narrow tubes of the kidneys.

The kidneys are not the only organs specialized for homeostatic excretion of chemicals. The liver, too, can extract materials from the blood and secrete them into tiny channels which come together to form the bile duct. Via this duct, the bile flows from the liver and drains (often after temporary storage in the gall baldder) into the upper portion of the small intestine. As we shall see in subsequent chapters, the bile constitutes a very important route for the elimination of a large number of endogenous and foreign chemicals, but its elimination of essential nutrients is mainly limited to some of the trace minerals.

Excretion from the body is the only route for elimination of the essential minerals, but catabolism within the body generally plays the major controlling role in the regulation of the essential amino acids, fatty acids, and some vitamins. These catabolic reactions are all catalyzed by enzymes and so, by controlling the synthesis of the enzymes and their overall activity, the body can regulate the rates of nutrient catabolism. If a large amount of a particular organic nutrient is being ingested, catabolism of that nutrient can be homeostatically increased; in contrast, if intake is low, then the catabolic machinery is partially shut down so as to retain more of the nutrient once it is in the body.

To summarize so far, stable total-body balance of a nutrient is maintained by homeostatic regulation of one or more of the input-output pathways. Just which pathway is the major regulated one varies from nutrient to nutrient. Based on the discussion of chapter 2, you should recognize that, as intake of the nutrient increases or decreases, the homeostatic responses minimize changes in total-body balance but cannot prevent them altogether. This means that the actual amount of the nutrient in the body when stable balance is reachieved varies over some range.

Now we shift our focus from the regulation of stable total-body balance to another group of mechanisms, those which determine just how effective any given amount of nutrient in the body will be in fulfilling its function. There are three general types of such mechanisms, the first being movement into or out of storage depots (the central "distribution" part of our generalized figure). Such movement often constitutes an important homeostatic mechanism for keeping the "pool" concentration of a nutrient from becoming too high or too low. For example, almost all the body's calcium is found in bones, and movement of this mineral into or out of bone is controlled by no less than three different hormones so as to keep the extracellular concentration of calcium relatively constant. Thus, if ingestion of calcium decreases, not only are the homeostatic mechanisms (enhanced gastrointestinal absorption and decreased urinary excretion) triggered which reestablish stable balance at this new level of intake, but so are these hormones which help maintain the pool concentration of calcium even though total body calcium is diminished.

The size of the storage reserves for a nutrient is a major determinant of how regularly it must be ingested. For example, there is very little storage of the B vitamins so that deficiency symptoms may show up within days when the diet is lacking in them; in contrast, the fat soluble vitamins such as vitamin A may be stored, dissolved in the body's fats, in quantities adequate to last for weeks or months.

A second "distribution" factor determining the effectiveness of any given level of body balance in supplying cellular needs is the ability of the most important cells to take up the nutrient from the pool and utilize it. Even though the total amount of the nutrient in the body or pool may be low, if the cells which require it most can improve their ability to obtain it, then relatively normal function can continue. An excellent example of this is iodine and the thyroid gland. Iodine is an important component of the hormone thyroxin, secreted by the thyroid gland, and thyroxin, in turn, exerts many important effects on various organs and tissues. Now, if iodine intake is reduced the thyroid cells may transiently not receive enough iodine to maintain their normal production of thyroxin. The resulting fall in blood thyroxin is detected by the brain which reflexly induces the release of a hormone (thyroid-stimulating hormone), which, in turn, travels by the blood to the thyroid gland and, as its name implies, stimulates the thyroid cells to enlarge and to transport iodine across their cell membranes more avidly than usual. This enlarged gland (the familiar goiter of iodine deficiency) thus becomes better able to obtain and utilize iodine so that it can manufacture an almost normal amount of its hormone.

Finally, the third internal factor is the cells' requirement for the nutrient. Overall balance of a nutrient might be achieved but at a level not adequate to permit the cells to function normally even after storage depots have been called upon and cellular uptake maximized. Now the only way to prevent deficiency effects from emerging is to cut down the cells' requirement for the nutrient, and that is just what occurs in a few cases. For example, deficiency of thiamine, the B vitamin which participates as a coenzyme in the metabolism of carbohydrates, causes a decrease in the appetite of experimental animals, the result being that there is less demand for the thiamine, and the deficiency symptoms will not appear even though the levels of this vitamin in the body fluids is less than usual. Another example is the decrease in total-body energy requirement that occurs in persons chronically ingesting diets low in total calories. Part of the decrease in energy utilization stems simply from the fact that these deprived people develop smaller bodies, and smaller bodies consume less energy, all other things being equal. But all other things are not equal: first, certain of their cells (the liver, for example) actually consume less energy per cell than do those of well-fed individuals (we do not know the mechanism); second, the people may cut down considerably in their level of physical activity. Thus, there is a large number of different mechanisms by which energy consumption can be diminished in response to a reduction in the intake of total calories.

To summarize, we have a multitude of homeostatic mechanisms for maintaining adequate nutrition in the face of changes in the dietary availability of essential nutrients. These reflexes culminate in adaptive changes in the seeking out and ingesting of nutrients, in their rates of absorption from the gastrointestinal tract, in their rates of excretion from the body or catabolism within it, in their rates of movement into and out of storage depots, in the cells' ability to take up and utilize them, and in the cells' requirements. These homeostatic mechanisms confer a considerable degree of adaptability to a wide range of nutrient intakes, but there are limits to their range of operation; when these limits are exceeded, symptoms either of deficiency or of toxic excess make their appearance.

Setting Nutritional Requirements

Quantitative assessment of our requirements for calories and all of the essential nutrients is one of the basic tasks of the nutritional sciences, but one which has proven extraordinarily difficult to accomplish. In many respects we know more about the nutritional requirements of our farm animals than of ourselves, and there are several obvious reasons for this. For one thing, it is much easier (from both a practical and an ethical point of view) to perform the required experiments in animals; for another, the criterion for assessing the adequacy of the diet is usually well defined for the animals—milk production by cows, egg production by hens, etc. But what should be the yardsticks for human beings? It is easy to answer "the optimization of health, well-being, and longevity," but the difficulties in measuring such end results in controlled experiments are enormous, compared to measuring the number of eggs a hen lays during her lifetime.

Let us begin our discussion of requirement setting by focusing on the Recommended Dietary Allowances (RDA) of the National Academy of Sciences/National Research Council (NRC), published first in 1943 and revised at approximately five-year intervals. The RDA are so frequently misinterpreted and inappropriately used that it is essential for the general public to understand what they really are and what kinds of experimental studies form their basis.

It cannot be emphasized strongly enough that the RDAs are *not* meant to be recommendations for an "ideal" or "optimal" diet. To avoid this common confusion, some have proposed that the designation "Recommended Dietary Allowance" be changed to "acceptable nutrient intakes," which emphasizes that these are the daily intakes of nutrients considered sufficient, within the limits of knowledge, to prevent nutritional inadequacy in most healthy persons. In other words, the RDAs are guides for preventing disease, not necessarily for optimizing health. This may sound like a purely semantic problem, but it is not, as you will see from the description of the types of information used by the expert committees which set RDAs and from subsequent sections and chapters.

A second point to be emphasized is that the RDAs are meant to apply only to healthy persons, not to individuals with disease. Thirdly, the RDAs are set high enough to meet the needs of most healthy persons in a population (97.5 percent to be exact), but not 100 percent. We will look at the implications of these guidelines as we proceed.

One major type of evidence used to set RDAs comes from so-called balance studies. The rationale for its use is easily understandable from the information presented in the previous section. If the intake of a nutrient is so low that stable balance cannot be achieved, then disease must sooner or later result. In principle, balance studies are simple to perform. Volunteers are placed on extremely low intakes of the essential nutrient under study, at least one of these levels being absolute zero or so low that stable balance is not achievable, i.e., the output of the nutrient is always more than the intake. This very low intake triggers the relevant homeostatic responses designed to conserve the nutrient, and so the rates of excretion and/or catabolism fall to their minimal values. These rates are determined by collecting all the individual's urine and feces (and often sweat and shed skin and hair, as well), and measuring how much of the nutrient and all of its breakdown products are present. In this way, the minimal output of the nutrient achievable by the body is ascertained, and this number is then assumed to represent the minimal intake required for maintenance of stable balance.

Balance studies of this kind have been performed for protein (essential amino acids) and several of the essential minerals, and theoretically could be applied to all of the trace elements. They are not applicable to the fatty acids and most of the vitamins since these substances are oxidized in the body and one cannot, therefore, measure the total amount catabolized.

However, even where applicable, the balance study has several major drawbacks. The first, the restricted length of time of almost all such studies, represents a purely methodological problem.

> It is difficult to carry out balance studies for prolonged dietary periods; such studies call for sophisticated facilities and a team of trained workers. The need to carefully control nutrient-intake levels requires that the daily menu be monotonous. Losses in the urine and feces (and ideally in sweat, skin, and hair as well) must be assayed quantitatively, which means additional inconvenience for the subjects and technical problems for the investigators, particularly when the subjects are infants, young children, or elderly people. For these reasons metabolic-balance studies are usually of short duration; a week or less in children and two or three weeks in adults. The long-term nutritional and health significance of these brief study periods has not been critically determined so that the adequacy of our current estimates of nutrient requirements, which have been based on short-term studies, is uncertain. This is not a satisfactory state of affairs.[5]

It is certainly not comforting to find, as will be described in chapter 5, that one of the very few relatively long-term balance studies (up to 100 days) demonstrated that daily provision of the amount of protein recommended as safe on the basis of short-term balance was not adequate to maintain body protein stores. This study is particularly disturbing since, based on the general theory of acclimatization described in chapter 2, it would have seemed more likely that the body's conservation mechanisms would have improved over the long term. That such was not the case only underscores our ignorance concerning long-term metabolic responses to threshold dietary deficiencies.

Methodological problems are not the only reason that balance studies should not constitute the sole source of information for setting requirements. I emphasized earlier that it is quite possible for balance of a nutrient to be achieved, but for the amount in the body to be inadequate to maintain normal cell function. Just because no further net loss of the nutrient is occurring doesn't mean that there is enough in the body for all the cells to obtain the amounts they require. Of course, any homeostatic mechanisms which improve the ability of the most important cells vis-à-vis the nutrient to obtain and utilize it will mitigate the problem, but cannot eliminate it altogether. For example, the body can achieve iodine balance even at extremely low levels of iodine intake, but the amount of iodine in the body at this balance point is simply too low to permit adequate thyroid function despite profound reflex stimulation of thyroid growth and capacity for taking up iodine; the result is thyroid deficiency in association with often gigantic goiters.

Because of all these problems with balance studies—lack of applicability to many nutrients, time constraints, likelihood of malfunction even at a balance point—another type of experiment is very commonly performed to help estimate requirements. Researchers, again using human volunteers, determine how low intake must be before some clearcut physiological or biochemical abnormality can be detected. For iodine, one would look for the earliest signs of thyroid deficiency; for vitamin C, those of scurvy, and so on. Such experiments obviously carry with them major ethical restrictions. A variant of this technique, really the reverse of it, which minimizes these ethical constraints, is to treat patients already suffering from a deficiency disease with progressively increasing amounts of the appropriate nutrient to determine just when the deficiency symptoms or signs improve or disappear.

These types of study are valuable when the variable being looked for is quite clear-cut and easy to measure—growth rate in children, for example. However, it is all too easy to miss a more subtle end point of deficiency, particularly in short-term experiments; for example, it is easy to spot a full-blown case of scurvy once it has developed but much more difficult to detect the mild form of the disease associated with slightly lesser degrees of vitamin C deficiency.

The two techniques described so far for obtaining information useful for RDA setting should make it quite clear why the RDA reflects an attempt to prevent disease, not optimize health. The balance study tells us what the lowest intake is, below which disease must result simply because a stable balance cannot be achieved. The second group of techniques actually uses the appearance (or disappearance) of disease as end points. Neither of these approaches tells us anything about whether intakes higher than those required for balance or prevention of detectable disease might optimize other physiological processes (increased resistance to cancer, for example) not associated with the diseases serving as end points.

For many essential nutrients (vitamins E and K, for example), neither of these two types of study has been performed, and reliance must be placed on other, less satisfactory forms of evidence. One is epidemiological; it is based on knowledge of the lowest intake of the nutrient by a population that shows no evidence of deficiency of that nutrient. Another is extrapolation from experiments using experimental animals, a risky procedure because of the frequent quantitative differences in metabolic pathways between animals and persons.

The third is perhaps the most arbitrary of all, determination of the intake which achieves a particular concentration of the nutrient in blood, urine, or some other body fluid. The concentration selected may simply be the average seen in a well-nourished population, some value lower than this average (but definitely not associated with deficiency symptoms), or, at the other end of the extreme, some maximal value which represents "saturation" of tissue stores with the nutrient. Such determinations are relatively worthless unless an attempt is made to correlate the targeted concentrations with some component of body function. Why should we aim for any particular blood or tissue concentration unless there is reason to believe that, below this concentration, malfunction results? I shall have much more to say about this question in chapter 5, in relation to iron.

These, then, are the basic research tools for obtaining the data required for the setting of RDAs. Once all available relevant data are in hand, the RDA committees must then evaluate them in order to come up with recommendations. This almost always requires a great many judgments on the part of the committee members, for rarely are the experimental data so ample and so consistent that only one value emerges as the obvious RDA. The degree of judgment which goes into formulation of the RDAs is emphasized by the fact that the allowances used by seventeen countries and international agencies differ by as much as threefold for some nutrients.

Now we must go into a bit of quantitation. I mentioned earlier that the RDA is set so as to meet the requirements of 97.5 percent of the population. Where does this number come from and how do the committee members meet this criterion? The first number that emerges from their evaluation of the relevant experimental data is an estimate of the nutritional requirement of the *average* individual in the population; if one assumes that in a population of healthy individuals, the distribution of requirements for each nutrient is symmetrical, this value covers the needs of 50 percent of the population (the individuals at dead center of the range of requirements for that nutrient and all persons whose requirements are less than this average value). Now the question is: How much should the requirement be increased to include an additional 47.5 percent of the population? As described in chapter 1, the statistical unit of variation from the mean is known as the standard deviation; adding two standard deviations to the mean gives a number which includes the requirements of 97.5 percent of the healthy population. For protein and the few other intensively studied nutrients, the standard deviation for the experimental populations studied turns out to be about 15 percent of the value of the mean; therefore, taking the mean plus 30 percent more (two standard deviations) gives the RDA.

There are several implications of this approach which require reemphasis. First, note that the RDA is not the minimal requirement for most people, but is at least 30 percent higher than that required by the average person and more than 30 percent higher than that required for persons at the lower end of the range; second, the RDA is too low to meet the daily requirements of an estimated 2.5 percent of the healthy population. Thus, the RDAs represent a statistical compromise set high enough to cover most members (97.5 percent) of a healthy population but not high enough to cover 100 percent, since trying to cover the needs of these last two or three persons per 100 would wastefully, and possibly dangerously, give far too much of the nutrient to the great majority of the population. Therefore, we must always keep in mind that, even if the RDAs were perfectly accurate, 2.5 percent of the population would get in trouble from following them.

How much confidence have we that the RDAs really are accurate measures of nutritional requirements for most of the population?

Perhaps the fairest conclusions are that they are, in general, the best we can do with our present level of information, but that many of them may turn out to be far off the mark when (if?) badly needed additional research is completed, and we ought to be very cautious about our use of them in the meantime. As we have seen, there are major weaknesses (short time span, few subjects, hazy end points, etc.) in the methods used to generate the data on which the RDAs are based, but even these considerations are dwarfed by perhaps the most difficult research problem of all in setting RDAs—the question of how to deal with variability.

Let us focus specifically on the assumption that the standard deviation for nutritional requirements within the population is about 15 percent of the mean value. Suppose that the actual variation in nutritional requirements for the American population were far greater than the committees have assumed, that the standard deviation were far greater than 15 percent of the average requirement. That would mean that the RDA, set by adding 30 percent to the average, would fail to cover the requirement of many more than 2.5 percent of the population. To that degree, its usefulness in building both personal and public-policy decisions concerning diet would be greatly diminished and perhaps even seriously misleading. Just how solid is this 15 percent value? "Not very" is the honest answer.

First of all, for many nutrients, the basic studies are so few and limited that no meaningful estimate of variability is available, and it is simply assumed that the variability for their requirements is essentially the same as those determined for the few nutrients, such as protein, which have been studied extensively.

Second, even when good data are available from appropriate human studies, they were obtained under highly standardized laboratory conditions (i.e., with all other environmental factors held as constant as possible) and from very small samples of persons who cannot possibly be representative of all healthy populations within a single country, let alone other countries of the world. Consider for a moment all the possible sources of variation in nutrient requirements—variations due to age, sex, body dimensions, and normal physiological state (pregnancy and lactation, for example); genetic variation among individuals; variation due to a host of environmental factors impinging on healthy individuals (environmental temperature, for example).

Attempts have been made to study some of these variables experimentally and to incorporate this information into distinct RDAs for the relevant populations. Pregnancy and lactation are two such variables. Age is another, although we still remain relatively ignorant of how nutrient requirements vary from birth to death.

> There is a tendency for investigators to regard [infants and young children] as little adults and, with a small allowance for their growth, to extrapolate their requirements proportionately by weight from studies of older individuals. This approach does not take into account changes in the metabolic activities of cells and in the rates of nutrient turnover with age.[6]

Our ignorance concerning genetic differences is almost total. The subjects used in balance studies and the other experimental models for determining nutritional requirements tend to be quite homogeneous in background, not covering a wide spectrum of the general population. Moreover, there are very few studies comparing the requirements of persons from different countries. This question of possible genetic differences is perhaps the most hotly debated aspect of nutritional requirements. Dr. Roger J. Williams has emphasized that, in some balance studies performed, the amounts of nutrient required to maintain stable balance has varied from twofold to sevenfold among different individuals.[7] He believes that even greater variability can be documented for the amounts of nutrients required to prevent deficiency disease. Indeed, he and his followers claim that the normal human requirements for many nutrients extend over as much as a fortyfold range. There is no precedent for such huge variability among normal persons so far as other physiological processes are concerned, and most authorities dismiss such claims as extremely unlikely. Yet the question is certainly deserving of careful study.

As for environmental factors which might influence nutrient requirements, it is simply impossible to evaluate, during a balance study, the effects of more than one or two. The tests are difficult and tedious enough without superimposing changes in environmental temperature, physical activity, psychological stress, and the multitude of other potentially important environmental variables, even if one could identify them all. Even the composition of the food in which the nutrient is ingested may exert profound effects on the utilization of that nutrient and, therefore, on its requirement. These antagonistic and synergistic interactions begin within the gastrointestinal tract itself. For one thing, the form of the nutrient in food may have a major effect on its absorbability; this is particularly true for the trace elements since the molecules to which they are bound in food may either enhance or impede their absorption. Moreover, nutrients may compete with each other for common transport pathways across the intestinal wall into the blood.

Nutrients interact not just by affecting each other's absorption from the gut, but by influencing almost any of the subsequent pathways in their utilization. An excess of one nutrient may hasten or impede another's catabolism or excretion, storage, uptake, and utilization by cells. Sometimes the interaction may be relatively nonspecific (for example, the ability of increased water intake to enhance urinary excretion of many minerals), whereas in others the interaction may be highly specific, stemming often from competition between two or more structurally similar nutrients.

With all these sources of variability, and with all the problems inherent in the basic methodology, it should be obvious that we must be cautious in applying the RDAs even to their targeted populations—healthy persons. As soon as one begins to consider the effects of disease on nutritional requirements, the RDAs are no longer applicable, since disease states may profoundly alter virtually any of the pathways involved in nutrient metabolism. Failure to recognize that the RDAs were never meant to apply to sick persons has led to extremely serious personal and public-policy mistakes, erring almost inevitably on the side providing too little nutrition.

Infection is certainly the most common disease influencing nutrient requirements, and it does so by a variety of effects, depending on the nature of the infection. It may diminish gastrointestinal function so that less nutrient is absorbed; it may increase the body's metabolism so as to elicit increased catabolism of nutrients; it may alter kidney function so as to enhance excretion; it may alter target-cell function so as to reduce the ability of cells to take up and utilize nutrients. In addition to altering the body's handling of nutrients, the infectious agent (intestinal parasites, for example) may itself drain off a large fraction of the ingested nutrient for its own purposes; for example, the fish tapeworm has a very high requirement for vitamin B_{12} and heavy infestations with this tapeworm (as may occur in persons consuming raw fish) may cause severe deficiency of vitamin B_{12} in the host simply because the tapeworms use up so much of the ingested vitamin.

Infection is certainly not the only disease process which influences nutritional requirements. Physical trauma, allergic responses, burns, and cancer may all do so, often in much the same manner (fever, decreased gastrointestinal function, increased catabolism or excretion, etc.). Genetic defects may also result in problems at various sites; an example of this is the genetic form of pernicious anemia, a disease in which vitamin B_{12} is not absorbed normally because of failure of the gut lining to synthesize the molecule required to transport the vitamin across the lining into the blood.

Disease processes do not always increase a nutrient's requirement, sometimes they lower it. For example, in some people the intestinal lining is lacking the mechanism which controls iron absorption; such persons are in danger of absorbing so much iron that toxic levels may be reached in the body. On a less specific level, disease may damage the liver or kidneys so that excretion or catabolism of a nutrient is diminished, thereby leading to a decreased requirement.

There are other environmental factors that the RDAs are not meant to take into account. Drugs and other chemicals to which we are exposed are one such important category. For example, oral contraceptives may strongly influence dietary requirements for certain vitamins and trace minerals.

All this should make it clear why the RDAs, estimates of the amounts of nutrients needed to meet the physiological requirements of almost all healthy persons, do not apply to situations characterized by illness or other unusual conditions. Under such conditions additional data from experiments designed to evaluate the effects of these specific situations on nutrient requirements must be used. There is simply no way that a single value can be applied to all persons under all conditions.

In conclusion:

> Recommended allowances cannot serve as an absolute indicator of the adequacy of a given intake for a given individual. They can justifiably be applied only to a reasonably healthy population. In spite of their limitations, however, estimates of caloric requirements and recommended allowances for essential nutrients must be supplied. They guide the design of diets for individuals, the evaluation of the relative adequacy of diets for populations, the content of nutrition-education programs and the planning by government of nutrition-intervention programs.
>
> There is no area of human health in which research is more urgently needed than the nutritional requirements of representative hu-

man populations over the full range of both health and disease. Clearly an adequate knowledge of the amount and kinds of food required by man is essential for food and nutrition policy planning and will be of major importance for the generations ahead.[8]

Optimal Nutrient Intakes and the Vitamin C Controversy

Ah, those were the days, those were the days when we doctors knew all about vitamins and the people who stuffed themselves with B and C were cranks and food faddists, not Nobel Prize winners! Those were the days, the lovely days when we could sit around the doctors' dining room and tell about examining some nutty woman who was taking 800 units of vitamin E daily, and not have to worry that some colleague across the table would reply that he took 1,600 units and had never felt better. Best of all, in those pre-Pauling days, when some steely-eyed patient fixed us across the consulting room table and asked if we "believed" in supplemental vitamins, we could look sympathetic-scientific and reel off a bit of vitamin tape from our minds, something to the effect that it wasn't really necessary to supplement a normal diet ("And I'm sure you eat a normal diet. . ."), but that if the patient felt better taking vitamins, there was no harm in them.[9]

I emphasized in the previous section that the RDAs are aimed at preventing disease, not optimizing health. For many years, we viewed most essential nutrients as bearing one-to-one relationships with specific diseases; vitamin D prevented rickets, vitamin C scurvy, and so on. Then came a radical reorientation of our thinking as it became obvious that, in addition to these quite specific effects, any particular essential nutrient often exerted widespread actions on a host of bodily functions; for example, vitamin C, in amounts larger than those specified by its RDA, enhances the activity of the liver enzymes which catabolize environmental pollutants, and vitamin D interferes with the transformation of cholesterol to other molecules. The inference from this knowledge (as well as the simultaneous recognition that virtually all diseases are multicausal) was that each nutrient might influence the development of a variety of diseases, perhaps with very different dose-responses. Thus, evaluation of the optimal intake of the nutrient requires the taking into account of all these different interactions and dose-responses.

If we look at the entire potential spectrum of nutrient effects, we can make several generalizations. At the opposite ends of the spectrum are the known beneficial actions (prevention of clear-cut specific disease) and the toxic effects. There is no question that, at high enough doses, many nutrients begin to cause damage; for example, iodine, which is essential for normal thyroid function, actually causes thyroid malfunction at high enough doses (this was first recognized when, soon after discovery of its physiological role, iodine became such a food fad that it was often carried by persons in little vials from which drinks were taken whenever the person felt sluggish or "down").

Between these two ends of the spectrum lies most of the dose-range over which most persons can maintain nutrient balance without obvious deficiency or toxicity. In this physiological range, the body's homeostatic mechanisms tend to minimize changes in total body content of the nutrient as intake changes, but as I emphasized in chapter 2, some change must occur, and this leads to the crucial question: Do these differences over the physiological midrange of the spectrum of bodily nutrient concentrations really matter? Is it better (or worse) to have a few percent more sodium in the body (the range of change of body sodium over the entire range of intakes compatible with the absence of frank disease)? A few percent more or less protein? 10 to 20 percent more zinc? 1,000 percent more vitamin C?

For such questions to have meaning, we must specify precisely those end points we will use in answering them: longevity, enhanced resistance to cancer or heart disease, increased ability to run marathons, and so on. The list is infinite as is the sister list for potentially harmful effects, and the experiments required to answer them are, for the most part, far more difficult to perform and analyze than those for setting RDAs. Just to perform such experiments for a single nutrient—say vitamin C—requires a massive outlay of funds and scientific personnel, and so we must choose carefully our priorities. Let us now use vitamin C as an example for illustrating certain of these points.

Many studies have demonstrated, in human subjects, that 10 mg of vitamin C per day is adequate to prevent almost all signs or symptoms of scurvy. Only maintenance of gum health seems to require more, and even here, 30 mg/day is adequate in virtually all cases. Studies using balance methods and measurements of pool size also document that 30 mg/day is more than adequate to maintain body stores of vitamin C at levels which prevent all the signs and symptoms of scurvy. Accordingly, the most recent National Research Council RDA for vitamin C has been set at 60 mg/day, the extra 30 mg/day being a safety factor added on to cover individual variation, losses in cooking, and other environmental factors.

There is unanimous agreement about the facts concerning vitamin C and scurvy; why then the controversy, led by Linus Pauling and Irwin Stone, who argue that the optimum intake of ascorbic acid—that is, the daily amount of this food that leads to the best of health—is somewhere between 250 mg and 10 g?[10] Pauling and Stone are emphasizing "optimum intake" and "best of health," not the amount adequate to prevent scurvy. They and their followers argue that scientists have been misguided in allowing scurvy—a dramatic, clear-cut disease—to dominate thinking about the role of vitamin C in bodily function. They believe that this vitamin, which is present in all body tissues, is a central substance in the functioning of these tissues and, as such, may be involved in a host of phenomena, including defenses against a wide variety of diseases. If all this is true, then basing our estimates of vitamin C "requirements" on experiments having only to do with scurvy is foolish. In short, they argue that scientists have been using the wrong end points in establishing recommendations for daily intakes of vitamin C.

There is no doubt that the furor over vitamin C and the fact that it has stimulated a large and rapidly growing number of studies is due mainly to the brilliance and achievements of Linus Pauling. The type of claims he has made for the efficacy of large doses of vitamin C in reducing the frequency of colds had previously been made by many others (and ignored) as Pauling was to emphasize. In addition to citing what he felt to be strong clinical data supporting the curative powers of vitamin C, Pauling buttressed his views with purely theoretical considerations of what was known about the normal physiology and biochemistry of vitamin C. As I pointed out in chapter 1, this is a perfectly sound way of pursuing a possible connection between an environmental factor and a disease.

Pauling particularly emphasized the intriguing metabolism of vitamin C. Almost all mammals except primates, the guinea pig, and the Indian fruit-eating bats are capable of synthesizing (in the liver) their own vitamin C, so that this substance is not an essential nutrient for them. Importantly, the amounts that they synthesize are usually considerably larger than those needed to prevent scurvy. Second, vitamin C is an example of a nutrient the plasma concentration and total body content of which changes markedly (compared, say, to sodium or protein) as intake is increased. This relation is at first almost a linear one. At an intake of 10 mg/day, plasma concentration is 1.4 mg/L and the pool size is about 300 mg; when intake is 100 mg/day, plasma concentration is 12 mg/L and pool size is 3,000 mg. So a tenfold increase in vitamin C intake produces close to a tenfold increase in its body content and plasma concentration.

How different this is from the case of sodium, the intake of which can be increased over a fiftyfold range with a resulting change in body sodium content of only a few percent. The major homeostatically controlled pathway for both sodium and vitamin C is urinary excretion, but obviously the control of sodium excretion is much more precise than that of vitamin C over the usual range of intakes. Within forty-eight to seventy-two hours after sodium intake has been doubled the kidneys have adjusted their handling of this mineral so as to double its excretion, because only a tiny increase in body sodium is required to trigger these sodium-losing reflexes. In contrast, a doubling of vitamin C intake does not lead to a doubling of urinary vitamin C until many days have elapsed and until body content has slowly built up until it is virtually doubled. In other words, a 1 to 2 percent change in body sodium can effect a 100 percent change in urinary sodium excretion, whereas a 100 percent increase in body content of vitamin C is required to drive a 100 percent increase in urinary excretion of this vitamin.

In terms of evolution, a possible inference is that there must be a strong selection pressure (survival value) for keeping the body's sodium content within very narrow limits but relatively little for keeping vitamin C unchanged over the almost tenfold range of plasma concentrations from 1.4 mg/L to 12 mg/L. Pauling, of course, draws a very different inference (with just as much justification), namely that the body is trying to conserve as much vitamin C as possible even at levels ten times greater than those needed to prevent scurvy.

But the pattern changes dramatically when vitamin C intake goes beyond approximately 100 to 150 mg/day, for then the concentration of vitamin C in the blood and the total amount in the body increase very little with increasing intake. For example, an intake of 2 g/day fails to produce a sustained rise in plasma concentration of vitamin C of more than a few percent over that seen at intakes of 250 mg (there is a rise of 20 to 30 percent during the first days after one goes on such an intake, but the plasma concentration soon is adjusted back toward its original values; this is probably also the case for body stores of the vitamin). There are two reasons for this. For one thing, absorption of vitamin C from the gut, close to 100 percent at low intakes, begins to decrease; only about 50 percent is absorbed when the intake is 2 g and still smaller at larger doses. Far more important, the kidneys resist the ability of large intakes of vitamin C to raise plasma concentration because they increase excretion very rapidly to match intake. Thus, the excretion of vitamin C in large amounts looks very much like that of sodium, in that no amount of ingestion (short of quantities so huge as to overwhelm the kidneys) can raise the plasma concentration or pool size of the nutrient by more than a few percent; the body is said to be "fully saturated."

Most nutritionists argue that it is logical (but not necessarily correct) to postulate two conclusions from these facts: (1) it makes little sense to ingest daily more than 100 to 150 mg of vitamin C since only a small sustained change in bodily concentration is achieved by so doing; (2) the presence of mechanisms which strongly resist elevations of plasma and pool vitamin C beyond intakes of 100 to 150 mg/day raise the suspicion that further increases might be harmful, i.e., that we have evolved protective mechanisms against large intakes.

Yet, flying in the face of these hypotheses, Linus Pauling and his followers have advocated daily intakes of 400 to 10,000 mg (0.4 to 10 g). It is this "megavitamin" approach which probably most upsets nutritionists and other scientists, who argue that such huge doses have nothing to do with nutrition, that human beings do not naturally consume these amounts, that Pauling is really advocating the use of vitamin C as a "medicine" not a nutrient, and that the likelihood of undesirable side effects at this dose is every bit as likely as that of beneficial effects. The distinction between "medicine" (or "drug") on the one hand and "nutrient" on the other is not trivial, for the label "nutrient" somehow connotes a beneficial "natural" substance (which explains the intense effort on the part of those who favor the use of laetrile to dignify it with the completely undeserved appellation, vitamin B_{15}). Moreover, a drug, unlike a nutrient, must be validated in carefully controlled animal and human experiments before it is advocated or allowed for widespread use by the public.

Pauling disagrees that his recommended doses are completely counteracted by decreased gastrointestinal absorption and increased kidney excretion or that they are really large and unphysiological, and he offers a variety of theoretical arguments to back up his position. For one thing, there is no question that the plasma concentration of vitamin C is quite elevated transiently after each ingestion of the recommended dose, and it is quite possible that the concentration of this vitamin in critical cells remains permanently elevated. Second, it is known that the utilization of vitamin C increases in a variety of stress situations, and it may be that large doses are required to maintain a high blood concentration of the vitamin at such times. Third, echoing Dr. Williams, Pauling believes that individual variation in nutrient requirements is so great that what seem to be extremely large amounts are required by many people (of course, by the same token, there ought to be the same degree of individual variation vis-à-vis toxicity so that some people might be highly susceptible to any toxic effects). Finally, and most important, Pauling argues that his recommendations are not large at all, when compared to the amounts synthesized or ingested by other mammalian species. When weight differences are taken into account, most of the animals which have retained the capacity to produce vitamin C do so in amounts equivalent to 2 to 15 g/day for human beings. The gorilla, only twice our weight, ingests 4 to 5 g of the vitamin each day, and, based on the amounts of vitamin C in purely vegetarian diets, our evolutionary predecessors were probably ingesting, Pauling believes, more than 2 g of vitamin C each day. Indeed, he reasons that it was this ample intake of vitamin C that permitted our distant ancestors to do without the machinery of synthesizing vitamin C. In this view the gene mutation resulting in loss of the enzymes needed for making vitamin C was selected because it saved the body the energy required to make a substance which the diet was already supplying in large quantities. Of course, this evolutionary guessing game is a double-edged sword, for one might argue a quite different view, that our ancestors never did ingest such large amounts of vitamin C, that these amounts are more harmful than beneficial, and that this accounts for the success of the mutation which prevented manufacture of vitamin C. Such games are great fun to play, but solve nothing. Nor do any of the other theoretical arguments, either pro or con. As I emphasized in chapter 1, theory alone can never by itself provide answers to questions of benefit and toxicity. The answer must come from research designed to answer the specific questions at hand. Do such doses of vitamin C really protect against the common cold (or cancer, arthritis, and mental disease, among others)? Do such doses exert harmful effects which would outweigh any beneficial effects?

Pauling felt, at the time he wrote the first edition of his book *Vitamin C and the Common Cold* (1970), that the existing human experiments were already adequate to answer those questions, that vitamin C definitely had been shown to be effective against the common cold.[11] However, of the five major studies he cited, only two meet even some of the criteria required for trustworthy human experimentation. The other three had no control groups at all, or were not double-blind, or presented no quantitative data which could be subjected to statistical evaluation.

A fourth study, performed in 1942, was not specified as being double-blind, but upon being contacted by Pauling (twenty years after the fact) one of the three authors stated that he recalled that "the study was double-blind in nature";[12] the other two authors did not comment on this question. I'd like to go into this study[13] in more quantitative detail than I will use for any other experiment to be described in this book, mainly because it is the first one we are encountering and should serve to emphasize how really difficult it is to perform valid experiments.

The most important data from this experiment are summarized in table 3–4. The average number of colds per person receiving ascorbic acid during the study period of twenty-eight weeks was 1.9 ± 0.07 (mean ± one standard deviation), whereas the value for the control group was 2.2 ± 0.08. This difference, one-third of a cold per person (representing a 15 percent reduction in number of colds per

TABLE 3–4   Data from 1942 Study of Response of Colds to Ascorbic Acid Therapy

	Ascorbic Acid	Placebo
Reported colds per person during year prior to study (no ascorbic acid or placebo given)	5.5 ± 0.12	5.9 ± 0.11
Colds per person during study (28 weeks)	1.9 ± 0.07	2.2 ± 0.08

Source: D. W. Cowan et al., "Vitamins for the Prevention of Colds," *Journal of the American Medical Association* 120(1942):1268–71.

person), was statistically significant ($P = 0.04$). The authors themselves questioned the practical importance of such a small "difference," but Pauling emphasized that 15 percent is really large, considering that the dose, 200 mg/day, was much less than those he believes are required.

However, is this difference really due to the vitamin C? Look at the data for the number of colds reported by the participants for the year *prior* to the study, and you will see that essentially the same highly significant difference (0.4 colds per person) existed for that period also (5.9 ± 0.11 versus 5.5 ± 0.12)! Thus, there is no reason to infer that vitamin C did anything.

This difference for the prior year not only gravely weakens the conclusion that vitamin C exerted any specific effect on the incidence of colds, but calls into question the procedure used to allocate subjects to the two groups for the study period. M. H. M. Dykes and P. Meier have emphasized that such a difference would be very unlikely to exist had the groups truly been chosen at random.[14] They point out that although a double-blind procedure might have been followed after the initial stages of the study, the methods described in the publication make it certain that the investigators were not "blind" at the time of subject assignment to the vitamin C and control groups, and so the opportunity for (unconsciously) biased allocation was present. Evidence that allocation could not have been by alternation (the claimed method) is the fact that there were 233 subjects in one group and only 194 in the other, despite the fact that alternation should yield groups of identical size.

Finally, the last problem in this study is that the dropout rate among the placebo group (20 percent) was twice that among the vitamin C group (10 percent). This difference not only could account for spurious differences in the final data analysis (as I described in chapter 1), but casts further doubt on the randomness of the selection procedure (Pauling argues that the smaller dropout rate of the vitamin C group reflects their satisfaction with having fewer colds).

In all fairness, it must be pointed out that Pauling gave most credence not to this study but to the fifth one, performed in 1961.[15] It was clearly double-blind, used a large dose (1 g/day) and revealed a significant reduction in the incidence of colds (45 percent) in the vitamin C group compared to the placebo group. This study is really the only one which could stand up to scientific scrutiny at the time of Pauling's first edition, but its study population and situation—

skiers on each of two week-long ski trips—are hardly representative enough on which to base strong inferences concerning the general population and everyday life.

Pauling's book created so much interest that a number of scientists launched controlled clinical trials aimed at evaluating the efficacy of vitamin C in the treatment and prevention of the common cold.

> In view of the fact that many controlled studies of ascorbic acid and the common cold have now been completed, it might be hoped that the matter of efficacy could be clearly settled one way or the other. In fact, because of the great variability in experience with colds from one subject to another, and because of the considerable subjectivity inherent in the evaluation of a cold, even a slight fault in experimental design or procedure may open the way to a bias of substantial magnitude. For most of the studies on which the arguments supporting efficacy are based, the measures taken to protect against such bias fall short of a satisfactory level, and the conclusions must therefore be accepted with great caution.[16]

These words were written at the end of 1974 and still apply five years later. The various studies have been reviewed by Pauling in the second edition of his book and by Dykes and Meier, and the interested reader would do well to read these and form his own opinion. Mine is that, based on a reasonable number of well-controlled studies, vitamin C may exert a small protective effect against the severity of cold symptoms, but that Pauling is wrong in his claim that large doses of vitamin C completely prevent or cure the common cold (Pauling certainly would not accept my conclusion!). Not atypical are the results of perhaps the most extensive study, performed in Toronto over fourteen weeks in the winter.[17] Approximately 1,000 volunteers were allocated randomly to receive either ascorbic acid or placebo (one of the reasons that such studies are so laborious, complex, and expensive is the need for large numbers of persons; with smaller numbers the results are likely to be inconclusive when only small changes are being looked for and when there is so much spontaneous variation in the end points being evaluated—the number and severity of colds per person). The subjects took 1 g of ascorbic acid or placebo daily and increased the dose to 4 g daily during the first three days of any illness. There were no statistically significant differences in the total number of episodes of illness or in the total days of recorded symptoms in the two groups. However, there were significant differences in the amount of disability experienced by the groups; the vitamin-treated group reported 30 percent fewer days "confined to the house" and 33 percent fewer "days off work" per subject. These figures may be put into better perspective by translating the percentages into absolute numbers—30 to 33 percent represented only one-half day per person for the entire 14-week period.

So far as the other much more serious diseases that vitamin C is hypothesized to be effective against, the data are far too few to permit any conclusions.

What about the other side of the coin—toxicity? Pauling has emphasized over and over again that vitamin C "is known to have extremely low toxicity," and it is certainly true that, other than diarrhea, no diseases have been proven to result from the use of large doses. But the fact is that we have not yet looked very hard, and if we have learned anything about toxicology in the past ten years, it is that subtle long-term toxicity is extremely difficult to determine without appropriate extensive testing, not merely the gross observation that people seem able to tolerate large doses without obvious harm. Such studies expressly designed to test long-term toxicity in experimental animals are in their infancy but are already yielding enough suggestive data to warrant caution.[18]

Perhaps the single most important effects to test for are those on the fetus, since so many pregnant women are now taking large amounts of vitamin C. In one fascinating but very inconclusive study, it was found that two infants born to such women developed scurvy postnatally despite normal intakes of vitamin C; the researchers hypothesized that the presence of high blood concentrations of vitamin C *in utero* had "imprinted" on the fetus an increased requirement for this vitamin.

I would like now to return to the issue I raised earlier about priorities. There are approximately fifty essential nutrients and testing all of them at supra-RDA intakes for specific beneficial (and harmful) effects to obtain data pertaining to "optimal" rather than merely "acceptable" intakes will be a massive, perhaps unachievable, but nonetheless worthwhile task. In the particular case of vitamin C, it seems to me a matter of high priority to investigate possible beneficial effects against serious diseases over the range of 45 to 150 mg (the "saturation" intake) daily intake. So far as higher intakes are concerned, I share the opinion of T. W. Anderson, a professor of epidemiology and a person quite friendly to Pauling's argument that the RDA is not the "optimal" intake for vitamin C.

> Higher intakes than those necessary to produce saturation may eventually prove to be desirable in certain situations, but until we have a clearer idea of the benefit/risk ratios involved, such "mega-vitamin" dosages should only be used on a short-term or experimental basis, or where the potential risk is far outweighed by the nature of the disease being treated [cancer, for example].[19]

These guidelines are probably appropriate for the search for optimal levels of most other nutrients as well, and it is important that such guidelines be set, since the controversy over "meganutrient" therapy is by no means limited to vitamin C. Nor did it really begin with vitamin C; the concept, now termed orthomolecular therapy, began about twenty-five years ago with the idea that massive doses of vitamin B_3 (niacin) might be effective in the therapy of schizophrenia. The concept has been, over the years, extended to many other nutrients and a host of diseases. Results claimed by its advocates were initially modest but, more and more, have become broad categorical statements and calls to action offered usually without much evidence; typical is the recommendation by Dr. A. Hoffer that "enrichment of our food with vitamin B_3 will prevent most cases of . . . schizophrenia from becoming manifest. I estimate that one gram per day started early in life will protect most of us."[20] The RDA for vitamin B_3, based mainly on the amount needed to prevent pellagra, is only 20 mg/day, and this vitamin is known to produce toxic effects at doses of 3 to 6 g/day. What makes this recommendation triply irresponsible is the lack of evidence that vitamin B_3 is effective at all in the therapy of schizophrenia, the good chances of toxicity in some people at the doses suggested, and the request that everyone in the population, not just patients with schizophrenia, be exposed to these amounts through the vehicle of enriching the food supply (I shall return to the general problem of food enrichment in chapter 5).

Unfortunately, the claims and recommendations made by disciples of orthomolecular therapy (including Pauling) have been so numerous, so varied, and so little supported in most cases by solid evidence that it is easy for nutritionists and other scientists to become exasperated and dismiss the whole subject of "optimal" intakes as nonsense. This would be throwing out the baby with the bath water. The problem could be minimized if a clear distinction were made between the levels of nutrient intakes achievable through normal dietary habits (i.e., by the ingestion of ordinary foods) and those which can be accomplished only by ingesting extremely large quantities of nutrient supplements. Studying potential beneficial effects of nutrients in the first instance really represents the pursuit of "ideal" or "optimal" nutrition, whereas the second instance (a perfectly legitimate one) is using nutrients as medication and should be subject to the usual constraints which apply to such research.

In conclusion, the quest for better means of determining RDAs and altered needs due to environmental factors, particularly disease, along with the just-beginning quest for optimal or ideal intakes as well as toxic effects of nutrients, establish nutrition as one of the most important areas of human health for future research efforts. It is to be hoped that such efforts will remedy the present situation, succinctly summarized by H. J. Morowitz:

> Most of what we are told about nutrition is neither true nor false; it is indeterminate. The experiments that have been carried out are often inadequate to develop conclusions within the ground rules of probability and statistics and the accepted notions of scientific verification. The information available to diet planners consists of a small body of universally accepted results such as the pathways of intermediate metabolism, a set of direct minimum requirements to avoid dietary deficiency, data on toxic substances and levels of acute toxicity, and a very large body of results—many of which do not measure up to the minimum standards of statistical acceptability.[21]

Chapter **4** | Protein Nutrition: The Problems of Setting Minimal Dietary Requirements

Protein Homeostasis

Protein is in many respects the single most important nutrient, for proteins form not only many of the structural elements of the body but also the enzymes which catalyze almost all biochemical reactions. When we talk of protein metabolism we are, in large part, really referring to the metabolism of the twenty-odd amino acids which are the building blocks for proteins. Only eight or nine of these amino acids are essential nutrients, since the body cannot synthesize them, at least not in adequate amounts, but this does not mean that only these amino acids need be ingested. The problem is this: Even though the body can synthesize the nonessential amino acids (mainly from carbohydrates), to do so it must have a source of nitrogen, not nitrogen gas, as in the air, but nitrogen atoms already incorporated into organic molecules in the form of amine groups (a nitrogen atom bound to two hydrogen atoms). The only really important source of these amine groups is amino acids themselves, so in order to form new amino acids, cells simply transfer the amine group from one amino acid to an appropriate carbohydrate, thereby forming a new amino acid. For example, transfer of the amine group from alanine, an amino acid, to the carbohydrate α-ketoglutaric acid, forms the new amino acid, glutamic acid. (There is never any problem having enough of the right carbohydrates around, for the body can make them in abundance.)

The end result of this ability to form the nonessential amino acids by transferring amine groups from one molecule to another is that, so far as the eleven or so nonessential amino acids (i.e., those the body can synthesize) are concerned, it doesn't seem to matter very much if each is ingested just so long as the total amount of all of them ingested is adequate to supply enough amine-group nitrogen for the body to do the required interconverting. Theoretically, all this nitrogen could be supplied by just a few types of amino acids; the cells could then transfer the nitrogen as needed to appropriate carbohydrates to form all the nonessential amino acids. In summary, protein requirements are specified by two criteria: (1) there must be adequate amounts of each of the essential amino acids; (2) there must be an adequate total amount of amino acids.

Figure 4–1 illustrates the major pathways for protein and amino acid metabolism in the typical balance form described in the previous chapter. We ingest some free amino acids but far more protein,

Fig. 4–1.   Pathways for amino acid and protein metabolism.

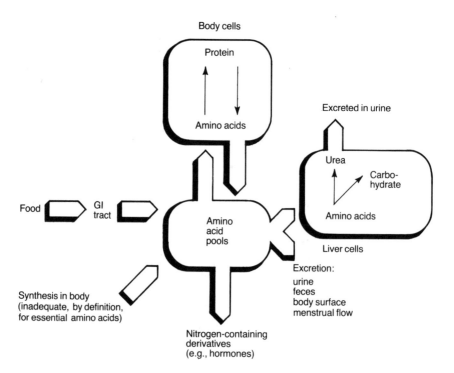

which is then degraded to free amino acids during gastrointestinal digestion. After their absorption, these amino acids enter the so-called amino acid pools, which is just a shorthand term for the body's total free amino acids. In the case of essential amino acids, ingestion is the only source of gain. In the case of nonessential amino acids, these pools are also supplied by synthesis of new amino acids within the body (again, remember that the nitrogen required for this synthesis must come from another type of amino acid so that the synthesized amino acid represents a new molecule of that particular amino acid type but not a net gain of total amino acids). Amino acids are constantly being removed from pools by the body's cells and strung together to form myriad proteins. Simultaneously, already existing proteins are being degraded to their constituent amino acids. Thus, there is a dynamic "turnover" of protein, a continuous building up and breaking down of almost all the body's proteins. The great majority of the amino acids participate in this protein turnover, but a small fraction is used for synthesis of certain nitrogen-containing molecules other than protein (several hormones, for example).

What about the output side of the balance—loss of free amino acids, proteins, or other amino acid derivatives from the body? Some of these molecules are always being lost from the body in the urine and feces, as well as in sloughed skin and hair. Menstrual fluid and milk are also sources of loss in women (and the developing fetus is, of course, a major protein and amino acid drain in a pregnant woman). These losses (except for those in milk and to the fetus) are extremely small in normal people, but may become very large in disease states such as burns, hemorrhage, and diarrhea.

Outright loss of intact molecules of proteins and amino acids is not the only way in which these molecules disappear from the body; of much greater quantitative importance in normal persons is the breakdown of the amino acid so that its nitrogen atom cannot be retrieved for incorporation into some other amino acid or useful amino-acid derivative. This type of catabolism occurs by a series of reactions in the liver. At an early point in the sequence, the nitrogen is removed from the amino acid to form a carbohydrate and ammonia (NH_3). This step, called deamination, is a one-way street, since the nitrogen in ammonia cannot be transferred to a carbohydrate to re-form an amino acid, and it is destined to certain excretion. Actually, ammonia is a relatively toxic molecule and so it is rapidly converted, also in the liver, to a much less toxic molecule—urea. Urea, therefore, is the end of the line for protein catabolism, and the kidneys excrete it via the urine as fast as it is formed.

Now let us backtrack and look again at all these pathways, asking this time not simply which pathways exist but which are homeostatically controlled so as to maintain a balance between input and output. We approach this using the tools developed in the previous chapter, so the first question is: Is there a specific appetite for protein, in general, or for specific amino acids? When we are protein deficient are we unconsciously driven specifically to seek out protein-rich foods or foods containing any particular deficient essential amino acid? The answer seems to be "no," and this means we cannot depend on intuition to guide our protein intake. Now, it is true that most cultures have developed over the years food preferences which are conducive to adequate protein nutrition, but within many of these same cultures are also taboos and social practices which predispose to protein malnutrition by forbidding the use of certain protein-rich foods, particularly by women and children.

How about absorption from the gastrointestinal tract? Is it physiologically regulated so as to favor absorption when protein supplies are low and reduce it when lots of protein is available? Again, the answer is no. In normal persons, the digestion of protein and absorption of the free amino acids formed in the process is virtually 100 percent complete all the time and is not subject to physiological control. Only in the presence of certain diseases, such as incomplete digestion due to inadequate secretion of digestive enzymes, does absorption of ingested protein fall significantly below 100 percent. Unfortunately, protein deficiency is itself one of the causes of such failure (for example, the digestive enzymes are themselves proteins and won't be formed normally in the presence of protein deficiency) and so a vicious cycle can develop.

The lack of a specific appetite for protein and amino acids and the lack of control over absorption means that no homeostatic control is exerted on the input side.* Accordingly, the output side must be the target of the body's reflexes for maintaining protein balance. The logical first place to look would be the kidneys, but we would not find them there. The urinary excretion of protein is always negligi-

---

*There does remain one other fascinating possibility, that the gut bacteria might act as nitrogen-fixing bacteria, attaching free nitrogen gas in the gut to carbohydrate to form new amino acids which can then be absorbed by the host. This may actually occur in New Guinea highlanders.

ble in normal persons (mainly because the blood proteins can't fit through the kidney's tiny filters), as is excretion of amino acids (the amino acids do pass through the filters but are reclaimed into the blood as the filtered fluid moves along the kidney's conduits). Even in persons eating huge quantities of protein, no protein or amino acids to speak of are excreted in the urine. In analogy to the gut, the kidney's conservation of protein and amino acids does not hold in a variety of diseases of the kidney; in some, the filters become leaky enough to spill protein and in others (mainly rare genetic diseases) the conduits do not have the ability to reclaim the filtered amino acids. In such diseases, of course, the excretion does not represent a physiological control mechanism but rather an abnormal loss which, itself, may produce deficiency of proteins or amino acids.

We are left, therefore, with catabolism by the liver as the dominant, indeed, the only really significant, control point in total-body protein homeostasis. The biochemical reactions for deamination and urea formation are catalyzed by enzymes, and the activity and concentrations of these enzymes are exquisitely controlled so as to achieve protein balance. When protein intake is high, these enzymes are "revved-up" so that the rates of deamination of amino acids and formation of urea from the ammonia generated thereby are greatly increased. The result is that the amino acids of the excess ingested protein are simply converted to carbohydrate and urea, the latter to be excreted in the urine.*

Conversely, when protein intake is low (or when protein loss from the body is increased by disease) the enzymes involved in deamination and urea formation become relatively quiescent. This permits most of the amino acids being ingested and absorbed to remain as amino acids and be incorporated into protein; in this manner intake and catabolism are brought into balance. A critical word in the previous sentence is "most," for the liver is unable to close down its deamination pathways completely, and so some amino acids are always being catabolized even when protein intake is zero. In other words, the minimal rate of deamination sets the lowest level of protein intake at which body balance of protein can be achieved. When intake is below this level, the inevitable consequence is pro-

---

*One of the implications of this phenomenon, frequently lost on athletic coaches, is that one cannot derive much of an increase in synthesis of protein in muscle or any other organ simply by eating large amounts of protein; the extra ingested protein is merely converted to carbohydrates and, thence, to fat if so much protein is ingested that total calories exceed energy expenditure.

gressive loss of endogenous protein and eventual death. It may take a long time for sickness to develop, even when a person is ingesting no protein at all, since there are considerable amounts of protein in muscle (and to a lesser extent in other organs) which can be called upon to supply the amino acids needed for continued replacement of other proteins more crucial for everyday function. But these are not really storage proteins in the sense that our fat cells are storage depots for fat, since the involved proteins perform important functions in the muscles; it is remarkable just how much protein can be lost before muscle weakness occurs, but there is, of course, a limit, and when other organs and tissues like the heart start losing their proteins, serious illness must result.

Given the world's shortage of protein and the huge number of persons who suffer from protein deficiency, one might imagine that the physiological controls over the enzymes responsible for deamination and urea synthesis would be among the most intensively studied fields in biology and medicine. If a way were found to reduce the activity of these enzymes to zero, then at least theoretically, adults would have to ingest only tiny amounts of protein, just enough to replace the losses in sloughed skin, hair, and external bodily secretions. (I say "theoretically" because such a "technological fix" on the problem of protein deficiency would almost certainly lead to unthought-of deleterious consequences; one can only assume that inability to shut off these enzymes completely carried some strong selective evolutionary advantage which outweighed the negative survival value such a mechanism carries with it in the face of deficient protein supplies.) Yet strangely, relatively little research has been done on the physiological control of this system. We know very little about the signals which act upon the liver to alter relevant enzymes. We don't know which hormones, if any, are involved and how they might interact with other blood-borne signals to integrate amino acid metabolism with that of carbohydrate and fat.

We do know several very important empirical phenomena. One concerns the interaction between the supply of protein and that of total calories, i.e., the energy content of all ingested organic nutrients. The exquisite coupling of protein catabolism to protein supply applies only to the case in which protein deficiency is an isolated nutritional problem, not accompanied by inadequate total calories. For whenever total calories are deficient this coupling breaks down, and regardless of how much protein is ingested, almost all of the amino acids will lose their nitrogen and be used for fuel. The importance of this fact cannot be too strongly stressed. One simply cannot remain in stable protein balance unless the total calories supplied by the diet are adequate to achieve caloric balance. We shall see later that this relationship makes it impossible to specify minimal protein requirements without simultaneously considering minimal total energy requirements.

The physiological responses to changes in protein intake have the same order of sensitivity as do those for sodium and water. It takes only 1 to 2 percent change in total body protein to trigger off the changes in deamination and urea synthesis which restore equality of input and output. For example (table 4–1), when an adult man is eating 90 g of protein daily, he loses about 12 g of protein or amino acids from the body surface (and to the synthesis of nitrogen-containing molecules other than amino acids) and he deaminates the conremaining 78 g, the overall result being no change in total body protein. If he were to go abruptly on a low-protein diet, say 40 g/day, we would find that the 12 g nondeamination loss remained relatively constant indefinitely but the amount lost to deamination and urea would change markedly in a stereotyped pattern. Probably no change would have occurred during the first day so that he would still lose 78 g by deamination. The result is that, by the end of twenty-four hours, he has gone into negative protein balance by 50 g (intake = 40 g and output = 90 g). This is really a tiny negative balance, since his total body protein approximates 12,000 g, but it is enough to trigger the required homeostatic response—inhibition of the deamination enzymes. Therefore, the next day amino acid catabolism may be down to 55 g, and by the fourth or fifth day to 28 g, at which point he has achieved a stable input-output balance. As

TABLE 4–1   Changes in Protein Balance During Transition from a High-Protein to a Low-Protein Diet

	Basal Days	Day 1	Day 2	Day 5
Intake (g/day)	90	40	40	40
Output (g/day)				
A. Loss from body surface	12	12	12	12
B. Deamination	78	78	55	28
Total	90	90	67	40
Net loss (g/day)	0	50	27	0

long as he stays on this 40 g/day intake, he will stay in balance, but don't forget he does so with a slight but unchanging reduction in his total body protein.

If he eventually returns to his 90 g daily intake, the entire series of events will be reversed as the activity and concentration of the deamination enzymes are increased to their original value. If he then were to go on a diet containing 120 g of protein the deamination enzymes would become even more numerous and active; he would have no difficulty achieving balance at this level of protein intake but would end up with a small, perhaps 1 to 2 percent increase in body protein over that which existed when he was eating 90 g/day.

If we were to make our examples more severe, a different picture would emerge. If intake were reduced below a certain level, say 20 g/day, he would never reachieve stable balance simply because catabolism could not be lowered enough. If he were to go to some extremely high level of intake (I don't really know how high one would have to go), the upper limit of catabolism would be reached, and amino acids would accumulate to even larger, eventually toxic, amounts.

But as long as he stays within the limits of homeostatic responses, balance is achieved, and the total body protein will differ by only a few percentage points between the high and low intake states. This brings us once again to the question which must be raised for every nutrient: Where within this range of intakes over which balance is achievable lies the "optimal" intake of protein, so far as health, well-being, and longevity are concerned? Does the additional few grams of body protein which high-intake persons carry around in their bodies confer any benefits? Does it perhaps increase one's resistance to infection or to environmental pollutants? Does it make one feel more energetic? Or might it actually have detrimental effects such as decreased longevity, as suggested by some data from experiments with animals?

The number of experiments dealing with this question of optimal, rather than minimal, protein intakes is incredibly small, yet the question is deserving of intensive study, since protein is such a scarce commodity. The average healthy American adult, for example, eats about twice the amount of protein specified by the RDA. There is no question at all that protein requirements are increased in the presence of infection or other diseases, as well as in children, and during pregnancy or lactation; in such situations, eating twice the adult RDA or even much more is almost certainly beneficial, but we simply have no idea whether, in the absence of these clear-cut drains on body protein, regularly ingesting large amounts of protein does either good or harm.

It has been argued on a theoretical basis that having "saturated body stores of protein" is a good thing because it allows a person to last longer in case he is suddenly faced with a long-term low protein situation (as in a famine, for example) or an infection. But this view makes no sense at all when one realizes that the extra body protein accumulated even on a very high protein diet is so small, only a few days' worth at most. All right then, our theoretician might argue, perhaps *total* body protein is up only a few percentage points but maybe certain specific very important proteins (antibodies, for example) might be elevated much more than this by a high protein intake. This is a perfectly sound hypothesis but experiments to verify it simply haven't been done. Indeed, several experiments have indicated that experimental animals chronically fed a high-protein diet do *not* survive as long during a period of fasting as do animals previously fed a low-protein diet. The average daily catabolism of protein during the period of starvation was much lower in the latter group of animals so that their total protein loss was considerably less than that of the former group. This result really shouldn't be too surprising for it almost certainly is a reflection of long-term acclimatization to low protein intakes, that is, the development of physiological responses which permitted those animals already acclimatized to low protein intakes to adjust better when the total shut off of protein occurred. It certainly demonstrates that theory alone simply won't do; we need the hard data.

Setting Protein Requirements

Those of us who live in a protein-rich society and who have the economic capacity to participate in the protein feast may be able to sit and ponder whether large amounts of protein are beneficial or harmful, but most of the world's population subsists at the other end of the spectrum. The question—What constitutes an adequate minimal level of protein intake?—is, therefore, perhaps the single most important question for world nutrition today. Seemingly small differences in the answer to this question can have extraordinarily important impact on long-range global agricultural planning, and on the health of hundreds of millions of people, as the events of the past decade illustrate.

To understand the problem of protein requirements you need one more helping of some basic biochemistry concerning the essential amino acids. The key ingredient left out of the discussion so far is that of protein *quality,* a reflection of the relative amounts of the different essential amino acids in the ingested protein. Each of the body's protein types contains all the essential amino acids in varying relative amounts, and so when a cell is stringing together different amino acids to form a new protein, each of the essential amino acids must be present in adequate amounts in order for synthesis to proceed. If even a single essential amino acid is in short supply the chain cannot be constructed. What is even more important, the other relatively abundant amino acids which would have gone into the protein had construction not been stopped, cannot be stored for later use (again, you see how critical it is that the body has no true amino acid stores), but are deaminated and lost for good. This is clearly a wasteful process for it means that deficiency of even a single amino acid will increase the catabolism (and, therefore, the requirement) for all the others.

For this reason, the requirement for total protein cannot be specified unless we know how successful the ingested proteins are in supplying the proper amounts of all the essential amino acids. The best proteins contain all the essential amino acids in approximately the same relative amounts found in the body. These nutritionally "complete" proteins—egg and milk proteins are the best, with meat proteins close behind them—are adequate to meet all the body's needs and are required in the smallest total amount. At the other end of the spectrum, proteins which are completely lacking one or more of the essential amino acids (as for example, corn protein, which lacks tryptophan and lysine) cannot, as the sole source of ingested protein, maintain growth or health. All their amino acids are simply deaminated, and no amount of them alone can maintain amino acid balance.

Between these extremes lie most proteins, not absolutely lacking any particular essential amino acids, but relatively deficient in one or more. If enough of such a protein is ingested, the job of synthesizing all the body's proteins can usually get done (at least in adults), but the process is quite wasteful since so much catabolism of the more abundant amino acids of the protein occurs.

Clearly, some quantitative index for comparing just how efficiently the body utilizes various proteins is needed, and that is the Net Protein Utilization (NPU). The NPU of a protein is determined by how closely its essential amino acid pattern matches that of the body's proteins, and its numerical value tells, quite simply, what percentage of the ingested protein is actually available for protein synthesis. No protein is 100 percent usable by human beings, but milk and egg proteins are the closest at about 94 percent and serve as the standard for all others. For example, if you were eating only one type of protein, one which had an NPU of 47 percent, you would require twice as much of that protein as of egg protein to maintain a stable balance. In general, plant proteins have considerably lower NPUs than do those from animal sources, because they are relatively deficient in one or more of the essential amino acids.

So far I have been talking only of individual proteins or those from a single food source, such as eggs. But, of course, we usually eat more than one food at a time and once the total meal has been digested, all the amino acids are absorbed together. This makes it possible to devise meals whose overall NPU is quite high by mixing foods, the individual proteins of which have low NPUs but complementary patterns of essential amino acids. By "complementary," I mean patterns which match like a jigsaw. For example, most cereal proteins are deficient in lysine but rich in methionine, whereas legumes have just the opposite pattern. Therefore, a meal containing cereal products and legumes would have a high NPU because each component of the meal makes up for what the other lacks.

As Nevin S. Scrimshaw and Vernon R. Young have pointed out:

> Every culture has evolved its own mixtures of complementary protein. In the Middle East wheat bread, which lacks adequate levels of lysine, is eaten with cheese, which has a high lysine content. Mexicans eat rice and peas. Indians eat wheat and pulses, and Americans eat breakfast cereals with milk. This kind of supplementation, particularly in infants and growing children, only works, however, when the deficient and complementary proteins are ingested together or are ingested separately within a few hours.[1]

Now you have enough basic science information to look at how protein requirements have been set and what the problems with this standard setting may be. The importance of these standards can be appreciated only by placing them in their global setting.

Figure 4–2 illustrates the calorie and protein supplies in selected areas of the world during the late 1960s. One obvious point is that calorie and protein consumption are closely related; the people who are ingesting the fewest calories are also ingesting the least protein. Second, there is approximately a twofold difference in per capita protein consumption between the highest and lowest areas. Third, the protein ingested by the wealthier nations is predominantly from animal sources (and therefore has a relatively high NPU), whereas the poorer nations are ingesting almost entirely proteins of plant origin, which have relatively low NPUs. This means that the effective nutritional difference for protein between areas is even more than twofold. Finally, it is important to recognize that these are average per capita values; many people in each area are eating considerably less and others much more than this average.

Figures like these demonstrate why virtually all experts agree that the major cause of malnutrition today is not an undersupply of total world food, but rather a maldistribution, both on a world scale and within individual countries and local communities. Barry Commoner has put it bluntly:

> The people who hunger and starve lack food not because it does not exist but because others have more food than they need. Some people, some nations, have more food than they need because they are rich enough to afford it. Other people, other nations, have less food than they need because they are too poor to buy it. It is just as simple as that. And just as complex.[2]

What then is the appropriate decision concerning the role of nutritional policy planning in combating malnutrition? I share the view of Erik Eckholm, of the Worldwatch Institute:

> Observing the strong correlation between poverty and nutrition, some analysts view adopting nutrition strategies as an unnecessary diversion from the overriding task of raising the incomes of the poor. According to various versions of this perspective, hastening economic growth, redistributing income, or both are the best defenses against undernutrition. While based on truths, such arguments can be dangerously incomplete. Setting minimum income levels is certainly a necessary part of any strategy for stamping out undernutrition, but it is seldom all that is needed. While the poor must have land, jobs, and decent incomes if undernutrition is to be obliterated, the positive impact of all three on diets can be enhanced when combined with careful attention to the nutrition factor. . . . Nutrition strategies, with which governments influence people's diets, are increasingly recognized as a public responsibility.[3]

Fig. 4–2.   Calorie and protein supply in selected areas of the world.
(Redrawn from *Population Bulletin* 29, no. 1, p. 19. Courtesy of the
Population Reference Bureau, Inc., Washington, D.C.)

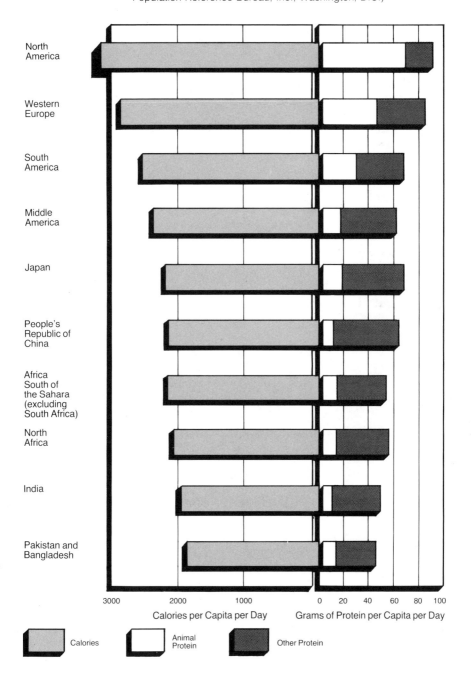

The first step, of course, in designing a strategy for the "nutrition factor" is to determine just which nutrients are the deficient ones. One major tool for doing so is simply to look for measurable signs of deficiency diseases. Another is the nutrition survey. The pattern of energy and nutrient intakes revealed by the dietary survey is then compared with "requirements," that is, the daily amounts considered to be necessary for health. Such evaluations in the world's poor nations invariably indicate that a large fraction (as many as half to two-thirds of all children, some believe) of the population suffers some degree of undernutrition for both total calories and protein. The real debate is over whether the protein deficit is relatively greater than the total calorie deficit.

For simplicity, let me state the two views in their most divergent form. View number one holds that the total-calorie and protein deficiencies are approximately of the same degree, that the most important reason for insufficient protein intake in developing countries is that people are simply not eating enough food. If more calories could be made available to them in the form of relatively inexpensively grown cereals (wheat, corn, and rice), then not only would total-calorie deficiency be taken care of but the additional protein represented by these foods would simultaneously eliminate protein deficiency as well. Thus, a single policy aimed at increasing total food production most efficiently would be the logical course to pursue.

The opposing view holds that the total-calories solution just described is based on an underestimate of minimal protein requirements, that ingestion of enough cereals to satisfy total energy requirements would not satisfy protein needs, because these foods are too low in total protein content and in NPUs. Rather, what is required are policies which emphasize provision of foods containing more protein and a wider variety of complementarity matchings.*

This latter course is a more expensive and complicated one to pursue but seemed to be the one called for by the estimates of protein requirements until the early 1970s. Dr. Nevin S. Scrimshaw, Institute Professor and Head, Department of Nutrition and Food

---

*Notice that this entire debate is couched in terms of the comparison between nutritional survey and presumed requirements. You might think that the other tool for nutritional evaluation—physical examination—would be able to settle the issue, but it is not, simply because we really are not confident of our ability to distinguish unique symptoms of protein deficiency as opposed to starvation. Some experts believe they can do so, at least in children, but most deny this. This explains why the two are usually lumped together clinically as protein-calorie malnutrition.

Science at Massachusetts Institute of Technology, has written most extensively on this topic and I have depended heavily on his approach and view points. He wrote in 1978:

> No issue of human nutrition in the last decade has occasioned more controversy and misunderstanding, nor been more significant to national and international strategies for dealing with malnutrition in developing countries than the relative importance of protein and energy deficits in the diets of the underprivileged...Throughout the 1960s there was increasing recognition by international and bilateral agencies of the problem of assuring adequate dietary protein for the rapidly increasing populations of the less developed countries of the world. It was emphasized that, while increased cereal production utilizing Green Revolution techniques might insure adequate dietary calories, there was a parallel need to assure production of foods providing more protein relative to calories.
>
> For populations where animal milks were unavailable, too costly, or culturally unacceptable as weaning foods, it was proposed that local food combinations be identified for preparation by the village mother as weaning foods. Particularly for populations in urban areas, processed weaning foods from local vegetable protein sources were recommended at as low a cost as possible for people who could not afford milk. It was also urged that, as a matter of agricultural and national development policy, support be given not only to cereal production, but also to the cultivation of legumes and oil seeds, to increased utilization of fish from fresh water and marine sources, to other animal protein production, and to the possibility of developing unconventional sources of protein such as those derived from fermentation processes, the so-called single-cell proteins.[4]

But this picture changed abruptly in the 1970s.

> In April, 1971, a Joint FAO/WHO Expert Committee on Energy and Protein Requirements convened in Rome, lowered the estimated safe allowances for protein [by approximately 20 percent], and thereby redefined dietary protein malnutrition [their formal report was published in 1973, but the conclusions were known in 1971]. Nutritionists working with the planning commissions of several developing countries suddenly found themselves preparing a vigorous attack on a problem that no longer existed as a priority issue, if the decisions of the Rome committee were applied to existing dietary intake data. . . .
> In many countries, medical and public-health workers, economists, and statisticians read of the new recommendations and adopted this conclusion.[5]

That this was the intent of the committee is clearly expressed in a letter written by three of its members in 1973.

The implication of the safe levels for the world's malnutrition problem is that *primary* [original italics] protein deficiency, even among young children, is most unlikely to be the cause of malnutrition in communities that have an adequate total supply of food energy even when cereal grains are the major source of protein.... A primary protein problem, if it exists at all, is likely to be confined to communities (probably no more than 5% of the world's population) where, because of ecological or economic constraints, people are obliged to subsist on starchy roots as staples. Even in these situations, the bulky nature of the food given to small children probably results in a deficiency of energy... as well as of protein.*[6]

In large part because of this report, there was a more single-minded emphasis during the seventies on cereal production, utilizing the Green Revolution techniques introduced earlier. The result, at least in Scrimshaw's view:

It is now well-recognized that concentration on improving yields of cereals... has been associated with a decrease in the per caput production and a rise in the relative price of legumes[†] in most developing countries in which Green Revolution techniques have made progress. Because legumes are important sources of more concentrated protein to complement cereal diets, and the poor in these countries have been able to afford less of them, their nutritional status has deteriorated in some instances.

If agriculturalists are encouraged by nutritionists and planners to believe that populations can subsist on cereal diets, there will continue to be a lag in the production or development of better sources of protein, and the diets of the poor will deteriorate further.... The narrow concentration of agricultural research, extension, and government subsidies on cereals is one unintended byproduct of the present wave of statements that protein is not a problem in the world if people receive enough calories.[7]

---

*A good example of the emotions generated by this change in viewpoint is given by the following quote from a 1974 article in *New Scientist*, the prestigious British journal somewhat analagous to our *Scientific American*: "Our view of malnutrition has changed considerably over the past few decades. By mistakenly concentrating on the so-called protein gap, which turned out to be largely a figment of their own imaginations, nutritionists have been responsible for one of the classic examples of non-appropriate technology.... We do not know how many millions of children have died over the past 30 years because food aid has wrongly concentrated on protein instead of energy" (J. Tinker, "The Green Revolution is Over," *New Scientist*, November 7, 1974, p. 388).

†Legumes, or pulses, constitute the family of food crops that includes peas, lentils, beans, chick peas, mung beans, pigeon peas, and broad beans. They are 18 to 25 percent protein, double that of wheat and triple that of milled rice. Moreover, their proteins are of better quality than those of the cereals. Widely accepted staples of the diet in most low-income countries, legumes production had been declining markedly ever since introduction of Green Revolution techniques. For example, in India, between 1961 and 1972, the per capita yield dropped 38 percent (while wheat yield was increasing 25 percent).

If Dr. Scrimshaw is correct, and there are many experts who feel he is not, then an underestimation of protein requirements promulgated by the 1971 committee will continue to have disastrous consequences for the world's poor. Let us look at the scientific basis for the 1971 committee's decisions.[8] Keep in mind that most nutritionists feel we know more about requirements for protein than for almost any other nutrient, so that the difficulties inherent in formulating a "safe allowance" (equivalent to the RDA) for protein should make us very cautious indeed concerning the accuracy of decisions by similar committees concerned with other nutrients.

The basic principles used to set nutrient requirements were outlined in chapter 3. The method given most credence by the 1963 FAO/WHO Joint International Committee was the so-called factorial (or balance) approach in which all nitrogen losses from the body via the skin, feces, urine, and menstrual flow are carefully measured while healthy volunteer subjects (young adults) are on a protein-free diet, and the sum of these losses provides an estimate of the amount of protein required for the replacement of these losses. Again, I must emphasize that nitrogen, when used in reference to protein balance, refers not to gaseous nitrogen but to nitrogen atoms bound up in organic molecules and ammonia. Since nitrogen accounts for one-sixteenth of the weight of most proteins, one need only multiply the amount of nitrogen lost from the body by 6.25 to determine the amount of protein which had to be catabolized to account for this much nitrogen.

Of course, the factorial method can only be as good as the experimental data gathered to make the calculation, and this was a real problem for the 1963 committee—there were simply not enough data on nitrogen losses for people on protein-free diets. The committee used what few data were available and also depended heavily on extrapolations from animal experiments. Once the committee had come up with a number, it added a small amount more to cover the increased protein catabolism presumed to occur as a result of everyday stresses in normal people, and then, since the goal of the recommendation was to cover 97.5 percent of the population, it added yet another 20 percent to cover the mean plus two standard deviations (at this time, 10 percent of the mean, rather than 15 percent, was thought to best approximate one standard deviation). After these additions, the grand loss total was 0.114 g of nitrogen per kg body weight. This is equivalent to daily total protein losses of 6.25 × 0.114 g/kg = 0.71 g protein per kg body weight.

Thus, the committee's estimate was that 97.5 percent of all healthy adults would break down no more than 0.71 g of protein for each kg body weight when ingesting no protein at all. If this represents the lowest level to which protein catabolism can be brought, then, so they reasoned, it also represents the minimal amount of protein which must be ingested in order to maintain protein balance, assuming the NPU of the ingested protein is 100 (a close approximation for egg protein). If the NPU of the ingested protein were only 50, then the total amount of protein which must be ingested to cover minimal losses is twice as great (1.42 g/kg body weight) and so on.

The diets of the wealthier nations such as the United States have an average protein NPU of 70 to 80, so that the "safe allowance" for adults in these countries is 0.8 to 1.0 g per kg body weight; adults of the poorer countries, with average dietary NPUs of 50 to 60, required proportionally more protein, 1.2 to 1.4 g per kg body weight. Recommendations for infants, children, pregnant and lactating women were then determined, as is the usual case, by extrapolations from these young-adult standards, using additional data such as those concerning growth, milk intake and production, fetal requirements, balance data for these groups, and efficiency of protein utilization.

Now we come to the 1971 FAO/WHO expert committee convened to reconsider the question of protein requirements on the basis of new research findings accumulated in the interim (one of the important results of the 1963 group's report, as should be the case for every nutritional committee's report, was to stimulate more research). By this time it was clear that the 1963 estimates of obligatory nitrogen losses from skin and in urine and feces had all been much too high. Careful measurements of all these values in human subjects had demonstrated that the actual grand total was only about half of the 1963 committee's estimate. This new research, accordingly, required a lowering of the FAO/WHO recommendation.

However, the story was not to be so simple, for yet another flaw in the 1963 committee's assumptions had surfaced, and this one had led that committee in the direction of underestimation of protein requirements. Remember that the members had assumed efficiency of egg protein utilization to be virtually 100 percent, an assumption backed up by many previous experiments. But since 1963 some strange results had been cropping up. Several of the groups of investigators who had performed the new studies of minimal nitrogen losses by persons on a zero-protein diet had then fed their subjects amounts of egg protein equivalent to these minimal losses, the first time this had ever been done. The expected result, of course, was that this protein would cause nitrogen balance to be reachieved, but that did not occur, for under these conditions, the egg protein was found to have an NPU of only 60 to 70, rather than the expected 90 to 100. Clearly, the latter NPU value, determined so many times by so many investigators under one set of standardized conditions, did not apply when the conditions were changed, specifically when protein intake was near requirement levels.

Thus (table 4–2), the 1963 committee had overestimated protein requirements by using too high an estimate of obligatory nitrogen excretion at zero protein intake, but had underestimated them by assuming a too high NPU value for egg protein at near-requirement levels of intake. These errors obviously tended to cancel each other out, but not completely, the former being the greater error, and so the final recommendation for healthy adults, based on egg albumin, was reduced by approximately 20 percent, from the 1963 value of 0.71 g egg protein per kilogram body weight to 0.57 g/kg. For ordinary diets, as opposed to egg protein, the safe allowance recommendation increased proportionally as the NPU of the diet (relative to the new value for egg protein) decreased.

TABLE 4–2   Errors and Problems in Committee Recommendations for Safe Protein Allowances

---

Major Inaccuracies of 1963 Committee Revealed by 1971

Error 1. Overestimated obligatory protein loss.

Error 2. Assumed NPU of egg protein to be 90 to 100 percent when protein intake is at the minimal level; it actually is 60 to 70 percent.

Error 1 was greater than error 2 and so the 1963 recommendation was too high; 1971 committee recommendation therefore was lowered by 20 percent.

Major Problems with 1971 Recommendation Revealed by New Data since 1971

Problem 1. Feeding volunteers the 1971 recommendation for 100 days resulted in significant and progressive net protein loss.

Problem 2. Previous use of high calorie diets in studies had led to overestimation of efficiency of egg protein utilization.

Problem 3. Poorer quality proteins show a much greater fall-off in percentage of utilization at replacement protein intakes than do high quality proteins.

Dr. Scrimshaw believes that the 1973 recommendations are definitely too low for many more than 2.5 percent of the normal population. Evidence for his view comes from the first really long-term studies of protein balance ever performed.[9] As Dr. Scrimshaw has pointed out, all the members of the 1971 committee were aware that the data they were using to prepare their recommendations were from balance studies of fifteen days or less; because of great cost and difficulty, no long-term studies had been done. Despite the extraordinary global significance of protein requirements, the funds for such a study, performed by Dr. Scrimshaw and his associates, ultimately had to come from a private nongovernmental source. The FAO/WHO "safe level" of egg protein, 0.57 g/kg, was fed to students for three months while complete balance studies and a variety of other indicators of physiological status were performed. The disturbing results: At the end of the three months, all six subjects had lost body protein, as evidenced by actual negative nitrogen balance, or by more indirect measures of muscle mass and nonfat body weight. This despite the fact that they were all given enough total calories to cause weight gain, the custom universally employed when performing nitrogen balance studies (so as to ensure that the protein is not catabolized for energy). Indeed, the protein loss was even greater when the study was repeated using only the number of total calories needed to hold body weight constant. Thus, the NPU value of 60 to 70 previously determined for egg protein when persons were ingesting near-replacement amounts of protein but excessive total calories must be lowered still more in order to apply to situations in which total calories are merely adequate for maintenance of stable body weight.

Although, as Dr. Scrimshaw has emphasized, the number of subjects in these experiments were few and were all previously well-nourished Americans, hardly a group representative of the world's population, the fact remains that these studies have confirmed several of the major fears of nutritionists. First, short-term balance studies are not sufficient as the sole criterion for assessing human nutritional requirements. They simply don't provide enough time for small, but in the long run very important, differences to become manifest or for delayed responses to occur. Second, certain time-honored experimental conditions may become so deeply ingrained that investigators virtually cease to recognize how different the results obtained using them may be from real-life situations. Trying to determine minimal protein requirements in persons receiving very high calorie diets is certainly an example of this type of blind spot, for most of the world's population face both calorie and protein deficiencies simultaneously.

Other new types of data have further contributed to the belief by some scientists that the FAO/WHO recommendations are inadequate, particularly for the developing countries. For example, it has been found that the discrepancy between NPU measured under standard conditions and the actual protein utilization at requirement levels may be much greater for poorer quality proteins than for egg protein. For the latter, you will recall, the discrepancy is approximately 30 percent (90 to 100 versus 60 to 70); for wheat protein it may be 75 percent, so that the FAO/WHO correction factor for mixed diets, based on egg protein, may be much too little. Here is another lesson—it is extremely dangerous to extrapolate from one type of substance to another, even when they belong to the same general family of molecules.

Dr. Scrimshaw has well summarized the overall lessons to be learned from these scientific events:

> It would seem prudent in the future to be somewhat more cautious about the limitations of our knowledge, not only of protein requirements, but for all nutrients, and to be willing to provide for adequate margins of safety. . . .We need constantly to remind ourselves that neither individuals nor committees are infallible, and that all scientific issues need to be addressed with some humility.
>
> As for human protein requirement, the pendulum is still swinging because our knowledge is so incomplete. In fact, for all nutrients, our knowledge of precise human requirements and the interrelations among them is far more fragmentary and tentative than generally realized. . . . More research is required, and for human nutritional requirements, it must be clinical research. This process must include long-term human feeding studies using as many measures of metabolic function and physical performance as possible to supplement nitrogen balance as a criterion.[10]

This last sentence has very important implications. The entire logic for setting protein requirements has centered on the concept of balance, and the grounds for criticizing the actual recommendations were whether the balance data in existence were adequate and correctly interpreted. Yet we know that, so far as some nutrients are concerned, stable balance can be achieved at levels too low to prevent deficiency disease. "Stable balance" must not be used synonymously with "absence of disease." For this reason, to be meaningful, RDAs or the FAO/WHO equivalent "safe allowances" must be based on measures of performance and on the presence of disease signs and symptoms. An example of the results of failure to do so will be described in detail in the next chapter.

I have gone into some detail on the scientific merits of the 1971 committee's recommendation, but probably of greater importance than the recommendations themselves was the misuse of them by planners, economists, and health workers. A major reason for misuse was an educational one—the failure to recognize that RDAs and "safe allowances" are for healthy persons. As I emphasized in chapter 3, such recommendations are simply not adequate for people suffering from acute or chronic diseases, the norm in developing countries. Nor are they adequate for catch-up growth in children whose growth has been stunted by previous malnutrition and disease, again the norm in most parts of the world.

The rationale for not including recommendations for other than healthy populations was stated clearly by three members of the expert committee writing in 1973, in answer to a highly critical report by the Protein Advisory Group (PAG) of the United Nations.

> The main contention of the PAG report is that the protein needs of populations suffering from repeated infections and parasitic infestations are higher than the recommended safe levels of protein intake. The Expert Committee recognized that infections increase the need for protein and other nutrients, but since the extent of this extra need is unknown, the only realistic course was to specify safe levels for healthy subjects.[11]

This is standard practice in the setting of requirements and so it is crucial that the mass media and those using such requirements recognize the problem. Moreover, it is incumbent upon the expert committees not to dismiss the problem in a few sentences (as was done in this particular expert committee report), but to emphasize how important it is to take variables into account even though no precise numerical estimates of the supplements required can be given. These expert committee reports are heavy reading, and it is very easy for everything else but the major quantitative conclusions to be lost on a general audience. Most important, we must come to grips with the fact that it will never be possible to devise any meaningful universal recommendations for nutrient requirements, and flexibility is badly needed in the application of any standard values proposed.

Chapter **5** | The Iron-Enrichment Controversy

This tentative order withdraws the stayed amendment that would have increased the added iron content [of enriched flour and bread products]. . . . The Commissioner of Food and Drugs has concluded that the increases are not proved to be needed, safe, or effective.

Donald Kennedy, *Federal Register*, November 18, 1977

With these words Food and Drug Administration (FDA) commissioner Kennedy concluded the debate (or at least effected a cease-fire) over iron enrichment, a debate which had lasted almost nine years and which was generally recognized as one of the most important nutritional issues of the decade in the United States. What began as a public-spirited and seemingly benign commonsense petition by the American Bakers Association and the Millers' National Federation to raise the standard of enriched bread and flour by tripling the amount of iron added to these products rapidly led to a vituperative dispute which impugned the scientific basis for the FDA's regulatory actions and raised grave questions concerning the basic intellectual principles underlying nutritional planning. It has prompted a reexamination of all food enrichment, that is, the concept of adding nutrients to the general food supply. The iron-enrichment battle may have been only the first engagement of a much more extensive war and it is critical, now that the smoke of confusing and often inaccurate public statements has cleared, for us to try to understand the scientific issues involved and their applicability to the broad question of food enrichment.

Perhaps the most poignant plea for such an analysis comes from former commissioner Alexander M. Schmidt:

> I heartily applaud this action by the Commissioner [Kennedy], even though I signed the order he reversed. In retrospect, this rather depressing regulatory episode holds several valuable lessons for the thoughtful observer.[1]

Some of the "lessons" Dr. Schmidt had in mind concern the inner workings of the FDA, the quality of its in-house scientists and research programs, and the ways in which it makes decisions. Although these issues all deserve a close analysis, they are not the ones I wish to deal with. Rather, what concerns me here is that the assumptions used by the proenrichment group and the FDA (until its turnabout under Commissioner Kennedy) were not scientifically defensible. The crucial questions relating to these assumptions not only could not be answered, but for the most part, had never even been properly subjected to scientific investigations. The FDA was proposing to mandate a major change in this country's diet on the basis of wholly inadequate evidence concerning necessity, efficacy, and safety.

First, a brief chronology. For almost thirty years, since the enrichment programs passed during World War II, the FDA had authorized the addition to flour of small amounts of iron, approximately 13 mg/lb (this queer notation of metric [milligrams] and English [pounds] units somehow got started and has persevered). This was really more of a restoration than an enrichment, for it approximated the amount of iron lost in the process of milling and in the production of our standard white bread. Since then, many respected nutritionists had continued to argue that consumption of iron by the general population was decreasing because of the increased use of "empty-calorie" foods (those containing much sugar or fat but few vitamins or minerals), decreased total food consumption (because of our more sedentary existence), increased refining of foods with attendant loss of nutrients, and the disappearance of cooking utensils made of iron. There was no way to really prove that dietary intake had diminished, but in any case, there was no question, they felt, that large numbers of people, particularly the poor (because of economic constraints on their purchasing of iron-rich foods) and women in their reproductive years (because of menstrual blood loss), were suffering from iron deficiency anemia. This view really "hit the headlines" as part of the scathing denunciation of the nation's nutritional status delivered by the famous 1969 White House Conference on Food, Nutrition, and Health. Indeed, the petition to the FDA by the millers and bakers was in response to a recommendation from the conference. In this atmosphere, it is understandable that the FDA was quite enthusiastic about the petition and published the original proposal (for an increase to 60 mg/lb) in the *Federal Register* on April 1, 1970.

Three objections, all to the effect that increased iron in the diet could be harmful, were received by the FDA following this publication, and the commissioner therefore requested the American Medical Association (AMA) Council on Foods and Nutrition to comment on the objections. The AMA council strongly supported the overall concept of the proposal. Moreover, by this time, the Preliminary Report of the Ten-State Nutrition Survey,[2] the largest nutritional survey ever conducted, was available, and the results were even more shocking than the nutritionists and the White House Conference had expected. Not only was there a very high prevalence of iron deficiency anemia among women, but unexpectedly, there was an even higher occurrence for men, 22 percent of those surveyed being characterized as having "below normal" levels of iron. Numbers such as these certainly qualified iron deficiency as a general public health problem worthy of attack with a full-scale preventive medicine program, and in the *Federal Register* for December 3, 1971, the commisioner again published an iron-enrichment proposal, this time lowering the recommended enrichment of flour from the original 60 mg/lb to 40 mg/lb in recognition of the previously expressed concerns over safety.

By this time many more persons had become aware of the proposal, and over 520 comments were received, the great majority opposing it, again mainly on the basis of safety. Most of these persons were physicians and researchers, particularly those specializing in the field of blood diseases and the physiology of iron. In contrast, almost all responding experts in nutrition favored the proposal. As Dr. Schmidt was to comment five years later, "it became apparent that the regulation, while supported by some who knew a lot about nutrition, was opposed by individuals knowing the most about iron metabolism!"[3] It was at this time that the controversy became known to the general public through coverage by the mass media. Charges of malfeasance were leveled against the FDA, and consumer groups which argued that adding anything to food is wrong suggested that bread was being made into a drug and should carry a warning label; even racism was injected into the public debate.

The FDA took little further action until a new commissioner, Dr. Schmidt, revised the proposal and promulgated it once more on October 15, 1973. The same objections were again raised, chiefly by the medical profession, and this time the commissioner called for a formal evidentiary public hearing while indefinitely staying the proposal. At the conclusion of these hearings, the hearing examiner reported that the weight of evidence favored the proposal; despite this, Commissioner Kennedy (who had replaced Dr. Schmidt in the meantime), in a strongly worded report highly critical of the proposal (the flavor of his report is given by the last line of the quote at the beginning of the chapter), decided to withdraw it, and that is where the matter stands today.

In order to understand the nature of the objections raised against the proposal, objections which Dr. Kennedy ultimately found convincing (but which, amazingly to me, the hearing examiner did not), one must know some basic information concerning the handling of iron by the body.

Iron is an essential nutrient and the characteristic which makes it so important to all living organisms is its ability to interact with oxygen. Most of the body's iron is contained in hemoglobin, the iron-protein molecules within our red blood cells responsible for carrying 99 percent of the blood's oxygen. Iron-protein molecules similar to, but quite distinct from, hemoglobin are also found in every cell of the body, and they function in the cells' utilization of the oxygen supplied to them by the blood.

In addition to all these iron-containing molecules which interact with oxygen, i.e., actually carry out the physiological functions of iron, other proteins exist whose sole function is simply to bind iron. The iron-binding protein in plasma (the liquid portion of blood) transports iron from one place in the body to another. The other major iron-binding proteins are found inside almost every cell of the body, but especially in the liver, bone marrow, and spleen; known as ferritin, these molecules serve as storage depots for iron. Ferritin is necessary both because free iron tends to form clumps if it is not bound to protein and because free iron will latch on to other proteins of the cell, altering their structure and causing damage. This last point is extremely important: Large amounts of iron are unquestionably highly toxic to living organisms.

Now, given the essential roles of iron, one can well predict that the body has evolved a variety of homeostatic mechanisms for preventing either a deficiency or excess of this element. The first requirement is that total-body losses and gains of iron balance out. It is impossible to avoid losing iron, since tiny quantities are lost each day in the urine, sweat, and pound or so of cells sloughed from skin, gastrointestinal tract, and genitourinary tract. This all amounts to only about 1 mg of iron each day. For comparison, this amount of iron is contained in only 2 ml of blood, so one can see that bleeding is a potentially much greater source of iron loss than any of these other routes. A woman loses about 30 to 60 mg of iron during each menstrual period; averaged over the month, this amounts to 1 to 2 mg/day. Add this to the 1 mg/day loss by the other routes, and you can see that normal women lose two to three times more iron than do normal men.

Obviously, in order for total-body balance to be maintained, the amount of this metal lost from the body via these routes must be replaced by absorption into the blood, across the intestinal wall, of an equivalent amount of ingested iron, and here is where the body makes the homeostatic adjustments required for achievement of balance. The percentage of ingested iron which is actually taken into the blood is subject to precise physiological control, the unabsorbed iron merely passing through the length of the tract to be lost in the feces. So far as total-body balance is concerned, evolution has placed all its regulatory eggs in one basket—control of intestinal absorption—for there are no active controls on the output side (loss in urine, sweat, sloughed cells, and menstrual flow). In this regard, iron, like some other trace elements, behaves very differently from the more familiar nutrients such as sodium, water, and the water-soluble vitamins. As described in chapter 3, these substances all have active controls over their excretion by the kidneys. An important implication of lack of excretory control is that iron, once in the body, cannot be excreted, to any great extent, by physiological means.

A few examples should help emphasize how this system functions. Let us take a normal man who is losing 1 mg of iron each day and ingesting 10 mg in his food; appropriate studies would reveal that only 1 mg of this ingested iron was being absorbed into his blood, the remaining 9 mg appearing in his feces, i.e., he is absorbing only 10 percent of ingested iron. Now suppose he suffers a single modest hemorrhage of 100 ml; this amounts to 50 mg iron and clearly upsets by a wide margin the daily balance between iron input and output. However, he has no trouble replacing the lost red blood cells by calling upon some of the iron attached to ferritin in his iron-storage depots. At the same time, the intestine is "informed" of the fact that iron reserves have diminished, and it responds by increasing the percentage of ingested iron which it absorbs from 10 percent to 25 percent (the pathways by which this information is transmitted and the response elicited need not concern us here). This means that he will start absorbing daily 2.5 mg of the ingested 10 mg and will therefore show a daily retention of 1.5 mg. If this is kept up for 34 days, all the iron lost in the original hemorrhage would have been replaced, the signal for increased absorption would then be completely eliminated, and the percentage absorbed would return to 10 percent.

Now apply this type of analysis to a normal 30-year-old woman who loses 100 ml of blood every month and has been doing so for fifteen years. It should be easy to see that if she were ingesting 10 mg iron each day, her iron stores would be partially depleted all the time, and the signal to her intestine to increase the absorption of ingested iron would be present continuously. If, averaged over the entire menstrual cycle, the increase in absorbed iron is great enough to precisely balance out the menstrual losses, she would maintain, from cycle to cycle, a stable level of iron balance. Her red blood cell count and hemoglobin concentration might be perfectly normal and unchanging, and the only evidence that she intermittently bleeds is the reduced iron reserves and the increased percentage of ingested iron absorbed. (The actual numbers I have used in these illustrations were selected quite arbitrarily for purposes of illustration and are not meant at all to indicate levels at which balance or normal blood values really are attained in any individual.) Such a woman can be said to have iron deficiency but not iron deficiency anemia.

Now, it should also be clear that if the blood loss of any woman (or man) increases enough, or if the dietary intake of iron decreases markedly, the level of iron reserves at which balance is achieved will get lower and lower, i.e., the degree of iron deficiency will get higher and higher. At some point in this sequence, there will simply not be enough iron in the body to maintain a high concentration of hemoglobin in the blood, and iron deficiency anemia will ensue. One must recognize that even under such conditions, a stable iron balance and hemoglobin concentration is usually ultimately achieved, but at lower levels of both variables; only when severe bleeding is caused by disease does the hemoglobin follow a progressive lethal downhill course.

This example emphasizes that there is a difference between simple iron deficiency and iron deficiency anemia. Only when negative iron balance is great enough to exhaust most of the body's iron stores, i.e., only when iron deficiency becomes quite severe, does anemia occur.

A third example—a normal man who changes his daily diet from one containing 10 mg of iron to one containing 100 mg. Let us assume he is losing 1 mg/day via the urine, sweat, and sloughed cells. Can he ever get into iron balance? Yes, simply by reducing intestinal absorption of the ingested iron to 1 percent, which amounts to 1 mg/day. When he first goes on the diet, his intestine is absorbing much more, say 10 percent, and the result is retention of some excess iron in the body. It is this resulting enlargment of iron stores that triggers the signal to the intestine to reduce its iron absorption to a value at which stable balance is reachieved. The important point is that stable iron balance can be achieved at very high iron intakes, but this new balance point will always be associated with increased total body iron.

Returning to the iron-enrichment debate, there were at least three different points of disagreement between the opponents and proponents of the iron-enrichment proposal: Was there a real need for iron enrichment? If so, would the method proposed to meet this need be effective? Was there any danger of such enrichment to significant numbers of the population?

Although the initial outcry against the proposal was based almost entirely on the third question, that dealing with considerations of safety, it soon became apparent that the first question, benefits to be expected, had not and could not be quantified at that time. Dr. William H. Crosby, a hematologist and professor of medicine at Tufts Medical School, and the most vocal (and effective) opponent of the iron-enrichment proposal, reiterated again and again that the data on iron deficiency used to justify the proposal were totally inadequate.[4] Dr. Crosby's particular target was the Ten-State Survey, which had revealed such high levels of iron deficiency. He emphasized that this epidemiological survey was not representative of the entire nation because it concentrated on only the poorest 25 percent of the population, i.e., the figures cited earlier for iron deficiency anemia did not apply to the general population, but only to this subgroup which almost certainly has a higher level of iron deficiency than the rest of the population. But even within this population, he argued, the number concluded to have iron deficiency anemia was much too high because of the misguided criteria used for its definition. The major indication of iron deficiency in the survey was the blood hemoglobin concentration, and any hemoglobin level below an arbitrarily selected "normal value" was automatically equated with iron deficiency anemia. Dr. Crosby pointed out that the "normal" value selected was too high, certainly higher than that recommended by the World Health Organization (WHO), so much higher that the use of the WHO standard in the Ten-State Survey would have reduced the prevalence of "deficient" and "low" values in males from 22 percent to 11 percent. Even more important, he argued, it is absurd to take any single cutoff value as "normal."

> First of all, it must be determined—by a committee—that the normal hemoglobin value for a man is 14 g or more per 100 ml. By irrefutable logic, it follows that any man with a level of 13.9 g is anemic. The committee must also decree that since most anemia is iron deficiency anemia, all anemia is iron deficiency anemia. Therefore, that poor fellow with the hemoglobin of 13.9 g has anemia and also, it is iron deficiency anemia.
>
> The report did not point out that men do not get iron deficiency anemia unless they have blood loss. Are 22 percent of American men bleeding? To nutritionists these figures have indicated something dreadfully wrong with the American diet. To physicians they indicate something dreadfully wrong with the Ten-State Survey.[5]

Dr. Crosby was attempting to impugn the survey's data for men, not because they were the target population for the enrichment program, but because showing how ridiculous the conclusions were for men would invalidate as well the conclusions for the real target population, women in their reproductive years.

But it was Dr. P. C. Elwood, Director of the United Kingdom Medical Research Council's Epidemiology Unit in Wales and probably the world's outstanding authority on the epidemiology of iron deficiency, who really placed the problem in focus. He stressed that the question of just how many men and women have subnormal levels of plasma iron or blood hemoglobin could be debated endlessly, but it is not really the important question, which is, plain and simple, So what?

> With regard to the importance of [iron deficiency] anemia, simple estimates of prevalence are, I believe, irrelevant. Prevalence estimates are, of necessity, based on arbitrary criteria—such as a circulating hemoglobin level of less than 12 g/100 ml—and these necessitate a prior judgment regarding importance.[6]

> There are obvious dangers in the "Humpty-Dumpty" principle ("Words mean what I want them to mean") . . . . The only reasonable and useful definition of a condition such as this [iron deficiency anemia] would be based on *valid evidence of harm to health or function which can be removed by treatment* [emphasis added]. One should not base the definition of a condition on some arbitrary level of a biochemical or hematological variate, the relevance of which to health has not been fully worked out. Diagnoses which are based on theoretical concepts of what is ideal are unlikely to be useful and may be misleading.[7]

In other words, although there is no question that an unknown number of persons have iron deficiency anemia, as defined simply by some arbitrary cutoff point for serum iron or hemoglobin, knowing this fact is of no value unless there is firm evidence that they are harmed by having the low iron or hemoglobin. (This is precisely the point I made in chapter 3 concerning the criteria used for setting nutritional requirements.)

And then came the shock: There had been almost no attempts to investigate whether low iron stores or mild-to-moderate iron-deficiency anemia really was harmful; it had always been an article of faith. The FDA, the Food and Nutrition Board, and the AMA had all declared categorically, without any qualification, that iron deficiency anemia is a major national nutritional problem, perhaps the most common one in the country, but all these proclamations were made on the basis of chemical measurements and assumptions that low values *must* be associated with symptoms and damage. Now, there is no question at all that *severe* iron deficiency causing hemoglobin to fall to below, say, 8 g/100 ml causes illness and, if severe enough, death, and it had simply been assumed that a diminishing continuum of negative effects existed all the way up to "normal" values. Dr Crosby pointed out this type of reasoning in Commissioner Schmidt's 1973 proposal, which began by acknowledging the "considerable lack of precise knowledge in the area of the clinical significance of mild to moderate anemia," went on to list only the symptoms and consequences of severe iron deficiency, and then concluded that "the preponderance of available evidence indicates that mild to moderate anemia is also deleterious to good health."[8]

Actually the few studies dealing with mild to moderate anemia did not support this view at all. As Dr. Elwood pointed out, although one older published study (and a large number of anecdotes) claimed that prompt relief from a variety of ill-defined symptoms (breathlessness, easy fatigability, loss of libido, etc.) followed a course of iron therapy in women, the placebo effect had been ignored, and several well-controlled more recent studies had failed to detect any benefits from therapy with iron in women with mild or even moderately severe anemia. Dr. Elwood's group had performed the most extensive and convincing of these studies, involving more than 15,000 subjects and a wide variety of tests of morbidity (sickness) and physiological function. Dr. Elwood had begun his studies convinced that mild iron deficiency anemia really was an important medical problem, and so he was, himself, surprised by the results. Not until hemoglobin levels fell below 8 or 9 g per 100 ml of blood did any evidence of harmful effects of anemia emerge. Above that point, work capacity, respiration, cardiovascular function, the ability to perform fine hand manipulation, brain function, and perhaps most important, how well the women felt, did not change at all as iron levels and hemoglobin concentration were raised by administration of iron. To a physiologist, none of this is surprising since the body has a variety of compensatory mechanisms which can easily maintain normal oxygen delivery to all organs and tissues despite modest degrees of anemia. (This is an important lesson; as emphasized by Lewis Thomas, we must stop treating the body as a fragile organism ready to fall into illness unless we maintain unending vigil over it.)

The nutritionists countered that the methods used to evaluate morbidity and malfunction in these studies were so crude that subtle changes could easily have been missed. Quite possible, responded Dr. Elwood, but the burden of proof ought to be on those who claim that malfunction is present, since they are the ones who wish to institute measures to correct the hypothesized problems.

But Elwood's studies and those of several other groups went much farther than merely questioning the presence of illness. They raised the rather astounding question: Are there any *beneficial* effects of having mild-to-moderate anemia? For one thing, microbiologists had for many years emphasized that the presence of an infection causes a rapid large decrease in plasma iron, as this metal moves into liver and other organs under the influence of hormones released in response to the infectious agent. This is beneficial to the individual because the bacteria are severely hampered in iron-poor plasma, and the body's defenses are better able to overcome them. (This is another example of how theory, although logical, may be completely wrong; some nutritionists, not recognizing the adaptive value of the fall in plasma iron had argued that the "stress" of infection was best met by increasing iron intake to ameliorate the fall.) The obvious, but unanswered, question is whether moderate anemia might actually protect against infection (and cancer, since some cancer cells also have a very high requirement for iron).

Even more interesting are the few epidemiological studies relating iron deficiency to a *reduced* risk of cardiovascular diseases in people. As Dr. Elwood has emphasized, the indirect evidence is controversial, but comes from widely different sources, and all of it is consistent with a protective effect.[9] Persons with iron deficiency tend to have lower blood pressure, lower plasma cholesterol concentrations, and more connections between blood vessels in their hearts (this is one of the compensatory mechanisms for maintaining blood flow to the heart in the face of decreased hemoglobin). Such random associations in retrospective studies are very difficult to interpret, but more enticing is a large prospective study in which mortality was related to an earlier measurement of hemoglobin level; over the period of this study, there were 40 percent fewer deaths from cardiovascular diseases in women whose hemoglobin levels were less than 12 g per 100 ml.

Now none of this means that we all ought to revert to the use of leeches and decrease our iron intake. The studies are few and the data not at all conclusive as yet. What it does mean is that construction of a real balance sheet of the harms and benefits of modest iron deficiency has barely been begun, and it was quite impossible during the debate (nothing has really changed since then) to conclude that the degree of iron deficiency in the overall population, whatever the number of persons involved, was (and is) a public health problem. It became more and more apparent as the debate dragged on that the proponents were arguing from intuition on this point, not from facts. One of the most revealing statements in this regard was made at a roundtable discussion by Dr. Grace A. Goldsmith, dean of the School of Public Health and Tropical Medicine at Tulane Medical School, and a principal advocate of the proposal.

> I think part of this is philosophy. I'd feel lots happier with some iron stores. I think this applies to a good many other nutrients besides iron. I wouldn't like to be running around with no extra ascorbic acid [vitamin C] and just right on the verge of scurvy, and if I go somewhere where I can't get ascorbic acid for a few months, I develop scurvy. . . . I think it's nice to have a little bit of reserve for times of stress and difficulty. And I feel the same way about iron. I grant you I can't prove having these stores is beneficial, per se.[10]

The second component of the overall debate concerned efficacy. Were iron deficiency shown to be a serious enough public health problem to warrant a preventive campaign, would the proposed iron enrichment of flour be an effective way of overcoming it? The proponents had common sense on their side. The proposed enrichment would raise the daily ingestion of iron in most people by approximately 50 percent and that certainly seemed adequate to get the job done. Their opponents argued that the targeted populations—women and children—generally ate relatively less bread than did men. More important, they emphasized (as I have in chapter 3) that iron is not at all like vitamins, since like other trace elements its absorption from the gut is subject to alteration by a large number of variables. The chemical form of the iron, unspecified in the proposal, makes a huge difference. The composition of the meal is important; meat and vitamin C, for example, enhance absorption, whereas eggs and phytates (found in certain grains) greatly reduce it. In support of their arguments, they cited a study carried out in Wales in which a community field trial had demonstrated no effect on hemoglobin concentration of adding iron to flour used for baking bread. The proponents of enrichment countered with a similar study from Newfoundland in which hemoglobin had increased. Of course, as Dr. Maxwell M. Wintrobe, an eminent hematologist, stressed, "neither observations in Newfoundland or in Wales necessarily apply to the United States, and even in the U. S., dietary habits differ in various parts of the country and in different economic groups and even according to age and sex."[11] The sad fact was that not a single field study had been carried out in the United States to determine whether the proposed regimen could achieve its purpose of raising iron stores and hemoglobin concentrations.

Finally, there was the question of safety. It was this issue which had first incensed Dr. Crosby and other hematologists, since these physicians had under their care patients with the iron-storage disease called hemochromatosis, a hereditary disorder of the intestinal control of iron absorption. Unlike normal persons, patients with hemochromatosis do not reduce intestinal absorption of iron as body iron increases; therefore, they may retain large enough amounts of iron to damage the liver and other organs. Clearly such persons would be placed at risk were the iron content of flour increased.

The proponents of enrichment, of course, realized the existence of this problem, but felt it was unimportant because, they claimed, the disease is very rare, affecting perhaps 10,000 to 20,000 persons in the entire country. Moreoever, these people could easily be warned by their physicians and precautions taken. Finally, Dr. Goldsmith argued that "these rare diseases of iron overload will occur regardless of dietary intake and are [already] medical problems."[12]

Nothing infuriated Dr. Crosby as much as this line of reasoning. The numbers cited, he emphasized, are estimates of *known* cases of hemochromatosis and are probably merely the tip of the iceberg. The disease exists in varying degrees of severity, and we simply do not know the true gene frequency. "In every study that has been done on ostensibly normal people, there have been 3 to 6 percent of people with very high serum iron levels."[13] Might these people have "preclinical" hemochromatosis, that is, be carriers of the gene, yet suffer no damage because of a relatively low iron intake?

The raising of this question was prophetic, for in 1978 a group of Swedish researchers published a sobering study.[14] In the previous two years they had seen ten patients with hemochromatosis in their hospital. This represented such a high incidence of a supposedly rare disease in their area that they looked for further cases. Their results: Two percent of the men in the district studied had early hemochromatosis! In Sweden, the average intake of iron is considerably greater than that in the United States because of generous iron enrichment programs (a difference which would have been obliterated by the FDA proposal). The Swedish authors quite rightly refused to conclude that the iron overload in the studied persons was the consequence of the iron fortification of Swedish food, but they left no doubt as to their suspicions. As Dr. Crosby concluded in an editorial review of their article:

The question of safety of iron fortification has not been resolved by this pilot study, but should not the matter of mandated fortification of American flour await the outcome of a definitive study from Sweden? In Sweden, 42% of the iron in the diet is fortification iron. In the United States, at the present time, an estimated 25%. . . derives from fortification. Perhaps we have come too far already.[15]

But the question of safety goes well beyond the issue of hemo-chromatosis (and the several other medical conditions associated with excessive intestinal absorption of iron). Dr. Elwood empha-sized that iron-storage disease should not be allowed to divert all attention from the very much larger problem which might arise from a general shift in iron balance in the general population. By this, he was really extending the same discussion raised earlier con-cerning possible benefits of mild iron deficiency. If such benefits really exist, then iron enrichment would be expected to eliminate them. Moreover, he argued, some evidence suggests that the unex-pected relationship between mortality from cardiovascular disease and low hemoglobin concentration extended to supranormal he-moglobin values as well. At levels of hemoglobin that are high (but well below those indicative of hemochromatosis) there is epidemio-logical evidence for increased mortality from cardiovascular disease in women. He was quick to emphasize both that it was impossible to predict whether iron enrichment would, in fact, raise the hemo-globin of some people with perfectly normal values to start with and that the relationship betwen hemoglobin and mortality might be spurious, generated by a third factor such as smoking, as was claimed by proponents of the proposal. Nonetheless, his conclusion was: "Once such an association has been detected, a very serious onus rests on those who propose to interfere to demonstrate, beyond all reasonable doubt, that the association is spurious. Mere opinion is inadequate."[16]

The final safety consideration raised by many physicians con-cerned not any direct harmful effect of iron but, rather, the likeli-hood that iron enrichment would interfere with the early diagnosis and treatment of cancers of the gastrointestinal tract. Blood loss in the feces due to the cancer may go unnoticed by the patient but be prolonged enough to lead to significant reduction of plasma hemo-globin. This anemia, then, is often the first clue as to the possible existence of the cancer. Opponents of the proposal argued (without real proof, it must be acknowledged) that iron enrichment would provide enough iron to delay the onset of this important signal that something is wrong.

What general lessons concerning nutrition can we learn from this eight-year debate, lessons which will help us deal with the overall question of food-enrichment programs and the role of the federal government in attempting to improve the nutritional quality of the American diet? For many years, vitamins and minerals have been added to food products—iodine in salt to prevent goiter and vitamin D in milk to prevent rickets are examples analogous to the iron-enrichment proposal. Not all additions are for avoiding nutrient deficiencies—salt in baby food and sugar in breakfast cereals are two examples of nutritional additives which ostensibly are to improve palatability. In the case of iron, an enormous number of foods—instant breakfasts, bakery products, and many convenience dishes, to name just a few—are already enriched with iron. We can expect much more of this, for nutrition has become a national craze, food companies are anxious to get on the bandwagon by adding more "goodies" to their products, and the FDA must decide how much regulation it wishes to impose on these enrichments, as well as the extent to which it wishes, itself, to use enrichment as a vehicle for public-health measures.

The first lesson to be learned is that until its turnabout under Commissioner Kennedy, the FDA and proponents of the iron-enrichment proposal treated this matter in a manner totally different from the way in which a proposal for a new drug would have been dealt with. The FDA demands extensive animal experimentation and pilot studies on human subjects concerning safety and effectiveness before a new drug can be released for public use. Moreover the drug, once released, is subjected to careful continuous scrutiny. In contrast, we have seen the FDA not only permitting but mandating the addition of a chemical—iron—to flour in amounts which would have made our bread the most iron-rich in the world, on the basis of completely inadequate information as to need, safety, and effectiveness, and with absolutely no program to monitor the effects of the enrichment, once in operation. As pointed out by the editors of *Nutrition Today*, the most widely read nutrition magazine and one which had responsibly covered the debate (indeed had greatly stimulated it through perceptive articles, editorials, and a roundtable discussion), "a convincing scientific case [for rejection of the proposal] was made by the FDA only when Commissioner Kennedy finally analyzed the question of iron metabolism in much the same way a physician would evaluate a new drug."[17]

Why is there a double standard for nutrients and drugs? The obvious answer is that nutrients are, by definition, "good" chemicals. Yet the fact is that virtually every nutrient can cause toxic effects if large amounts are ingested (ironically, included in the very same package calling for increasing iron enrichment was a proposal for dropping the level of enrichment with vitamin D because clear-cut cases of vitamin D toxicity had begun to appear). The public has the right to demand that the benefit-risk analysis for a nutrient to be added to food be even more rigorously scientific than that for a new drug since enrichment programs affect the entire population. Moreover, in the analysis of risk, looking only for gross toxicity or specific diseases known to be associated with too little or too much of the nutrient is probably missing the real point, which is that more subtle forms of harm may exist at lower levels of intake than those required for gross toxicity, and in perfectly normal people. This may take the form of an increased incidence of infection, cancer, heart disease, or other chronic disease not previously known to be assoiated with the nutrient in question.

This leads us to a second lesson, one already raised in chapter 3. A convincing benefit-risk analysis could probably not be developed presently for any nutrient, not just iron, because the nutritional sciences are in a very primitive state of development. It cannot be emphasized too strongly that the opponents of the iron-enrichment proposal did not argue that the claims of the proponents were wrong, only that they had not been proven, that they were indeterminant, not indeterminable. We simply do not know the optimal level of any nutrient. We don't know whether what we have arbitrarily labelled as the "normal" values for iron (or hemoglobin, the product derived from it), really are the most healthy values to have. The same can be said of vitamin C, thiamine, protein, or any other nutrient. Intuition may tell us that it is absurd for a mild "anemia" to be more conducive to a long life, but intuition and preconceptions won't test the validity of such a possibility, or the possibility that the amounts of vitamin C known to prevent scurvy are too small to give maximal protection against other diseases (or, to reverse the example, the statement that very large amounts of vitamin C are not toxic, as the proponents of megavitamin usage claim).

Dr. Crosby has written: "The powerful nutritionists of this country, in government and out, behave, unlike scientists of other disciplines, as though their hypotheses required no testing."[18] I believe Dr. Crosby's statement is too strong and too sweeping, for there is no question that a good deal of excellent research is performed by nutritional scientists. Yet, unhappily, the shoe does fit in this case. Most scientists are delighted when an important health issue involves their particular field, for they smell research dollars. But in this case, amazingly, over the entire period of the debate, as the editors of *Nutrition Today* pointed out, "the advocates of superenrichment did not initiate or support research necessary to meet the criticisms of their iron proposal despite the fact that the endorsers were persons of high repute in nutrition who are experienced in obtaining research grants."[19]

The nutritional sciences, rather than having completed their task, as was assumed some years ago, are really just getting started, for the task of optimizing health, rather than merely preventing gross deficiency diseases, is an enormous one. As Dr. Morowitz has emphasized, "the first step to remedy these problems [of present nutritional research] consists of a probing examination of the problems of obtaining valid results within these fields of study."[20] The iron-enrichment controversy certainly spotlighted many of these problems and I'd like to reemphasize only one of them, the one pointed out over and over again by Dr. Elwood. Measurements of the amounts of nutrients (or the products, such as hemoglobin, derived from them) in the blood or body cannot, alone, serve as indicators of health or disease, until it has been shown by valid experiments that such levels really correlate with well-defined changes in physiological function, well-being, morbidity, and mortality. Dr. Elwood's admonishment is worth repeating: "Diagnoses which are based on theoretical concepts of [biochemical levels that are] ideal are unlikely to be useful and may be misleading."[21] At the risk of overkill, here is one more example of how deeply ingrained is this use of arbitrary chemical measurements. In an experiment described by Dr. Howard A. Pearson, professor of pediatrics at Yale, a member of the Nutrition Committee of the American Academy of Pediatrics and a supporter of the proposal, it was shown that "although significant degrees of anemia were unusual, about a third of indigent black children 4 to 6 years old showed substantial increases in their hematocrit [the percentage of blood which is red cells] levels when they were given nutritional supplements including iron. *This indicated that their hematocrit levels had been less than optimal"* [emphasis added].[22] No, it doesn't, one might almost hear Dr. Elwood replying, unless Dr. Pearson had conclusive evidence that bodily function and health, not just the hematocrit, had improved, or unless others had previously shown that specific measures of health improve when hematocrit rises over the range observed in this study.

This is not a trivial issue (nor is it universally accepted, as evidenced by Dr. Goldsmith's belief that one can have a nutritional "disease that is biochemically apparent and not clinically apparent at all"[23]), for recognition of this point must be a guide to experimental design. For example, as we shall see in chapter 6, it is one thing to demonstrate that certain diets can lower plasma cholesterol by 15 percent, but quite a different matter to show that such a drop has any influence on the frequency of heart attacks. But such experiments—long-term controlled animal experiments followed by even longer-term studies of large numbers of people, involving extensive measurements of a large number of physiological and medical variables (difficult to perform and crude, compared to simple measurements of nutrient concentrations), are, as Commissioner Schmidt emphasized, "tedious, expensive, [and] not of the type leading to Nobel or other prizes. Some mechanism for performing such work must be found, if we are to avoid arguments even more serious than those surrounding the iron-in-bread regulation."[24]

The last major lesson I would like to draw from this episode is that we must be very cautious in deciding whether the appropriate solution to a medical problem should be a preventive program involving the entire population. All throughout the debate the opponents of the proposal kept demanding to know exactly at whom the program was directed. In the roundtable discussion sponsored by *Nutrition Today*, a particularly illuminating exchange occurred between Dr. Goldsmith and Dr. Elwood.

> *Goldsmith:* You [speaking to Elwood] said you wanted to be able to show morbidity and mortality before you decided this was a real community health problem. From my standpoint I consider it serious if there is a loss of iron stores and a stress situation arises such as hemorrhage or if the woman becomes pregnant. I think this is serious and that she ought to have iron stores.[25]
>
> *Elwood:* It is a reasonable assumption to make and I am sure it is true. [But], one would question to what extent in this day and age, with advanced hospital services, how important this is to a community, because, after all, one is considering preventive measures which

will be applied to the whole community. If one's justification simply relates to those people who may have low iron stores and will [also] become pregnant or . . . have an operation, then this, I think, is a very different argument from those that are usually advanced about the whole community.[26]

In other words, Dr. Elwood and other opponents of the proposal were trying to point out that, if pregnant women are the real target, then this can easily be handled by treating this specific group. Likewise, if patients are to have an operation, treat them with iron or blood, as appropriate.

I should like to permit Dr. Elwood the last word in this regard, an admonition not to be taken casually:

There are several ways in which preventive medicine differs from clinical practice. One of these differences is of great importance in the present context. In clinical practice a doctor acts in good faith on the best evidence known to him. Both he and the patient who originated the contact know that in most situations evidence is limited, but advice is given and taken with a high level of trust. In public health preventive medicine, action is taken without the agreement by all the individuals to be affected and usually without any attempt to tailor the measure to the needs of each individual. At the same time, there is a high level of trust on the part of the community—trust in those who recommend the measure. Therefore, if a measure is introduced without certainty that benefit will ensure to a high proportion of subjects and that the chance of danger to anyone is trivial, that trust is betrayed.[27]

Chapter 6 | Cholesterol, Fats, and Heart Disease

In 1909, a Russian army physician, A. Ignatowski, made an inspired intuitive connection when he wondered whether the heavy meat intake of army officers might account for their having many more heart attacks than the near-vegetarian peasants. He followed up this hunch by feeding rabbits animal products and finding that they developed atherosclerotic lesions, the fatty thickening in arteries which leads to heart attacks. Several years later, two other Russians, N. Anitschkov and S. Chalatow, noted that rabbits fed cholesterol and fat in pure form showed both a rise in plasma cholesterol and the appearance of severe atherosclerosis, both of which gradually disappeared when the dietary lipids were discontinued.

The past seventy years have witnessed a vast number of similar experiments on virtually every species of laboratory animal. Species differ in sensitivity, but if enough cholesterol and animal fat are fed, the qualitative results are always the same—increased plasma cholesterol and an enhanced rate of development of atherosclerosis and heart disease. Animal experiments have also shown that it is extremely difficult to produce atherosclerosis by any other method (for example, by physically damaging vessel linings) unless plasma cholesterol is simultaneously raised by diet (or other means).

Forty years after Ignatowski's pioneering work, scientifically performed epidemiological studies began to extend his observations on army officers and peasants to include many population groups worldwide. They revealed a definite association between the amount of animal fat ingested by a population and the population's mean plasma cholesterol and incidence of heart attacks.

These findings, coupled with those for the animal experiments, and the simple fact that cholesterol is a major component of atherosclerotic lesions, led to the formulation of the so-called diet-heart hypothesis: Cholesterol and saturated fat in the diet raise plasma cholesterol, which in turn, promotes development of atherosclerosis and increases the likelihood of a heart attack. A protective role for certain plant fats and oils was later added to the theory. Note the word "likelihood" in the hypothesis. Adherents to the diet-heart hypothesis do not claim that diet is the only causal factor in atherosclerotic heart disease, only that it is an important one, but almost certainly one among many.

All this time, the absolute number of persons dying from heart and blood vessel diseases was rising rapidly in all Westernized countries, and in 1961 the pleas of scientists like Paul Dudley White, Irvine Page, Ancel Keys, and Jeremiah Stamler, for a public health approach to this number-one killer resulted in a recommendation by the American Heart Association (AHA), through its Nutrition Committee, that the American population modify its usual diet by eating fewer foods rich in cholesterol and animal fat, with some replacement of the latter by foods higher in fats of plant origin. Ten years later, the National Heart and Lung Institute of the National Institutes of Health also came out in support of these recommendations for the general public. Even Congress, as expressed in a document published in 1977 called *Dietary Goals for the United States* and in several pieces of legislation, has given its official sanction to the diet-heart hypothesis and urged a massive educational campaign, aimed primarily at the young, on the dietary prevention of heart disease and strokes. The United States Department of Agriculture has expressed its full agreement with this proposal as have a large number of other governmental and private groups.

Many scientists do not believe that the government should be pursuing such a course. Some officials at the National Institutes of Health have emphasized that the diet-heart hypothesis is just that— a hypothesis, the evidence for which is ambiguous and far from conclusive. They believe it is premature to call for a radical change in the American diet that may prove useless (and, some would add, possibly even harmful). As recently as May, 1980, the Food and

Nutrition Board of the National Academy of Sciences issued a report which stated that the evidence for the diet-heart hypothesis was inadequate enough that there was no need for the average American to cut down on dietary cholesterol.

The key point in this debate was stated by *Science* magazine in 1975:

> A national obsession with dietary fats and cholesterol seems to have developed despite the fact that there is as yet no convincing evidence that people can voluntarily decrease their risks of heart attacks by changing their diets.[1]

This same point has been made more emphatically by Dr. George V. Mann, a distinguished researcher at Vanderbilt University and one of the most outspoken critics of the diet-heart hypothesis.

> A generation of research on the diet-heart question has ended in disarray. The official line since 1950 for management of the epidemic of coronary heart disease has been a dietary treatment. Foundations, scientists and the media, both lay and scientific, have promoted low fat, low cholesterol, polyunsaturated diets, and yet the epidemic continues unabated, cholesteremia [high blood cholesterol] in the population is unchanged, and clinicians are unconvinced of efficacy.... [The] oil and spread industry advertises its products with claims and promises that make these foods seem like drugs. The vibrant certainty of scientists claiming to be authorities on these matters is disturbing.... [Yet] no one has been able to prove that dietary treatments either prevent or modify the behavior of coronary heart disease. It is useful to review the evidence that the diet-heart hypothesis is wrong. That demonstration must be accepted before it can be abandoned for some more useful proposition.[2]

The problem referred to by the above quotation is that there are no conclusive data from controlled human experiments documenting that dietary alterations of the kind proposed by the AHA really reduce the incidence of coronary heart disease in the general public, and do so without increasing the risk of other diseases. Such experiments simply have not been done, although they are presently in the works. Therefore, while awaiting the outcome of these direct tests of the diet-heart hypothesis, we must base our present actions on the circumstantial evidence provided by existing epidemiological and controlled studies. In this controversy, in contrast to the situation for the iron-enrichment debate of the previous chapter, there is an immense number of such studies.

Dr. Mann believes the data from these studies warrant the conclusion that, although our plasma cholesterol concentrations are high enough to cause heart disease, diet is not a major contributor to these high plasma cholesterols. Therefore, he feels that the possibility of preventing heart disease through alteration of dietary cholesterol and fats has already been adequately disproven, that no direct experimental evaluation of this question is needed, and that we should spend our time and manpower on looking for the real causes. In contrast, many more scientists believe that the data, while not conclusive, are strong enough to warrant prediction that dietary manipulation really will reduce heart disease.[3] They hope that the direct studies will be done, but recognizing that the completion of the experiments may require many years, they urge that we take action now, particularly since (they believe) we have nothing to lose by doing so, i.e., such diets carry no increased risk from other diseases. There is yet a third group of scientists who straddle the fence between these two positions, arguing that no public policy action be taken until the results of the direct studies are in. This last group's view of the diet-heart hypothesis spans the range from skepticism to qualified belief; what unites them is their feeling that getting people to change their life-styles is extremely difficult to achieve even when the evidence is beyond doubting (as in cigarette smoking, for example) and calling for a population-wide change in the American diet that might prove to be unwarranted could have grave effects on public confidence.

Before we tackle the scientific evidence, we must first become familiar with the cast of characters (blood and dietary lipids), the nature of the disease process they are reputed to facilitate (atherosclerotic cardiovascular disease), and the metabolism of the central character (cholesterol).

Lipids

Lipids (Greek *lipos*, fat) are molecules which are relatively insoluble in water but are soluble in organic substances such as acetone and ether. The members of this class thus share a physical property rather than a particular molecular structure. The fats belong to this class, and sometimes the term fat is used interchangeably with lipid, but this usage is not correct. Cholesterol, for example, is a lipid but its ringlike structure bears little resemblance to fat molecules. It belongs to the subclass of lipids called steroids, and to go one step further, to the subfamily of steroids termed sterols (a sterol is a steroid bearing a hydroxyl [O–H] group). Cholesterol is found in most foods from animal sources (meat and dairy products), particularly in egg yolks.

Cholesterol is probably viewed by most Americans as a foreign toxic substance which, following its ingestion, heads straight for the large blood vessels of the body, particularly those of the heart, and clogs them, bringing on heart attacks and strokes. In our hierarchy of demons, it occupies a position at the right hand of the arch-fiend cancer. Yet, the fact is that cholesterol is an extremely important, normally occurring molecule, so far as our biochemistry is concerned. It is synthesized by almost all the body's cells, for it is an integral component of their membranes. It is a precursor for the synthesis of a variety of other specialized molecules, including several hormones and the bile acids so important for the intestinal digestion and absorption of ingested fat. If you eat no cholesterol whatever, the body will go ahead and synthesize whatever it needs (and then some), so that cholesterol is not classified as an essential nutrient in the jargon sense of that term. In short, there is nothing inherently toxic about cholesterol and if this nutrient is really involved in the genesis of cardiovascular diseases, it is one more example of the fact that too much of a good thing may be harmful.

The other type of lipid important for atherosclerosis is the fatty acid content of triglycerides, the major ingredient of animal and plant fats and oils. Each triglyceride consists of a molecule of glycerol to which are attached three fatty acids, chains of carbon atoms containing a carboxyl group (C–O–O–H) at one end of the chain. Carbon atoms form four chemical bonds with other atoms, and for each interior carbon atom in a fatty acid chain, two of these bonds must always be with the two carbon atoms adjacent to it in the chain. What happens to the remaining two bonds is very important in determining the chemistry of the fatty acid. One possibility is that, instead of two adjacent carbon atoms being joined by a single bond, they form two bonds. Another, the most common, is that the remaining bonds are with atoms of hydrogen. These possibilities are, of course, mutually exclusive; when adjacent carbon atoms form double bonds with each other, there are fewer bonds left to form with hydrogen atoms. Therefore, when double bonds between carbon atoms are present in a fatty acid, it is said to be unsaturated (with regard to hydrogen atoms). If only a single double bond is present, the fatty acid is monounsaturated; if multiple double bonds, then polyunsaturated; if no double bonds, at all, then saturated. In general, fatty acids of animal origin (meat and dairy products) tend to be saturated (in cow's milk for example, 60 percent of the fatty acids are saturated), some are monounsaturated, and very few are polyunsaturated. The opposite distribution tends to hold for fatty acids of plant origin, but there are exceptions, as we shall see. The consistency of fat is usually an indicator of its degree of saturation—the softer it is at room temperature, the more unsaturated; thus, butter is very hard whereas corn oil is a liquid. The commercial soft margerines are made by partially hydrogenating plant oils such as corn oil, the result being the formation of fatty acids which are still relatively polyunsaturated but less so than the parent oil.

Finally, a fatty acid may combine via its carboxyl group to a molecule of cholesterol. The resulting molecule is called a cholesteryl ester.

Because lipids are relatively water-insoluble, they do not, by themselves, dissolve in blood plasma (blood plasma is 94 percent water). To solubilize them, they are coated with proteins (made mainly by the liver), and so virtually all the plasma lipids are carried in the form of lipoprotein complexes.

There are four main types of lipoproteins, classified according to their size and density, the latter property reflecting both the relative amounts of lipid and protein in the complex (lipids are less dense than proteins), and the particular types of lipid. The largest and least dense (size and density go in opposite directions down the types of lipoproteins) are the chylomicrons, followed by the very low density lipoproteins (VLDL), the low density lipoproteins (LDL), and the high density lipoproteins (HDL).

The chylomicrons are really emulsification droplets with a very thin surrounding protein coating. They are the form in which ingested lipids are absorbed from the gastrointestinal tract, and they are present in the blood of normal persons only during ingestion of a fat-containing meal. In contrast, the other lipoprotein classes, while their concentrations may vary somewhat with meal eating, are present in the plasma at all times. It is mainly the LDL with which we shall be concerned, for this class carries most of the cholesterol found in blood, and plays key roles in the development of cholesterol-containing lesions in blood vessels as well as in the regulation of cholesterol metabolism by cells.

Atherosclerotic Cardiovascular Diseases

Diseases of the heart and blood vessels—cardiovascular diseases—are the leading causes of death in the United States and all other industrialized nations. The great majority of these diseases are attributable to the process known as atherosclerosis, the progressive occlusive thickening of blood vessel walls with cholesterol, cells, and other substances. The end result of this thickening, often made worse by the formation of blood clots at the affected sites, is damage or death to the area supplied by the vessel because of reduced blood flow. The blood vessels which supply the walls of the heart are known as coronary arteries, and so atherosclerosis of these vessels leads to coronary heart disease, which may take the form only of intermittent chest pain on exertion (angina pectoris) or ultimately of a heart attack. The presence of angina pectoris signifies that the heart muscle (myocardium) is getting enough oxygen at rest but not during exertion, whereas a heart attack occurs when the damage to the heart muscle secondary to reduced blood supply is permanent. The damaged area is called an infarct, and myocardial infarction, heart attack, and coronary occlusion are all synonyms. Coronary thrombosis denotes that the heart attack was precipitated by a clot within the arteries, usually at the site of the atherosclerotic lesion. Heart attacks are fatal when the damage to the myocardium is very extensive or when there is a disruption of the conduction of electrical signals throughout the myocardium so that the various parts of the ventricles—the chambers which pump blood to the lungs and rest of the body—beat in a totally uncoordinated manner (ventricular fibrillation). In either case, the heart can no longer function adequately as a pump. Coronary heart disease claims the lives of approximately 600,000 Americans each year.

Atherosclerosis can affect any artery, not just the coronaries. For example, if the lesions block the arteries to the legs, the result is numbness, pain in the legs on exertion, and ultimately gangrene if the blockade to blood flow becomes extreme. If the arteries to the brain are blocked, brain damage or "stroke" may occur. (Stroke also can occur when a brain blood vessel ruptures, rather than is occluded, an event more common in persons suffering from high blood pressure.) Stroke causes about 200,000 deaths annually in this country.

Atherosclerotic cardiovascular diseases thus claim the lives of almost one million Americans each year, approximately half of all deaths. It affects both sexes, although women are relatively protected until after menopause. The mortality rate from coronary heart disease is ten times greater for men in their 30s and 40s than for women of the same age, and males are the victims in 75 percent of all fatal heart attacks in persons under the age of 65. This is why almost all the studies I will discuss pertain to men only; what data there are for women indicate that precisely the same principles apply.

Because the incidence and severity of atherosclerosis is clearly correlated with advancing age, it has been tempting to regard it as a normal inevitable physiological consequence of the aging process. There is an element of truth in this view, for almost anyone who lives long enough will eventually manifest some evidence of atherosclerosis, since the bodily events which constitute the aging process and those that lead to atherosclerosis interact with each other. Yet, we now know from the types of evidence described in chapter 1 that these processes are to a large degree distinct from one another and separable. This accounts for why heart attacks strike the young and middle-aged as well as the elderly (one-fourth of all heart attacks in American males occur before 65 years of age) and why some populations exhibit almost no evidence of atherosclerosis even in the extremely old.

Surely a disease which affects so many persons would seem to deserve the term often applied to it of "epidemic," but, generally unknown to the public, this epidemic may be waning. The most striking manifestation of this phenomenon occurred in 1975 when the absolute number of annual deaths from all major cardiovascular diseases went below one million for the first time in a decade; the 1977 total, 960,000, was the lowest since 1963. But looking only at absolute numbers of deaths underestimates what has really been occurring. The percentage of old people in our population has, of course, been progressively increasing and because cardiovascular diseases are more common in the aged, we would expect the absolute incidence of these diseases also to be increasing. To take this into account, we must look at age-adjusted mortality rates (see chap. 1), for these numbers are the meaningful ones for gaining insight into the rise and fall of diseases. The encouraging fact is that the age-adjusted mortality rate from all cardiovascular diseases had been declining for many years before 1975, indeed by 32 percent in the past thirty years! Even more encouraging is that the trend is accelerating. The rate for coronary heart disease declined by 23.4

percent from 1968 through 1977, and for stroke, the fall was even greater, 32 percent.[4]

Before we all decide that, if these patterns continue, within another thirty years coronary heart disease and stroke will go the way of smallpox, we must focus on the "catch" in all these numbers. We have been speaking of death rates, not incidence. These numbers tell us only that fewer people are dying from atherosclerotic diseases, but we don't know whether these declines are due to the diseases themselves becoming less common or, alternatively, to better patient care. It is quite possible that the incidence rates could be stable, or even on the rise, but that better therapy is lowering the percentage of afflicted persons who actually die of the diseases. The answer to this question is crucial to any assessment of preventive programs (such as dietary alteration) or of the aggressive curative therapy of the past few decades (including coronary care units and heart surgery). Most experts believe that both prevention (which decreases incidence) and therapy (which decreases mortality at any given incidence) have played a role in lowering mortality rate, but in fact, the real relative roles of these factors are not known.

Development of Atherosclerosis

When a normal artery from a young person is looked at microscopically, three distinct layers are discerned: the intima, media, and adventitia (fig. 6–1). The intima is the innermost layer, i.e., the layer adjacent to the blood flowing through the artery. It is a narrow region, bounded on its inner surface by a one-cell-thick layer of endothelial cells that line the opening (lumen) of the tube. Thus, the endothelial cells are the only part of the normal artery in direct contact with the blood flowing through the artery. The intima is bounded on its other side by a perforated sheet of elastic fibers, called the internal elastic lamina; between the endothelial cells and the internal elastic lamina is a relatively homogenous noncellular matrix with an occasional smooth muscle cell (so-called because these cells lack the striated appearance of skeletal muscle fibers).

The media, or middle layer, of the normal artery is much thicker than the intima. Its most conspicuous component is large numbers of smooth muscle cells, each surrounded by small amounts of connective tissue matrix, particularly the fibrous proteins elastin and collagen, and several long-chain sticky carbohydrates. These connective tissue elements are all secreted by the smooth muscle cells.

Fig. 6–1. **Structure of normal artery.** (Redrawn from R. Ross and J. A. Glomset, "The Atherogenesis of Atherosclerosis." *New England Journal of Medicine* 295 [1976]:370. Reprinted, by permission of the *New England Journal of Medicine* [vol. 295; p. 370, 1976].)

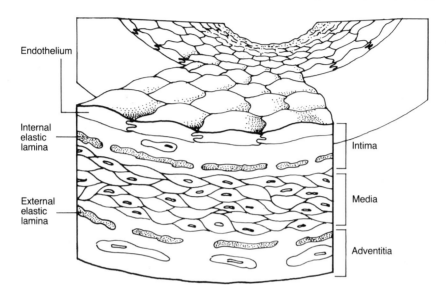

The adventitia, or outermost layer, is mostly connective tissue, and we will not be concerned with it at all.

The lesions of atherosclerosis are found in the intima, but their formation involves participation of cells from the media. Let me first merely describe the types of lesions and then face the controversial problem of how one type of lesion proceeds over time into the next.

The first classic type of lesion is the fatty streak. There is some question as to whether the fatty streak should really be called a "lesion" at all, for it can be found in the arteries of almost all young children in all countries, but it is felt by many to represent the foundation upon which later lesions are built. Fatty streaks are yellowish, relatively flat regions in the intima. The color is due to lipid deposits, mainly cholesterol,* found primarily in very small congregations of smooth muscle cells which have a foamy appearance be-

---

*Some of the cholesterol is in the form of cholesteryl esters. Although there are important differences in mobility and effects between cholesterol and its esters, I shall, for the sake of simplicity, lump these distinct molecular types together as "cholesterol" in the remainder of this chapter.

cause of their lipid content. They may also surround small amounts of extracellular lipid, but there is very little connective tissue matrix in the fatty streak and it in no way occludes the lumen or impairs function.

In those persons prone to atherosclerosis, fatty streaks begin to enlarge, often as early as the second or third decade of life, thereby leading to the second type of lesion, the fibrous, or "true," plaque (fig. 6–2). Fibrous plaques are whitish in appearance and are elevated so that they protrude into the lumen of the artery. They contain large numbers of lipid-containing foamy smooth muscle cells in association with a large quantity of extracellular lipid as well. As in the fatty streak, most of the lipid is cholesterol, and large amounts of LDL are present. The extracellular components of the plaque are not only lipid but very large quantities of dense collagen fibers, usually admixed with some elastin and carbohydrate. The cells, lipid, and connective tissue fibers form a cap which covers a large deeper deposit of lipid and debris from dead and dying cells. It is

Fig. 6–2. **Advanced atherosclerotic plaque.** There is an ulcer on the surface, and the interior is filled with fatty debris and smooth muscle cells. (Redrawn from E. P. Benditt, "The Origin of Atherosclerosis," *Scientific American*, February, 1977, p. 81. Copyright © 1977 by Scientific American, Inc. All rights reserved.)

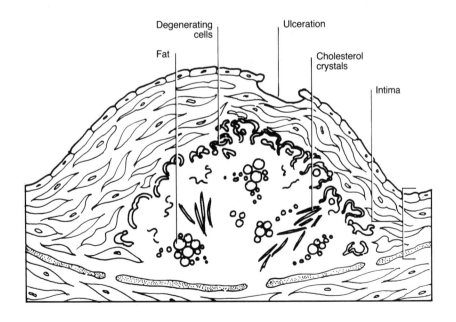

this soft fatty debris that suggested the name atherosclerosis (Greek *athera* [gruel] and *sclerosis* [hardening]).

The third stage—complicated lesions—are fibrous plaques that have become even more extensive and have been altered by rupture of the plaque into the lumen, hemorrhage into the plaque, laying down of calcium, extensive death of its smooth muscle cells, or formation of clots on the luminal surface of the plaque. These are all predictable consequences of plaque progression once true plaques are formed.

What causes the progression from fatty streak to true plaque (or from normal intima to true plaque, if, as some claim, the fatty streak is neither a lesion nor a precursor of the true plaque)? At present, all major theories of the genesis of atherosclerosis, based on examinations of human plaques and studies of experimentally induced plaques in laboratory animals, share the belief that the critical event is the localized excessive accumulation of smooth muscle cells in the intima, presumably by proliferation of smooth muscle cells in the media and their migration from the media into the intima. These cells then take up large quantities of lipid and also secrete all the connective tissue elements (collagen, elastin, etc.) found in the plaques. Given agreement on these points, the real current debate is over what causes this proliferation of smooth muscle cells. One's answer to this question in large part determines one's views concerning the precise roles of the risk factors for atherosclerosis and how best to prevent or reverse the atherosclerotic process.

The two major competing theories for explaining smooth muscle cell proliferation and plaque formation are as follows: (1) plaques form in response to frequently recurring injury to the arterial wall; (2) plaques are benign tumors, each of which is formed by offspring of a single cell whose growth is out of control.

The first theory has been around a long time, originating in its simplest form with the great German pathologist, Rudolf Virchow. The strongest evidence in its favor comes from many studies demonstrating that almost any kind of repeated damage to the arteries of laboratory animals induces the development of atherosclerotic plaques quite similar to those seen in humans, particularly (and often only) when the animals are fed a high-cholesterol diet. The damage must be frequent; if not, the lesions eventually regress and disappear. The key event is injury to the endothelial cells lining the artery. This layer of cells normally offers an effective barrier to the passage of large molecules, such as lipoproteins, from the blood into the vessel wall. Once this barrier is broken, the plasma lipoproteins—bearing their cholesterol—can enter the wall and act as a source of lipid both for deposition in the expanding plaque and for use in the formation of cell membranes by the proliferating smooth muscle cells.

Even more important, high concentrations of LDL have been shown in animal experiments to exert a powerful stimulatory effect on the proliferation of smooth muscle cells. LDL is not the only stimulant to reach the smooth muscle cells at an injured site. Platelets, the small blood cells which play such an important role in blood clotting, have an extraordinary tendency to adhere to underlying tissue once the endothelium is gone, and they release a variety of substances known to stimulate proliferation and migration of smooth muscle cells. So important are these factors that treatment of animals with antibodies against their platelets completely prevents the development of atherosclerotic plaques upon subsequent endothelium damage.

This theory nicely explains the role of the most important factors hypothesized to play causal roles in the development of atherosclerosis (to be described below). High blood pressure damages the endothelium, as do many of the powerful chemicals in cigarette smoke. Cholesterol, too, in high concentrations, has been shown, in laboratory animals, to damage endothelium. Moreover, cholesterol-LDL, as we have seen, is a stimulant of smooth muscle cell proliferation.

The competing hypothesis—the plaque as benign tumor—is much more recent, and is based pretty much on a single fascinating line of evidence, developed by Earl Benditt and his colleagues at the University of Washington School of Medicine.[5] They had become disenchanted with certain of the animal models of atherosclerosis when they found that, at least in the chicken fed large amounts of cholesterol, the cells of the enlarging plaque were not, unlike the human case, smooth muscle cells. In doing these experiments they discovered that some chickens spontaneously developed atherosclerosis with no treatment at all, and they began to study the earliest stages of this naturally occurring plaque. Their most important finding was that the intima cells in the plaque, while undeniably smooth muscle cells, were subtly different from the normal cells of the media, both in their anatomic features and their enhanced capacity to secrete collagen. Did these unusual cells represent the progeny of a previously normal media cell which had undergone a mutation and then was stimulated to proliferate? In other words, did the plaque constitute a tumor (a benign one because it did not invade and destroy surrounding normal tissue)?

Fortunately, the question of whether all plaque cells are derived from a single original cell is susceptible to testing, in human plaques obtained at autopsy. Here is the logic: All cells (excepting the mature ova) of women have two X chromosomes, and it is generally accepted that only one of these chromosomes in a given cell actually expresses itself (by coding for messenger RNA), the other being completely inactive. Just which X chromosome it is to be is decided randomly during embryonic development, and all the progeny of that cell will also express only the genes from that X chromosome. If there were in the maternal X chromosome a "marker" gene, one which codes for a particular enzyme that is different from the corresponding gene in the paternal X chromosome, then by looking for the enzyme, scientists could distinguish between populations of cells in which one or the other of the chromosomes is active. Such a "marker" gene is present on the X chromosome of many black women, and codes for one of the two forms of a particular enzyme, depending upon which X chromosome is active. Benditt and his colleagues studied atherosclerotic plaques obtained at autopsy from four black women and found that the cells from each plaque produced one or the other form of the enzyme but not both. In contrast, plaque-free sections of arterial wall from the same women produced equal mixtures of both enzymes.

Although, as other investigators have pointed out, alternative explanations of these data are possible, the finding that all cells of a plaque are monoclonal, that is, are descended from a single cell, is certainly consistent with the view of plaques arising as benign tumors. If true, then the essential ingredients for development of a plaque would be an initial mutation in a media smooth muscle cell (see chap. 9) followed by a stimulus for its rapid proliferation. In keeping with this hypothesis, Benditt has emphasized that both cholesterol and chemicals found in cigarette smoke are known mutagens (or give rise within the body to mutagens, as described in chap. 8) and that LDL are major carriers for mutagens or mutagen-precursors. Moreover, diets high in fat have been strongly associated, in epidemiological studies, with various tumors as well as with atherosclerosis. Finally, the DNA of persons with high blood pressure, the other major risk factor for atherosclerosis, is known to be more susceptible to breakage by mutagens than the DNA of persons with normal blood pressure.

And so on down the list of other hypothesized causal factors in atherosclerosis. Both the damaged-endothelium and benign-tumor theories provide a plausible framework for explaining the ways in which these factors might facilitate the development of atherosclerosis. In closing this section, I'd like to emphasize that the theories are not at all mutually exclusive. To take one scenario, for example, a mutation might be required to confer upon a smooth muscle cell the capacity to undergo rapid proliferation, but the actual triggers for this proliferation might be the chemicals (like LDL) allowed in or released as a result of endothelial damage.

Cholesterol Metabolism

Figure 6–3 summarizes the average plasma cholesterol concentration in American males of different ages. At birth, the value is ap-

Fig. 6–3. Average plasma cholesterol concentrations in healthy males of different ages.

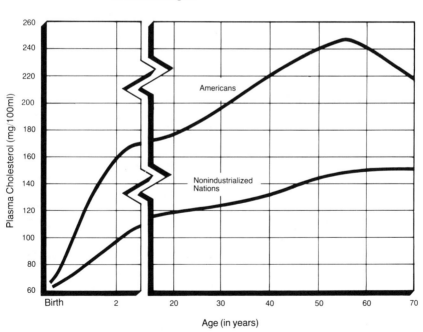

CHOLESTEROL, FATS, AND HEART DISEASE

proximately 50 mg/100 ml, but then rises very rapidly to reach 165mg/100ml by the age of two. There is relatively little change until late adolescence, at which time, in men, the mean value begins a progressive rise to reach a peak of 245 mg/100ml in the 50s. Women show less of a rise until after menopause (this has been hypothesized to explain why premenopausal women are relatively protected from atherosclerotic cardiovascular diseases). Now, compare this pattern to that seen in persons of nonindustrialized nations. At birth, the value for these people is essentially the same as ours, but the early rise of the first two years is much less pronounced, so that by the age of two, American children have plasma cholesterols, on the average, 50 to 100 mg/100 ml higher than those of children in nonindustrialized countries. Similarly, the rise throughout life is much less steep, the value for men in their 50s generally being only 140 to 160 mg/100 ml, the same as our two-year-olds, and 40 percent less than Americans of the same age.

There is no question that genetic factors do not explain the majority of such population differences for plasma cholesterol. It has been shown frequently that emigrants and their children rapidly take on the cholesterol pattern of their adopted countries (and the pattern of mortality from atherosclerotic cardiovascular diseases as well). So do persons who remain in their original countries but take on Western ways. Clearly, environmental factors must be the major factors. In order to understand just how such factors could operate, it is essential to know the basic pathways whose rates of activity ultimately determine plasma cholesterol.

If cells could synthesize all the cholesterol they required for building cell membranes, there would theoretically be no need at all for any cholesterol in the blood. But such is not the case; despite the fact that virtually all cells can synthesize some of their required cholesterol, most cannot do so in adequate amounts (what the adaptive value of such a state of affairs is remains in the realm of pure speculation). This means that most cells depend, to some extent, upon the cholesterol brought to them via the bloodstream from the liver and the intestinal tract.

The actual concentration of cholesterol in the plasma reflects the relative rates of inputs and outputs and can be analyzed by the balance methods which should be old hat to you be now. The scheme for cholesterol is illustrated in Figure 6–4. The sources of cholesterol addition to the body are shown on the left. Our dietary cholesterol comes from food from animal sources, egg yolk being far the richest in this lipid; a single egg contains about 250 mg of cholesterol. The average daily per capitum intake of cholesterol by Americans is 550 mg. However, much of this ingested cholesterol is not absorbed into the blood but simply moves the length of the gastrointestinal tract to be excreted in the feces.

The second source of gain is synthesis of cholesterol within the body. This occurs mainly in the liver but also in cells lining the gastrointestinal tract and in other locations.

The central portion of the figure does not denote net loss or gain from the body but rather distribution within it. Thus, cholesterol leaves the plasma to enter cells and be built into cell membranes while, at the same time, old membranes are being broken down with release of some of their cholesterol back into the blood.

The sources of net loss from the body are shown on the right; because of recycling processes, they appear more complex than they really are. First of all, some plasma cholesterol is picked up by the liver cells and secreted into the bile, which flows through the bile

Fig. 6–4. Pathways for cholesterol metabolism.

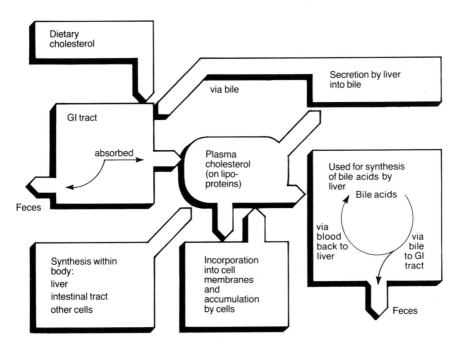

| CHOLESTEROL, FATS, AND HEART DISEASE

duct, usually after temporary storage in the gallbladder, to enter the small intestine. Here it is treated pretty much like ingested cholesterol, some being absorbed back into the blood, and the remainder being excreted in the feces. Second, much of the cholesterol picked up by the liver cells is metabolized into bile acids. These substances are not waste products, like urea from protein, but are important for aiding the digestion and absorption of fats. After their production by the liver (and temporary storage in the gall bladder), they too flow, during ingestion and digestion of a meal, through the bile duct into the small intestine. Most are then reclaimed by absorption back into the blood across the wall of the lower small intestine, only those escaping absorption being excreted in the feces. This is an important point because the drain on plasma cholesterol represented by its conversion to bile acids will depend upon how many of these bile acids are ultimately lost in the feces.

It should be clear that the liver is the center of the cholesterol universe. At one and the same time, it may be synthesizing new cholesterol, secreting old cholesterol from blood into bile, or transforming it into bile acids. The controls on all three of these processes are to a large extent independent of each other.

One of the most fascinating aspects of this entire picture is the newly emerging picture of just how cholesterol is taken up by nonliver cells. As I mentioned earlier, most of the cholesterol in plasma is carried by LDL, and we now know that almost all nonliver cells have on their surfaces molecular configurations (receptors) which "recognize" and specifically bind LDL. The binding of LDL to the outer membrane then triggers the invagination of the cell membrane and the engulfment of the bound LDL, just like an amoeba engulfs extracellular fluid or a white blood cell engulfs a bacterium. Once inside the cell, the LDL-containing membrane vesicle merges with one of the cell's little pockets of powerful enzymes called lysosomes, and these enzymes break down the LDL, liberating free cholesterol in the process. The real beauty of this system is the multiplicity and preciseness of its controls. When a cell is short of cholesterol, it begins synthesizing its own but it also synthesizes more LDL receptors and deposits them on its outer membrane. This allows the cell to bind more LDL, imbibe it, and liberate its cholesterol, which is preferentially used over the cholesterol synthesized by the cell itself. Indeed, the acquisition of cholesterol from plasma LDL inhibits, in some manner, the rate-limiting enzyme in the cell's own cholesterol-synthesizing machinery.

Remarkable events also occur as old membranes break down, releasing their cholesterol. It appears from present evidence that this cholesterol is preferentially picked up not by LDL but by HDL, the high-density plasma lipoproteins. It looks like the HDL are specialized for carriage of cholesterol from cells to the liver for excretion into the bile or conversion into bile acids. In contrast, LDL are specialized for cholesterol transport from the liver and intestinal tract to the other cells of the body. What is exciting about this is that persons with unusually high plasma levels of HDL, due to genetic mutation, have an extraordinarily low incidence of atherosclerotic cardiovascular disease.

To return to our balance figure, the next question to be asked should be on the tip of your tongue: What are the homeostatic control mechanisms which operate to keep plasma cholesterol relatively constant? They are multiple, indeed so redundant that one can only conclude that there is a strong adaptive value in preventing any increases (that makes sense in light of the effects of high cholesterol on atherosclerosis) or decreases!

The first control operates on the absorption of cholesterol from the gastrointestinal tract. Only a relatively small fraction of ingested cholesterol (or cholesterol secreted by the liver via the bile into the small intestine) is absorbed, the rest being excreted in the feces. As dietary cholesterol increases, the percentage absorbed decreases quite sharply and may actually reach an absolute maximum. This process, the mechanism of which is unknown, partially offsets the ability of increased dietary cholesterol to raise plasma cholesterol. On the other hand, this relationship also opposes the ability of low cholesterol diets to reduce plasma cholesterol.

Our next homeostatic response operates on cholesterol production: The synthesis of cholesterol by the liver is inhibited whenever dietary cholesterol is increased. This is because cholesterol, itself, inhibits the enzyme critical for cholesterol synthesis by the liver (a lovely example of the principle of end-product inhibition described in chap. 2). Thus, as soon as plasma cholesterol starts up because of increased cholesterol ingestion, hepatic synthesis is inhibited, and the plasma concentration remains close to its original value. Conversely, when dietary cholesterol is reduced, and plasma cholesterol begins to fall, hepatic synthesis is stimulated (released from inhibition) and this increased production opposes any further fall. This homeostatic control of synthesis is another major reason it is difficult to alter plasma cholesterol in either direction by altering only dietary cholesterol. However, as you should be able to predict from the material of chapter 2, there must be some change in the expected direction, since a finite perturbation from the original operating point is required to drive the compensatory alteration in hepatic synthesis. We'll look at some actual numbers after adding two more homeostatic controls.

These controls operate on cholesterol loss. An increased plasma cholesterol stimulates the liver to secrete more cholesterol into the bile and to convert more cholesterol into bile acids. These are important responses but neither is quantitatively as important as the alterations in cholesterol absorption or synthesis just described.

This summary of cholesterol metabolism leads us to two very important generalizations. The first, that a variety of homeostatic responses oppose the ability of changes in dietary cholesterol to influence plasma cholesterol, has already been emphasized several times, and our last task in this regard will be to provide some actual numbers. The second, equally important, is that altering dietary cholesterol is not the only way to change plasma cholesterol; other environmental (and genetic) factors can influence plasma cholesterol by inhibiting or facilitating any of the pathways for cholesterol metabolism. We now look at these two generalizations in turn.

Just how effective are the homeostatic controls in opposing the ability of changes in dietary cholesterol to alter plasma cholesterol? There is still some disagreement (simply because different scientists have obtained different results) over the answer to this question. However, you can assume that, on the average, reducing your cholesterol intake from 550 to 300 mg/day (equivalent to eating one fewer egg per day) would lower your blood cholesterol about 3 to 5 percent (conversely, raising intake from 550 to 800 mg/day would increase plasma cholesterol 3 to 5 percent); going all the way down to zero intake would drop off another 5 to 10 percent.

Now to other environmental and genetic factors. Those that have received the most attention are the quantity and quality of dietary fats (remember that the first causal link in the diet-heart hypothesis specifies not just cholesterol but the dietary fats as well). Many experiments have conclusively demonstrated that the composition of fatty acids in the diet influence plasma cholesterol. This is not because the fatty acids are precursors for cholesterol but because they influence one or more of the metabolic pathways affecting cholesterol balance. Saturated fatty acids, the dominant fatty acids of animal fat, tend to raise plasma cholesterol both by stimulating cholesterol synthesis and by inhibiting cholesterol conversion to bile acids. Just how the saturated fatty acids influence these pathways is not yet clear, but probably involves alteration of the critical enzymes mediating them. In contrast, most polyunsaturated fatty acids tend to lower plasma cholesterol, at least in part by increasing the fecal excretion of both the cholesterol and bile acids secreted by the liver into the bile (loss of the bile acids contributes to lowering of plasma cholesterol because the liver must then convert more cholesterol into bile acids to replace those lost). To finish the general picture, monounsaturated fatty acids generally exert little or no effect on plasma cholesterol. There are exceptions to all these generalizations; for example, the fatty acids in peanut oil are unsaturated but, for unknown reasons, raise the plasma cholesterol and enhance atherogenesis in experimental animals. Much remains to be learned about the contributions of specific fatty acids.

To summarize, there are two potential culprits in diets rich in animal fat—saturated fatty acids as well as cholesterol. Indeed, most experts believe that the former is more responsible than the latter for raising our plasma cholesterol. The American diet, with its heavy emphasis on animal sources, is very rich in total fats (43 percent of all calories), a large fraction of which are saturated (19 percent of total calories) with relatively few polyunsaturated (5 percent), the remaining 10 percent being monounsaturated. Diets consisting mainly of plant products have a cholesterol-lowering effect; not only are saturated fats and cholesterol avoided, but the intake of polyunsaturated fats is increased.

Many environmental and genetic factors other than fats are also known or suspected to influence plasma cholesterol. A few examples should suffice to reinforce this point.

Familial Hypercholesterolemia. This is a group of genetic diseases characterized by an extremely high plasma cholesterol and an extraordinary propensity toward atherosclerosis and coronary heart disease, some of these people dying in their 20s. The defect in at least one of these diseases has been identified: Because afflicted persons lack the gene which codes for LDL receptors on cell membranes, their cells cannot remove LDL from the blood at a normal rate, and so these lipoproteins, loaded with cholesterol, build up to very high concentrations in the blood. As emphasized earlier, genetic defects such as these account for only a small fraction of persons with atherosclerotic heart disease and do not explain the relatively high plasma cholesterol concentrations which are the norm in this country.

The Masai. These herdsmen of Tanzania provide an example of how one homeostatic mechanism can overcome not only diet but an opposing homeostatic mechanism. Their dietary staple is milk, often mixed with blood. They drink, on the average 3 to 5 liters of milk per day, 65 percent of their total calories comes from animal fat, and their daily cholesterol intake is 1,500 to 2,000 mg (the average American intake is 550 mg)! Yet their mean plasma cholesterol is extremely low, 135 mg/100 ml, and shows almost no tendency to increase with age. What would you predict about their cholesterol metabolism? The first scientists to study them logically predicted that the Masai would show marked inability to absorb the cholesterol, but they couldn't have been more wrong. The Masai were absorbing about 650 mg cholesterol per day, almost twice the maximal capacity observed for Americans given equivalent amounts of cholesterol and saturated fat to eat. The real answer came when cholesterol synthesis by the liver was studied. The Masai liver is exquisitely sensitive to inhibition by dietary cholesterol, much more so than ours, so that the decrease in hepatic synthesis is easily a match for the increase in cholesterol ingested and absorbed. We do not know whether this phenomenon represents a genetic trait or an acclimatization induced by a lifetime's exposure to such huge amounts of dietary lipid. At least one other herdsmen tribe, the Samburu of Northern Uganda and Kenya, manifests a similar picture.

Drugs and Surgery. A variety of drugs has been developed to lower plasma cholesterol. Most work in one of two ways—they block cholesterol synthesis or they increase the secretion of cholesterol and bile acids. Unfortunately for therapeutic purposes, the homeostatic responses to the reduction in plasma cholesterol induced by these drugs are so great that 10 to 20 percent is about the largest reduction that can be expected from their use alone.

Surgery is another matter, for the operation presently being used therapeutically to lower cholesterol in patients who have coronary heart disease and very high plasma cholesterols has been found to lower plasma cholesterol by 30 to 60 percent. The principle of this operation is easy to understand, for it is based on the fact that the absorption of cholesterol and bile acids occurs mainly in the last third of the intestine, the ileum. Disconnection of this segment from the rest of the tract causes the fecal loss of these substances. This operation is so effective because it leads to multiple interferences in cholesterol metabolism, thereby limiting the efficacy of the homeostatic responses. Cholesterol is directly lost because its major site of absorption is gone; cholesterol must be used to replace the similarly lost bile acids; and deficiency of bile salts interferes, because of failure of normal emulsification, with whatever cholesterol absorption can occur in segments other than the ileum.

Environmental Pollutants and Dietary Factors Other than Cholesterol and Fats. Here we enter into the realm of speculation based on relatively scanty evidence. Nevertheless, there is a growing body of evidence suggesting that many nutrients and environmental pollutants may influence plasma cholesterol by inhibiting the conversion of cholesterol to bile acids. Vitamin D, which is often consumed in very large amounts in our culture because of excessive levels of enrichment, and carbon monoxide are two examples given by Dr. Mann, who is convinced that somewhere in the environment of Western man there is a noxious agent that causes trouble by inducing high blood cholesterol via inhibition of cholesterol synthesis to bile acids. Indeed, he believes the evidence is already adequate to establish such inhibition as the dominant cause of our high cholesterol. Needless to say, there is no general agreement on this point.

Now we are ready to evaluate the diet-heart hypothesis. We will do this by evaluating the data from our usual three types of experiments—epidemiology and controlled human and animal studies.

Laboratory Animal Data

We can dispose of these experiments rather briefly, for the key findings were presented at the beginning of this chapter. In essentially all species studied—rabbits, dogs, chickens, pigs, rats, guinea pigs, hamsters, and nonhuman primates—the feeding of large amounts of cholesterol and animal fat has resulted in elevations of plasma cholesterol and enhanced rates of development of atherosclerosis and coronary heart disease. In most cases, the disease processes appear to be very similar to those seen in people, and the fact that they are generally reversible is extremely important, for it is consistent with the hypothesis that dietary changes might cause already existing atherosclerotic lesions to regress.

The major criticism of these animal experiments is that the amounts of dietary cholesterol and fat used have often been so large as to produce astronomic levels of plasma cholesterol. However, as I described in chapter 1 (and will analyze in much greater depth in chap. 9), such use of large doses is acceptable practice in animal experiments to insure the development of enough disease to be detectable in a small number of animals, particularly since the species used may be much less sensitive than human beings to the agent administered. Perhaps the most important experiments have been on nonhuman primates. Simply feeding the animals a typical American diet was adequate to cause severe atherosclerosis. However, these animals are clearly more susceptible to the cholesterol-raising effects of diet, since their plasma cholesterol concentrations rose to 380 mg/100 ml on this "typical" American diet, a value much higher than those manifested by all but a very few people.

In short, the laboratory animal experiments are qualitatively quite consistent with all aspects of the diet-heart hypothesis.

Epidemiological Data

Epidemiological studies, more than any others, have molded our thinking about the way in which coronary heart disease arises and made it absolutely clear that this disease is due to the interaction of a number of environmental and host factors. It is the classic multifactorial disease in that no single factor causes the disease in the sense that the measles virus causes measles. Epidemiologists have had a field day attempting to isolate individual risk factors for coronary heart disease by studying the characteristics of individuals and populations with high and low incidences of it. Keep in mind as we delve into these studies that the term risk factor simply refers to a characteristic which is associated with an increased incidence of a disease (and/or mortality from it), i.e., has predictive value for the likelihood of the disease occurring. The burning question for every risk factor is whether the association is fortuitous or represents a cause and effect relationship. This is the question we are trying to answer for both plasma cholesterol and the ingestion of animal fat, but let us spread our net a bit wider for the moment and include several other risk factors as well.

The "Big Three" Risk Factors

The three risk factors which emerge consistently in study after study as strongly associated with coronary heart disease are a high plasma cholesterol, cigarette smoking, and the presence of another distinct disease—high blood pressure (hypertension).* Figure 6–5 illustrates data from the National Cooperative Pooling Project of the American Heart Association, a ten-year prospective study of middle-aged (30 to 59 years of age at the outset of the study), white males in Framingham, Albany, Los Angeles, Chicago, and Minneapolis.[6] Note first of all that a dose-response exists for each risk factor. Secondly, as shown by the last panel of the figure, the risk factors are additive, i.e., the likelihood of having a heart attack increases as the number of risk factors increases. For the sake of simplicity, the analysis of additivity shown in this figure is based not on the actual dose-responses, but on arbitrary cutoff points for what constitutes a "high" value for each risk factor, as established at the outset of the study. The cutoff for plasma cholesterol was 250 mg/100 ml, that for hypertension was 90 mm Hg diastolic pressure,[†] and that for cigarettes was any use at all. Such an analysis clearly shows that risk increases as the number of risk factors increases, so much so that when all three are present, the incidence of heart attacks is increased almost ninefold.

The full impact of this analysis can only be appreciated when one realizes how common the presence of one or more of these risk factors is in our population. In terms of the definitions listed above, only 17 percent of the men in this study were classified as "not high" on all three factors, about 45 percent were at risk from one factor, and 38 percent from two or more. This 38 percent of the

---

*Hypertension, at least in its chronic well-established phase, is not itself a disease of the large arteries, as is atherosclerosis, but rather of the small vessels (arterioles) which connect large arteries to capillaries. Because the smooth muscles surrounding these vessels contract too strongly, blood is "dammed up" in the large arteries and creates an abnormally high pressure. Sometimes, the cause of the excessive contraction is known, but in the great majority of cases it is not.

†Arterial blood pressure is routinely measured as the high point (systolic pressure) occurring during heart contraction and the lowest pressure (diastolic) existing just before contraction; the latter is the better measure of the severity of hypertension. The units (mm Hg) refer to the height (mm) of a column of mercury (Hg) which could be supported by the pressure of the blood.

Fig. 6–5. **"Big–three" risk factors for coronary heart disease.** These data are from the national cooperative Pooling Project, a ten-year prospective study of men aged 30 to 59 at the outset of the study and free of evidence of coronary heart disease at that time. "Major coronary event" includes all fatal and nonfatal heart attacks and sudden death due to coronary heart disease. The criteria used for defining the presence or absence of each risk factor for the lower right-hand graph are described in the text. (Redrawn from figure by A. Miller from J. Stamler, "The Primary Prevention of Coronary Heart Disease," *Hospital Practice,* September, 1971, pp. 53–54. Reproduced with permission.)

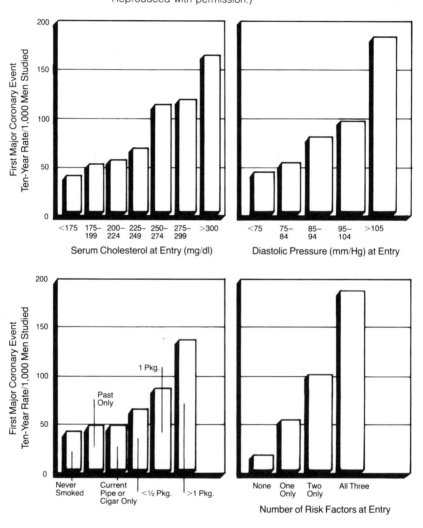

population accounted for 59 percent of the heart attacks. Of course, the choice of other arbitrary cutoff points, i.e., definitions of what constitutes a "high" value for that factor, would yield different re-sults. For example, if simply the upper third of plasma cholesterols and blood pressures were called "high," and smoking again was defined as any use at all, then approximately 25 percent of the test population would be at risk from all three factors and account for almost 50 percent of new heart attacks.

As impressive as these numbers are, the other side of the coin must also be emphasized. These three "traditional" risk factors do not account entirely for differences in the rate of coronary heart disease, indeed for only about 50 percent. For example, depending on one's definition of "normal," somewhere between 15 and 25 percent of men with coronary heart disease do not have even one of these risk factors. Just as important, about the same numbers of men who are at risk from one or more of these factors do not suffer from coronary heart disease. I point this out not to denigrate the importance of these "big three" but only to emphasize that other important risk factors (and antirisk factors) remain to be newly discovered or, in the case of already implicated factors, more fully documented.

There certainly is no dearth of candidates. The following are only a sample of factors which have been associated with coronary heart disease in one or more epidemiological studies: obesity, intake of animal fat, intake of sugar, lack of dietary fiber, lack of physical activity, behavior patterns, psychosocial stress, diabetes, living in cities, polluted air, coffee, water hardness, and elevated plasma con-centration of uric acid.

This list offers excellent illustrations of why it is often so difficult to disentangle risk factors from one another. Take obesity, for ex-ample. Epidemiological studies definitely incriminate it, but obese persons are more likely to have high plasma cholesterol, be dia-betic or hypertensive, and have an elevated plasma uric acid. Does obesity, per se, contribute to coronary heart disease, or is it one of these other variables that really is the causal factor, in which case obesity might have nothing at all to do with coronary heart disease or might be a risk factor for a risk factor (for example, for the development of diabetes)? Such distinctions are important in the planning of preventive and therapeutic programs directed against coronary heart disease.

Now let us look more closely at the cholesterol data, with particular regard to the strength and consistency of the association, the two most important characteristics for inferring that a risk factor really is causal. It would be hard to ask for a more consistent association. The association between plasma cholesterol and coronary heart disease has been observed not only for American communities but for almost every country and population group for which data have been collected. For example, figure 6–6 summarizes the findings for thirteen population groups in six countries; like the strictly American Pooling Project described earlier, it too was prospective, following for five years men who had been between 40 and 59 years of age and free of heart disease when the study began.[7] Note that the indi-

Fig. 6–6. **Association between serum cholesterol and age-standardized incidence of coronary heart disease.** The subjects were all men who were age 40 to 59 at the outset of the study and free of evidence of coronary heart disease. The "median" serum cholesterol is that value below and above which equal numbers of values occur. (Redrawn from figure by A. Miller from J. Stamler, "The Primary Prevention of Coronary Heart Disease," *Hospital Practice*, September, 1971, pp. 53–54. Reproduced with permission.)

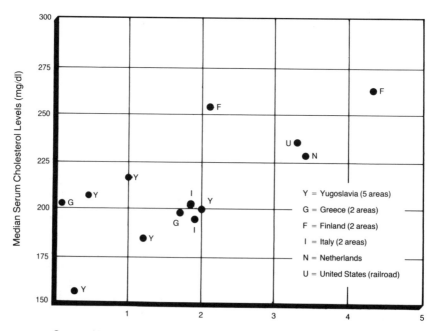

vidual points scatter about a single line, their deviation from this line presumably providing some indication of noncholesterol factors at work in causing the disease.

Are there any major exceptions? Yes, a few (for example, Italian-American men of Roseto, Pennsylvania, have the usual American level of plasma cholesterol but a very low mortality rate from coronary heart disease), but this is only to be expected when a disease has as many contributing causes as coronary heart disease seems to.

The existence of a clear dose-response is another important characteristic suggesting causality. Look again at the cholesterol data of figure 6–5. When plasma cholesterol is greater than 300 mg/100 ml, the incidence of coronary heart disease is more than four times greater than at cholesterol values less than 175 mg/100 ml. This is a very strong association, and there is virtually universal agreement that plasma cholesterol really plays an important causal role in the relatively few persons with such high values. In contrast, there is relatively little increase in risk at values less than 225 mg/100 ml, with a small jump between 225 and 250 and then a very large increase beyond 250 mg/100 ml. What this might signify for the average middle-aged American male can be appreciated by looking at figure 6–7, a frequency distribution curve for the plasma cholesterol concentrations of American men in their 40s and 50s.[8] Approximately 40 percent of all such men have values above 250 mg/100 ml and so would be at considerable risk according to our analysis.

To summarize, the consistency and strength of the association between plasma cholesterol and coronary heart disease revealed by both international studies and those carried out purely within the United States add greatly to the likelihood that the association is a causal one. The next question, then, is whether diet is a major determinant of plasma cholesterol.

Association Between Dietary Lipid and Coronary Heart Disease

If dietary lipids are a major determinant of plasma cholesterol concentration, then the epidemiologic association between diet and coronary heart disease should be very similar to that between plasma cholesterol and coronary heart disease. For most interpopulation studies, this is the case; there is a striking direct correlation between a population's percentage of calories ingested as animal fat and both its mean plasma cholesterol concentration and its coronary heart disease incidence or mortality rate. Thus, the great majority of non-Westernized populations have low intakes of animal fat, low plasma cholesterol, and low incidences of coronary heart disease, whereas Westernized nations have, to a greater or lesser extent, higher values for all these variables. Very importantly, the association also holds when Westernized nations are compared to one another.[9]

However, there are important exceptions in these interpopulation comparisons, i.e., populations who consume large amounts of ani-

Fig. 6–7. **Frequency distribution curve for serum cholesterol concentrations in American men in their forties and fifties.** (Redrawn from R. B. McGandy, D. M. Hegsted, and F. J. Stare, "Dietary fats, carbohydrates, and artherosclerotic vascular disease," *New England Journal of Medicine* 277 [1967]:4. Reprinted by permission of the *New England Journal of Medicine* [vol. 277; p. 4, 1967].)

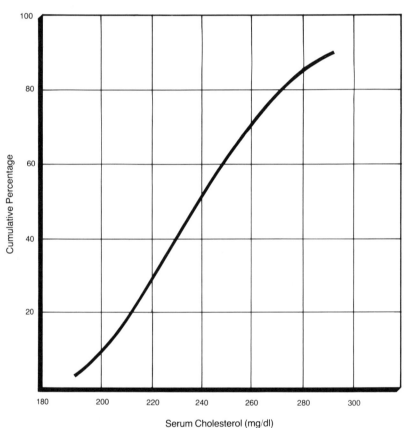

mal fat but have low values for both plasma cholesterol concentration and incidence of coronary heart disease. One such exception is the Masai; others are Eskimos, Swiss Alpine villagers, and Navajo Indians. Other exceptions are groups that eat fairly large amounts of animal fat but have much higher mortality rates from coronary heart disease than do most populations eating essentially the same diet. For example, the Finns living in the eastern half of Finland eat the same amount of cholesterol and animal fat as the Finns living in the western half of the country, but have twice the incidence of coronary heart disease. Perhaps the most famous example is the "Boston brothers" study; a large number of Irish immigrants to Boston were compared with their brothers who had remained in Ireland and were found to suffer twice as many heart attacks despite the fact that they ate somewhat less cholesterol and animal fat than their brothers did.[10]

The numerous exceptions, of course, weaken the diet-heart hypothesis but not lethally so, for its adherents do not claim that diet is the sole cause of elevated plasma cholesterol and coronary heart disease, or even the major one, only that it is an important one. Certainly, for some populations and environments, genetic differences and nondietary environmental factors may be far more prominent than diet and obscure the diet-heart relationship altogether. Moreover, it is very important to note that all these deviations involve populations who eat moderate or large amounts of animal fat. At the low end of the spectrum there are no exceptions; no populations habitually subsisting on diets low in animal fat have an appreciable amount of coronary heart disease! This fact (which has its counterpart in the animal experiments described earlier) suggests that a diet relatively high in animal fat is an absolute prerequisite for a high incidence of coronary heart disease. In other words, such a diet may not itself cause the disease, but in its absence, other causal factors are much less effective.

A much greater problem than these interpopulation exceptions for the diet-heart hypothesis, one that critics like Dr. Mann do consider lethal, is that the often impressive epidemiological associations seen when one compares whole populations breaks down completely when one studies single populations in this country (or any other). For the communities of Framingham, Massachusetts, and Tecumseh, Michigan, there was absolutely no association between dietary habits and either plasma cholesterol or coronary heart disease; at the same time, plasma cholesterol and coronary heart disease did correlate quite well with each other.[11]

Adherents to the diet-heart hypothesis do not believe that this constitutes a refutation of their theory. They argue that the lack of association stems from the documented fact that, in these communities, as almost everywhere in America, people vary little in their dietary habits, compared to the very large differences in dietary habits between whole populations throughout the world. Because of this, they argue, the effect of diet on plasma cholesterol cannot be demonstrated against the background effects of nondietary influences (other environmental factors and genetic differences in sensitivity to dietary effects). Moreover, if some critical threshold exists for dietary contribution to plasma cholesterol, most of us probably ingest quantities of cholesterol and saturated fats above this threshold.

Critics of the theory retort that all this might possibly be true but smacks of after-the-fact rationalization. They believe it is more likely that diet simply is not an important factor in the setting of plasma cholesterol for most Americans, and therefore, not a causal factor in atherosclerosis. Profoundly different diets (near-vegetarianism, for example) might make a difference but this has little relevance for the preventive dietary alterations being suggested by the AHA. Finally, they argue, this lack of intrapopulation association suggests that the good interpopulation associations between diet, on the one hand, and plasma cholesterol and coronary heart disease, on the other, may be completely fortuitous; populations which do not eat very much animal fats differ in many other ways from those who do—low incidence of obesity, high levels of physical activity, very low sugar intakes, very high intakes of complex carbohydrates and fibers, and low exposure to air pollutants, to name just a few. Any of these might be the true causal factor(s) rather than dietary lipid.

Clearly, the lack of intrapopulation association between dietary lipid and coronary heart disease constitutes the single greatest source of uncertainty for the diet-heart theory. The adherents' proferred explanation for this discrepancy is not, in fact, just rationalization, and given the well-known limitations of epidemiological surveys in diseases characterized by multiple causal factors, could very well be true. On the other hand, so might the opposing view. The point is that this is as far as the epidemiologists, alone, can take us.

Controlled Human Experiments

Does Diet Influence Plasma Cholesterol?

The direct way to determine whether the Western diet has a significant effect on plasma cholesterol is to submit the question to controlled research on human beings. The information one hopes to gain from the experiment dictates how much dietary change is employed. Thus, if the question asked is how much of the total world-wide differences in plasma cholesterol concentrations are due to diet, then the studies must employ very severe dietary alterations. The only really extensive, long-term study involving such dietary manipulation was performed on middle-aged prisoners, European and Bantu, fed a "Bantu-type" diet (15 percent of total calories as protein, 15 percent fat, and 70 percent carbohydrate) for thirty-nine weeks.[12] At the end of this period, plasma cholesterol was very low in both groups, essentially at the same level as that of free-living Bantu natives. For the next year, the carbohydrate intake was reduced to 45 percent of total calories and the fat raised to 40 percent, using either polyunsaturated fat (sunflower seed oil) or butter. With the oil, plasma cholesterol remained low, whereas the addition of butter raised it, in both European and Bantu, to levels seen in Westernized countries. This study has provided a strong indication that dietary lipid may, indeed, be one of the most important determinants of plasma cholesterol, but it is, after all, a single study performed on very few subjects under highly artificial conditions.

In contrast, a large number of dietary-manipulation studies have been performed asking a very different question, the one most germane to the preventive dietary proposals put forward by the AHA and other diet-heart enthusiasts. These studies have evaluated quite specifically the changes in plasma cholesterol induced by relatively modest alterations of the usual American diet in the direction of less total fat, saturated fat, and cholesterol, but increased polyunsaturated fats. Typical of such diets is the so-called prudent diet recommended by the American Heart Association: (1) a caloric intake adjusted to achieve and maintain ideal body weight; (2) a reduction in calories as fat from the usual 40 to 45 percent of total calories to no more than 35 percent; (3) of this fat, less than 10 percent of the total calories should come from saturated fatty acids and up to 10 percent from polyunsaturated fatty acids, the remainder being from monounsaturated fatty acids; (4) daily intake of cholesterol of approximately 300 mg. Such a diet would represent, for most Americans, relatively minor and easily achievable alterations. The results of this type of dietary alteration (sometimes supplemented with much larger amounts of polyunsaturated fats such as sunflower seed oil) have been quite consistent. In most subjects, plasma cholesterol falls, on the average, 10 to 15 percent.[13]

In summary, controlled human experiments clearly document that dietary lipids account for at least a fraction of the population differences in plasma cholesterol and that relatively modest dietary changes can result in a small but significant decrease in plasma cholesterol. They leave completely unsettled the question of whether other factors also play important roles in causing our plasma cholesterol concentrations to be higher than those in non-Westernized populations.

Will a 10 to 15 Percent Decrease in Plasma Cholesterol Reduce Risk?

This is the central question of the entire diet-heart debate, the one to which our previous discussions have been leading, so let us apply the relevant information gleaned so far in this chapter to the question. We know that, regardless of what the major cause of our high plasma cholesterol concentrations really is, the recommendations embodied in the prudent diet will predictably lower plasma cholesterol concentration 10 to 15 percent. Further, we are reasonably certain that a very high plasma cholesterol, say around 300 mg/100 ml, plays a causal role in atherosclerosis. Putting these two facts together, it is reasonable to conclude (and there is virtually total agreement on this point) that the prudent diet will help persons having such high values. However, only a small number of people are in this highest bracket, and they usually require extensive therapy, not just a preventive diet. At the opposite end of the association between plasma cholesterol and coronary heart disease, persons whose values are 200 mg/100 ml or less bear relatively little risk from their plasma cholesterol, and little improvement would be expected from a 10 to 15 percent reduction.

This leaves us with the 65 to 85 percent of the middle-aged male population with values between these extremes. Looking at figure 6–5 again, and assuming that the associations are really causal in this range, you can see that if a person's original value were 260 and the prudent diet lowered it 15 percent to 221, that person's risk would have diminished by almost 50 percent. This kind of number juggling has led to the generalization by diet-heart adherents that only a 10 to 15 percent average decrease in plasma cholesterol might cut the incidence of coronary heart disease in this country by approximately 20 to 25 percent in young and middle-aged men, no mean accomplishment.

This is, of course, all based on the assumption that the observed association between plasma cholesterol and coronary heart disease is really causal in this range and that moving a given individual down along the dose-response curve in this range lessens his risk as much as if he had been in the lower group to start with. These are reasonable assumptions but they may not be valid; in this range the association is not so strong as to establish causality with any degree of confidence, and the total lack of success in establishing an intra-population association between diet and coronary heart disease weakens the inference of causality.

Therefore, the only way to achieve a greater degree of certainty upon which to base public policy and personal decisions is to do the appropriate controlled clinical study—take a group of relatively young people, feed half of them the prudent diet and the other half the usual American diet, and follow them for many years, determining their incidence of and mortality from heart attacks.

Such clinical trials are easy to propose but incredibly difficult, laborious, and expensive to perform. One way to diminish the number of subjects required as well as the length of the study is to use elderly people, particularly those known to have coronary heart disease at the onset of the study. Several such studies have already been reported, but the results are really quite inconclusive. The trend certainly has been toward a decrease in mortality from coronary heart disease, but the differences were usually very small and sometimes not statistically significant.[14]

Predictably, how one evaluates the overall significance of these studies of elderly people depends on one's original leanings. Dr. Mann states: "the better the trial design, the less well the diet treatment seems to work. . . . No diet therapy has been shown effective for the prevention or treatment of coronary heart disease."[15] Dr. John F. Mueller, professor of medicine, University of Colorado, and a diet-heart enthusiast, writes: "Admittedly, in all of these heroic attempts . . . there are flaws and in some, statistical significance is either lacking or barely present. This is not surprising. Rather it strongly supports the argument in favor of dietary modification for one compelling reason: All the studies showed the same trend."[16]

Considering the subjects' ages (most experts agree that, if cholesterol is a causal factor, it has already done most of its damage by one's late years) and their relatively small numbers, I believe that Dr. Mueller's appraisal is the fairer of the two. Certainly, these studies do not *disprove* the diet-heart hypothesis.

Surprisingly, perhaps the most consistent finding in these studies was that, regardless of the trend in mortality from cardiovascular diseases, the total numbers of deaths from *all* causes in the experimental and control groups were essentially the same. Indeed, in two, the number of deaths from cancer was significantly higher in the group fed the diet high in polyunsaturated fatty acids and low in cholesterol and saturated fatty acids.[17] This finding must be taken seriously in light of experimental evidence that very large quantities of polyunsaturated fats cause cancer in experimental animals and exert other toxic effects as well.[18]

A second shortcut has been to use drugs to lower the plasma cholesterol by the same amount achievable through use of the prudent diet. One such study, performed in elderly men, provided no evidence of a protective effect. More recently (1978), a much longer, larger trial, this time beginning with healthy men, aged 30 to 59, was reported.[19] A highly significant 25 percent decrease in the number of heart attacks was observed for the group given the cholesterol-lowering drug during the four to six years of the study (the average fall in plasma cholesterol in this group was 9 percent over the same period).

The importance of this study can be felt from the exclamation of an editorial writer in the *New England Journal of Medicine*: "What is clear, at last, is that reduction of serum cholesterol concentrations is relevant to the prevention of coronary heart disease."[20] Alas, what was also clear from this study is that the drug used is unsafe; the number of heart attacks may have been down, but the deaths from all causes was significantly greater in the drug-treated group (seventy-seven versus forty-seven)! The excess deaths were due to diseases of the liver, gallbladder, and small and large intestines. The gallbladder was particularly affected, the drug-treated group showing a threefold greater incidence of gallbladder diseases serious enough to require its surgical removal. These results and other types of evidence from less extensive studies with this or similar drugs make it clear that no safe drug exists today for the lowering of plasma cholesterol. Nevertheless, if one assumes that these noncardiac illnesses and deaths were due to the drug, not to the lowered cholesterol, this study does suggest that a modest reduction of plasma cholesterol in middle-aged men may reduce coronary heart disease significantly.

So we are left with the need for the "big" studies if any completely convincing answer is to be forthcoming. The National Heart, Lung, and Blood Institute (NHLBI) is presently sponsoring two such blockbusters. Both will follow healthy men, one looking only at the effects of lowering blood cholesterol concentration through dietary manipulations, the other at the effects of reducing all three major risk factors. Planning for these studies began in 1972, and it will be at least 1981 before any results are available. They are going to cost a lot of money, at least $200 million (and probably much more), so much that some critics believe it was a mistake ever to begin them. They point out that the irreversible committment to them (no knowledge at all would be gained if they were terminated early or if corners were cut) means that larger and larger portions of the NHLBI budget are being drained away from studies of other risk factors and from basic research, which many feel has a better chance of guiding us to the major causes of atherosclerosis than do studies such as these. Dr. Mann, for example, points out that despite the growing indirect evidence that physical activity may be an extremely important antirisk factor, no systematic controlled trials of this possibility have been done—"a commentary on the lost generation of diet-heart enthusiasts."[21] Others answer these critics by pointing out that the cost of conducting such large trials is trivial compared with the economic (and human) costs of atherosclerotic cardiovascular diseases to this country, and that these types of trials are the only present way of obtaining the information needed to determine the direction future preventive programs should take.

There is another extremely important rationale for doing these studies. I have restricted this discussion of the role of cholesterol and dietary fats in disease entirely to a consideration of atherosclerosis. Yet, emerging over the past ten years has been a variety of epidemiological studies suggesting an equally prominent association between these factors and cancer. One gets a profound feeling of déjà vu in reading these reports, for one need only substitute "cancer" for "cardiovascular diseases" to make them almost identical to previous studies. There is also a growing basic science literature dealing with the mechanisms by which diets rich in cholesterol or saturated fats might predispose to cancer. This is very confusing in at least one respect, since as I mentioned earlier, polyunsaturated fats have also been implicated in carcinogenesis. The controlled studies now underway should, therefore, do double duty in providing an answer as to just what the effect of dietary manipulation might be on cancer incidence and mortality as well as coronary heart disease.

Conclusion

What do we do while waiting for the results? There are two quite different dimensions to this question—the individual one and that pertaining to public policy, such as the campaign visualized by Congress and the Department of Agriculture. The latter requires complex value considerations, a few of which were presented at the beginning of this chapter. In contrast, the personal decision facing each of us requires only an evaluation of how convinced you are of the health consequences of your present diet by the existing data, as ambiguous as they may be, and how much pleasure, if any, you foresee giving up by switching your dietary habits. So far as the scientific aspects of the discussion are concerned, the most cogent case I have encountered for opting for the prudent diet has been expressed by Dr. Mueller.

> To take the negative point of view, I am not aware of any evidence that raising serum cholesterol protects against progressive atherosclerosis or of any evidence that low polyunsaturated fat diets increase the risks of myocardial infarction. All available evidence points in the opposite direction and that fact is worth keeping in mind. Until the federal government or a local government is willing to invest in a large scale, prospective diet-heart study, absolute proof will remain lacking. . . .
>
> Can we afford to wait? The answer to this question lies in the final major arena of disagreement, namely, relative risks. If the arguments in favor of the cholesterol-heart theory are considered to be unproved, then the counter-argument, that fat-modified diets are harmful, should be labeled conjectural.
>
> . . . An analysis of all published long-term fat-modified dietary studies, in which morbidity and mortality were documented, failed to reveal any significant correlation between diet and cancer. Perhaps the most compelling fact relevant to this concern lies in the epidemio-

logical observation that large population groups around the world routinely ingest diets that are comparable in fatty acid patterns and cholesterol content to those recommended for coronary-artery-disease prevention. There is no evidence that neoplastic disease [tumors] occurs oftener in such groups than it does in those ingesting diets high in saturated fatty acids and cholesterol.

Those of us who have supported and personally subscribe to the fat-modified dietary approach to coronary artery disease have never claimed to have proved it beneficial or attempted to rank diet against other known risk factors in a rating scale of relative importance. What we have said is, that, on the basis of existing scientific data, there is reason to believe that reducing dietary saturated fat and cholesterol will likely retard progressive atherosclerosis. We have also held that when coupled with other risk-factor modification programs, it represents the most practical and safest preventive approach to the problem of coronary artery disease that we know of.

Only time will prove the soundness of this theory. To wait for that proof may mean waiting forever. Such a wait is unacceptable as long as the potential for harm from diet modification is negligible.[22]

Dr. Mueller is, in effect, saying "go along with the odds," and I believe his case is solid, but only if one accepts his view that there is no real evidence for toxicity of polyunsaturated fats in reasonable amounts. He dismisses one of the studies I cited earlier which demonstrated increased cancer mortality in elderly men on the fat-modified treatment diet by quoting the author as later stating he (the author) did not believe the correlation to be significant. Moreover, his reference to the lack of increased cancer in the non-Westernized world, while correct, overlooks the likelihood that the many risk factors for cancer existing in our industrial environment could easily obscure any positive association of cancer to saturation or unsaturation of the dietary fats.

The fact is we really don't know whether raising intake of polyunsaturated fats to 10 percent of total calories carries any health risk in our environment, or whether any such risk might be specifically related only to certain polyunsaturated fats but not others. There is particular concern over the partially hydrogenated soft margarines prepared commercially, since many of the molecules formed do not occur normally in nature and so deserve the same kind of suspicion we reserve for other synthetic chemicals. Of course, one can always strike a middle path by cutting back on cholesterol and saturated fat while not going overboard on polyunsaturated fats and avoiding the soft margarines altogether. But somewhere off in the distance, you will hear a voice saying, "Yes, but what is the effect of all the additional carbohydrate that such a diet requires?"

What else shall we do while waiting for the answer? Keep funding basic research. It would be a disaster if funds for research into the basic physiology of plasma lipids and the arterial wall really were sacrificed to foot the bill for these mammoth human studies. Just one example: Many scientists believe that the emerging information on HDL (mentioned earlier) may turn out to be more crucial to our understanding of atherosclerosis than the previous work on LDL. Already, data coming from Framingham suggest that HDL might be a better predictor, particularly in people over 50, than plasma cholesterol or LDL; yet we know very little about the basic physiology of HDL or the factors which raise or lower it.

Part **III** | Stress

Chapter 7 | Psychosocial Stress and Disease

No other question of environment-disease interactions generates as much controversy and confusion as: Do the stresses of our psychosocial environment play an important causal role in the development of major diseases, including coronary heart disease and cancer? The great majority of the lay public seems convinced that the answer is "yes," whereas most physicians have been reluctant to accept the proposition. In the middle are growing numbers of researchers slowly accumulating data in this most difficult of research areas and laying the basis for a scientifically sound answer. My own opinion, the basis of which forms this chapter, is that the data are already adequate to answer the question in the affirmative but not to quantitate the precise contributions of psychosocial stress to different diseases or to establish with certainty the physiological links leading from one to the other.

The confusion over psychosocial stress and disease begins with the very definition of the word "stress." Many scientists use it to denote those environmental stimuli, both physical and psychological, acting upon us to elicit a particular group of responses, whereas others define stress as the bodily responses, themselves, calling the stimuli "stressors." I believe the debate over this question is a distracting "tempest in a teapot," for there is little obvious advantage to either terminology. Except where explicitly stated, I'll routinely use the former definition because it is the more familiar of the two.

There is also no universally agreed-upon definition of the adjective "psychosocial," but most scientists in the field would accept something like the following: "Psychosocial" denotes stimuli originating in the social environment and affecting the individual through the mediation of processes residing in the brain. We'll put flesh on this skeleton definition as we proceed.

Hans Selye, the Montreal scientist who is one of the fathers of this research area, has been most influential in popularizing the response definition of stress (the one I am not using). Selye's great contribution was in hypothesizing and documenting that diverse environmental challenges (increased external temperature and toxic chemicals, for example) not only called forth *specific* responses which maintain homeostasis in the face of the challenge, but elicit a relatively stereotyped *nonspecific* set of neuroendocrine responses, which he collectively termed "stress." (In the terminology I am using, these nonspecific bodily responses constitute the "response to stress," the stress being the environmental stimulus which elicits them.)

Selye had studied mainly one such group of responses, those due to the outpouring of hormones by the endocrine gland known as the adrenal cortex, in response to noxious physical stimuli such as severe cold and trauma. In hypothesizing both that this adrenal-cortical response was only one of several components of the stress response and that psychosocial stimuli elicit virtually these same nonspecific responses, he was standing on the shoulders of a scientific giant, Walter B. Cannon, the Harvard physiologist who, we saw in chapter 1, had been instrumental in documenting the concept of homeostasis. Cannon had done a great deal of research on the physiological responses of experimental animals associated with arousal and behaviors which seemed analogous to those exhibited by human beings experiencing rage and fear; for example, the responses of a cat to a barking dog. He had documented that such responses were inevitably accompanied by activation of the sympathetic nervous system (including its hormone-secreting component, the adrenal medulla), and he labeled this the "fight-or-flight" response, signifying that it prepares the animal either for actively resisting a real or perceived threat, or for fleeing from it. Cannon had not studied the response of the adrenal cortex, the gland which would so occupy Selye, to such psychosocial stresses.

Selye connected Cannon's findings and his own, and made an intuitive leap to the hypothesis that a host of threatening physical and psychosocial stimuli would all prove to elicit, nonspecifically, the same battery of neuroendocrine responses, notably activation of the adrenal cortex and the sympathetic nervous system. These nonspecific responses are in addition to and distinct from the homeostatic responses specifically elicited by the various stimuli; thus exposure to low temperature or low oxygen concentration elicit completely different specific responses (shivering and increased breathing, respectively), but both activate the sympathetic nervous system and the adrenal cortex ("activate" is a shorthand term I'll use for "increases the activity of"; in the complete absence of stress, there is always a finite amount of activity by the sympathetic nervous system and adrenal cortex, so stress does not produce something out of nothing, but rather increases the rates at which these systems function).

The past twenty years have witnessed both a confirmation of much of the central core of Selye's hypothesis and an expansion of the list of neuroendocrine responses elicited by stress (to mention it one last time, the list of responses constitutes the stress itself in Selye's terminology). The secretion of almost every hormone in the body has been shown to manifest a relatively stereotyped response to many acute physical stresses and psychosocial stimuli, and we shall go into some of these later. On the other hand, the mushrooming research into stress physiology has also made it quite clear that the concept of a homogeneous totally nonspecific stress response is too simplistic. This was really predictable, for variability is the rule in biology, not the exception. The magnitudes of responses of the different hormones and their time courses may vary considerably depending upon the nature of the stimulus and may even change direction. For example, rage is almost always associated with increased activity of the sympathetic nervous system, whereas extreme fear, in some people, is accompanied by the inhibition of sympathetic nervous system activity which results in fainting. Even within the purely psychological realm, some degree of specificity almost certainly occurs. For example, there is some evidence for a dichotomy of responses, social interactions which lead to defeat and feelings of frustration and depression eliciting mainly activation of the adrenal cortex, whereas the sympathetic nervous system is called into play in situations associated with arousal and aggressive attempts to maintain status. Nevertheless, there is enough consistency in the general pattern of most stress responses to warrant survival of the concept of nonspecific stress responses and evaluation of the role these bodily changes play in health and disease.

The Fight-or-Flight Paradigm

Let us look first at the sympathetic nervous system. This communication system so consistently activated by stressful stimuli, both physical and psychosocial, consists of neurons (nerve cells) whose fibers leave the middle portions of the spinal cord and make contact with the cell bodies of second neurons, the fibers of which ramify throughout the body. They innervate glands, the heart, and the smooth muscles surrounding blood vessels, the gastrointestinal tract, the bladder, the pupils of the eyes, and still other components. The effects at all these sites are mediated by a chemical, norepinephrine (noradrenalin is a synonym), released from the terminals of the second nerve fibers. There is also a hormone-secreting (endocrine) component of the sympathetic nervous system—the adrenal medulla. There are two of these glands, both of which receive sympathetic nerve fibers from the spinal cord. In response to stimulation via these nerve fibers, the cells of the adrenal medulla release some norepinephrine (just like the second nerve fibers in the purely neural parts of the sympathetic system) but much more of a closely related substance called epinephrine (or adrenalin). This hormone, which exerts effects similar to those of norepinephrine, enters the blood flowing through the adrenal medulla, goes to the heart via the venous blood, and is pumped all over the body. So epinephrine released from the adrenal medulla exerts widespread effects whereas the individual sympathetic nerve fibers influence, via their released norepinephrine, only those structures they end upon.

This arrangement permits a good deal of specificity in the responses controlled by the sympathetic nervous system. For example, exposure to cold elicits, via the sympathetic nerves, profound constriction of the skin blood vessels, a specific homeostatic response which serves to conserve heat, but little increased sympathetic discharge to other blood vessels of the body. I point this out to emphasize that the sympathetic nervous system is one of the major mediators of specific homeostatic responses. Its much less specific, widespread activation by stress represents a quite different phenomenon. Thus, if the cold exposure is so severe as to become painful or frightening, then activation of the sympathetic nerves to other blood vessels, the heart, the gastrointestinal tract, etc., along with massive discharge of epinephrine from the adrenal medulla, may supervene.

What is the adaptive value of such a widespread activation? Walter Cannon's concept of fight-or-flight remains, to this day, an excellent explanatory paradigm. Table 7–1 is a list of the major effects resulting from a generalized increase in sympathetic activity; they constitute a splendid guide on how to prepare for emergencies. The heart's rate and force of contraction increases, resulting in the pumping of more blood; breathing is stimulated, providing more oxygen and eliminating carbon dioxide more rapidly; the blood vessels of the internal organs (like the gastrointestinal tract and kidneys) constrict while those going to skeletal muscles dilate, thereby distributing blood preferentially to the latter; the central nervous system is aroused, becoming more alert and responsive, and less cognizant of fatigue; both glycogen, the storage form of carbohydrate, and fat depots are broken down (to glucose and free fatty acids, respectively), supplying fuels for exercising skeletal muscles and preparing the body for a period of fasting (a fleeing or fighting animal obviously is not eating); the blood becomes more coagulable (mainly because of a change in blood platelets), reducing the potential for wound-induced blood loss.

The role of the increased adrenal cortical hormones released during stress also can be fitted to this paradigm, as is evident from Selye's terms—"alarm reaction" for the acute phase and "general adaptation syndrome" for the entire multistage responses he strove to identify. Before describing the actions of these hormones, we might take care of a few technical terms which may have already caused you some confusion. There are two adrenal glands, one sitting on top of each kidney, but each adrenal gland consists, itself, of two distinct glands, one surrounding the other. The inner gland is

TABLE 7–1   **Effects of Increased Activity of the Sympathetic Nervous System**

---

1. Increased pumping of blood by the heart
2. Stimulation of breathing
3. Redistribution of blood from internal organs to exercising muscles
4. "Arousal" of central nervous system and decreased perception of fatigue
5. Breakdown of carbohydrate and fat stores
6. Increased coagulability of the blood

the adrenal medulla, which, as we have seen, secretes mainly epinephrine. The outer gland, the adrenal cortex, is totally different in structure, and it secretes ring-structured lipid-soluble steroid hormones collectively known as adrenal corticosteroids.* The major ones are cortisol, aldosterone, and dehydroepiandrosterone. Cortisol (the public is more familiar with a commercially made substance, cortisone, which has essentially the same effects as cortisol and is often used therapeutically) has a large range of effects, many of which are related to the regulation of organic metabolism in general and glucose handling in particular; for this reason it is known as a glucocorticoid. Aldosterone controls the kidneys' excretion of sodium and potassium, and is termed a mineralocorticoid. Dehydroepiandrosterone is one of the family of hormones called androgens, all of which exert effects similar to its most potent member, the male sex hormone, testosterone. The adrenal cortex of both men and women secrete dehydroepiandrosterone; its effects in men are not important because they are dwarfed by testosterone, but in women, who make little or no testosterone, this hormone is important for growth, sexual drive, and possibly other bodily processes as well.

Cortisol is the classic "stress hormone" secreted by the adrenal cortex. (One more detail: Certain species of experimental animal, like rats, produce as their major glucocorticoid and stress hormone not cortisol but a closely related hormone called corticosterone which is made in only relatively small quantities by the human adrenal cortex. The effects of cortisol and corticosterone are so similar that much of what we presume concerning actions of cortisol in people has been gleaned from experiments actually involving corticosterone in other species.) The pathway by which cortisol secretion is increased by stressful stimuli is illustrated in figure 7–1. The immediate stimulus for its secretion is another hormone from the pituitary gland known appropriately as adrenocorticotropic hormone (ACTH, literally "hormone which stimulates the adrenal cortex"). The secretion of ACTH is regulated by yet another hormone produced by nerve cells in the hypothalamus, a small brain area at the base of the skull immediately above the front (anterior) portion

---

*For years, physiologists have puzzled as to why the adrenal medulla and cortex were packed together into a single gland. At least one reason now seems likely; some of the blood leaving the adrenal cortex flows into the adrenal medulla, and the major hormone (cortisol) secreted by the adrenal cortex in response to stress activates the key enzyme catalyzing the synthesis of epinephrine (from norepinephrine).

of the pituitary and connected to it by small blood vessels. This hormone, known as adrenocorticotropin-releasing hormone (CRH, for corticotropin releasing hormone), is released from the hypothalamic nerve cells into the small blood vessels which carry it directly to the pituitary. Obviously we are dealing with a chain of hormones—CRH → ACTH → cortisol—but the pathway is not yet complete since I have not given the first component, the input to the hypothalamus controlling the secretion of CRH. It constitutes mainly neural input from all parts of the body and this explains why many different physical and psychosocial stimuli can all elicit cortisol secretion. The neural pathway into the hypothalamus for any particular situation depends upon the nature of the stress— pain pathways in the response to trauma, visual pathways via brain association areas for the response to seeing one's enemy approaching with a gun, higher brain centers for the response to emotional distress, and so on. The destination is always the same, connections with the hypothalamic neurons which secrete CRH, and the hormonal chain then takes over—CRH stimulating the release of ACTH, which then stimulates the release of cortisol. The neuronal pathways converging on the hypothalamus to regulate CRH secretion also often give off branch pathways which connect

Fig. 7–1.   Pathway which controls the secretion of cortisol.

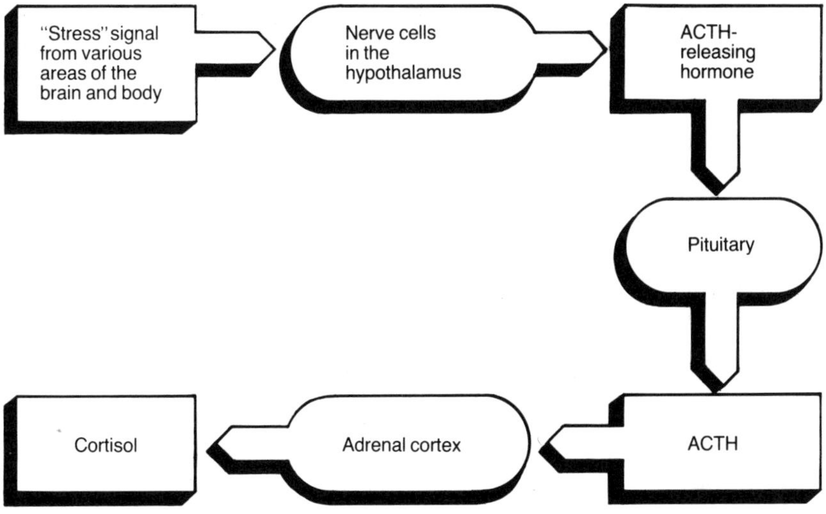

with the origins of the sympathetic nervous system, activating it at the same time.

What does the secreted cortisol actually do upon reaching its targets throughout the body? This hormone has a bewildering array of actions, many of which fit nicely into the "fight-or-flight" or "preparation for emergency" paradigm. It stimulates the catabolism of protein and the liberation of free amino acids into the blood; these amino acids can serve as a pool for protein synthesis elsewhere in the body, for example, in damaged tissues undergoing repair. In addition, many of these amino acids are converted by the liver into glucose which is then released into the blood. Thus cortisol, like epinephrine and norepinephrine, causes the blood glucose concentration to rise, although by a totally different mechanism. A second major way that cortisol raises blood glucose is by blocking its entry into various tissues (an anti-insulin action). Now this may seem antithetical to a fight-or-flight response, since you would imagine that it is maladaptive to prevent glucose from getting into muscle at a time when the muscle may require fuel for contraction. However, exercising muscle is not very much affected by cortisol (or any other hormone), and what is much more important, free fatty acids, not glucose, are the major fuel during prolonged exercise. Remember that the sympathetic neurons cause the mobilization of these fatty acids by stimulating the breakdown of fat deposits; cortisol greatly enhances this process by synergizing with epinephrine and norepinephrine at the level of the fat cells.

Cortisol has major effects other than those on organic metabolism. Indeed, pehaps the single most important of all cortisol's actions in stressful situations is to permit small blood vessels to remain partially constricted for long periods of time. A patient lacking cortisol and faced with even a moderate stress may develop low blood pressure and die if untreated. This is because, for unknown reasons, stress induces a tendency for small blood vessels throughout the body to dilate, despite the fact that increased activity of the sympathetic nerves is generally opposing this dilation, and only a high concentration of cortisol can prevent this tendency from becoming a reality. If it should occur, the blood pressure would fall because not enough blood would be retained in the large arteries, and blood flow to the brain and heart muscle would be drastically reduced with potentially lethal results. We don't know how it is that cortisol exerts this "permissive" effect on blood vessel smooth muscle, although at least a fraction of it may represent yet another synergism between it and the sympathetic nervous system. The really critical point is that the blood concentrations of cortisol which exist in the unstressed state are not adequate to get the job done when the same individual is stressed; thus, cortisol secretion must increase during stress for normal survival. The CRH-ACTH system, of course, mediates this increase.

I mentioned earlier that the secretion rates of hormones other than cortisol and epinephrine are frequently increased during stress, and several of these, too, make sense in terms of the fight-or-flight paradigm. Aldosterone, the other major adrenal corticosteroid, is increased (ACTH is probably the major stimulus for its increase during stress) and, by minimizing the urinary excretion of sodium, this hormone retains salt in the body and blood. Water is also retained because another hormone (vasopressin or antidiuretic hormone), produced by the hypothalamus, is secreted in large amounts and acts on the kidneys to cut down their excretion of water. These salt and water responses are adaptive in the face of potential fluid loss through sweating, tissue damage, or hemorrhage.

Two other hormones, both of which help regulate organic metabolism, are usually increased during stress: glucagon, a hormone secreted (like insulin) by the pancreas, and growth hormone by the pituitary. Both raise the blood glucose in several ways and facilitate the mobilization of fat stores, actions similar to those induced by epinephrine and cortisol. Insulin, which has precisely the opposite actions on blood glucose and fat mobilization, is either unchanged during stress or is decreased. The control of the secretion of both glucagon and insulin during stress offers a good example of neuroendocrine coordination; there is a rich supply of sympathetic neurons to the pancreatic cells secreting these two hormones, and increased activation of these neurons during stress stimulates the cells which secrete glucagon and inhibits those which release insulin. Growth hormone secretion is controlled by a hypothalamic-pituitary interaction analagous to that for ACTH.

There are still other hormones the secretion rates of which change during stress, but in these cases, we have real difficulty explaining the adaptive significance of the changes in terms of preparation for an emergency. Prolactin, the hormone which stimulates milk synthesis in lactating women (and whose function in men is unknown) is almost invariably elevated by stress, but for what conceivable reason? The male and female sex hormones, testosterone and estrogen, have not been studied much in persons subjected to stress, but what little evidence there is suggests that their blood concentrations are decreased. I'll return later (in the section on "crowding") to the question of how these changes might be adaptive.

Obiously, then, stressful stimuli elicit a host of neuroendocrine responses, and this might be a good time to summarize just which ones scientists tend to use as indicators that a stress response is actually occurring in the person or animal being studied. Looking only for changes in glucagon, growth hormone, aldosterone, vasopressin, or prolactin would not give a very good indication of stress since the secretion of all of these hormones, while responsive to stressful stimuli, is controlled mainly by other types of input (aldosterone by salt balance, glucagon by blood sugar, etc.). In contrast (and really by circular reasoning), physiologists have come to accept changes in the activity of the sympathetic nervous system and ACTH-cortisol pathway as being virtually synonymous with stress.

The most direct measures of the levels of activity in these two systems are the plasma concentrations of epinephrine, norepinephrine, and cortisol. The disadvantages of using these parameters are that they require blood sampling (itself a potential stress), and the chemical analyses are time-consuming and expensive. Moreover, in the case of the two sympathetic transmitters (which belong to the chemical family called catecholamines), the chemical analyses for them have, until recently, not been accurate enough for blood measurements (in contrast to urine). Finally, the plasma concentrations of these substances, like those of many other hormones, bounce around a good deal, often from minute to minute. Because of these problems, scientists more often use a timed urinary excretion of these substances or their metabolites as indicators of their secretion rates. Most of cortisol's metabolites are in a form known as 17-hydroxy-corticosteroids, and so this term appears frequently in the stress literature as an indicator of adrenal cortical secretory activity.

Once we move away from chemical measurements of hormones, neurotransmitters, or their metabolites, we are getting on somewhat shakier ground in inferring the presence of a stress response. Nevertheless, many other indicators are used, mainly because they are convenient, and are generally acceptable as components of the stress response. Some of these are the results of increased sympathetic activity: increased heart rate, blood pressure, pupil diameter, blood concentrations of lactate, cholesterol, and free fatty acids. Another indication of enhanced sympathetic activity is the so-called galvanic skin response (GSR), which measures changes in the ease with which electric current can flow through the skin; it is familiar to us as the lie detector. Two small wires are placed on the skin of the hand or forearm, and an extremely small electrical current is passed between them; when the sympathetic nerves to the skin become more active, the needle on the recording apparatus deflects downward (the precise reason for the change in current flow is still debated).

Another indicator of arousal is the appearance of particular brain wave patterns in the electroencephalogram (EEG). Also, since stress often causes people to tense their muscles, electrical changes in muscle (EMG) may be used as a marker.

Beyond Fight-or-Flight: Stress and Learning

To reiterate, the fight-or-flight or "preparation for emergency" concepts have proven quite useful in analyzing the adaptive value of the neuroendocrine responses to psychosocial stress. However, the psychosocial situations which elicit the stress response are so varied that one becomes uncomfortable in pushing the use of this paradigm too far.

Look, for example, at table 7–2, a partial listing of the large number of psychosocial situations known to elicit increased secretion of cortisol (or corticosterone, in rats) as evidenced by increases either in plasma concentrations of the hormone or the urinary excretion of its metabolites. With few exceptions, the same list would apply to the sympathetic nervous system. Note that many of these situations certainly are threatening or could be perceived as such, but many others simply don't fit this description. Many are so benign that the very term "stress" seems inappropriate, and the neutral term "stimulus" is preferable. For example, adrenocortical activity, in both people and animals, tends to be decreased on weekends. This is true for people even when the person is not, himself, working on the weekdays but is merely exposed to others who are; for example, a hospitalized patient experienced a drop in his adrenocortical secretion every weekend when he was transferred from a busy surgical ward to a quiet hospital across the street. Presumably, just the hustle and bustle of the work place (or the animal housing quarters, with its constant comings and goings of

TABLE 7–2   Psychosocial Situations Shown to be Associated with Increased Plasma Concentration or Urinary Excretion of Adrenal Cortical Steroids

Experimental animals

1. Any "first experience" characterized by novelty, uncertainty, or unpredictability.
2. Conditioned emotional responses; anticipation of something previously experienced as unpleasant.
3. Involvement in situations in which the animal must master a difficult task in order to avoid or forestall aversive stimuli. The animal must really be "trying."
4. Situations in which long-standing rules are suddenly changed so that previous behavior is no longer effective in achieving a goal.
5. Socially subordinate animals. (Dominant animals have decreased cortisol.)
6. Crowding (increased social interactions).
7. Fighting or merely observing other animals fighting.

Human beings

I. Normal persons
   A. Acute situations
      1. Aircraft flight
      2. Awaiting surgical operation
      3. Final exams (college students)
      4. Novel situations
      5. Competitive athletics
      6. Anticipation of exposure to cold
      7. Workdays, compared to weekends
      8. Many job experiences
   B. Chronic life situations
      1. Predictable personality-behavior profile: aggressive, ambitious, time-urgency
      2. Discrepancy between levels of aspiration and achievement
   C. Experimental techniques
      1. "Stress" or "shame" interview
      2. Many motion pictures
II. Psychiatric patients
   A. Acute anxiety
   B. Depression, but only when patient is aware of and involved in a struggle with it

Source: A. J. Vander, J. H. Sherman, and D. S. Luciano. *Human Physiology: The Mechanisms of Body Function,* 3d ed. (New York; McGraw-Hill, 1980).

personnel, cleaning of cages, etc.) is adequate to stimulate the hypothalamic-pituitary-adrenal pathway. In one experiment, rhesus monkeys were being housed in individual cages in the same room; when the cages were simply removed to separate rooms, adrenocortical secretion decreased.

Moreover, the evidence is that the "weekend-weekday" phenomenon does not reflect the pleasantness or unpleasantness of the subject's work. Indeed, there is clear-cut evidence that many stimuli which elicit a classic "stress" response are not at all distressing to the individual but are highly enjoyable. For example, simply watching the delightful musical comedy, "Charley's Aunt" caused a considerable rise in epinephrine secretion similar (although smaller in magnitude) to that induced by movies producing fear, anger, or frustration in viewers.[1]

Hans Selye has made much of this.*

> From the point of view of its stress-producing or stressor activity, *it is immaterial* whether the agent or *situation we face is pleasant or unpleasant* [Selye's emphasis]; all that counts is the intensity of the demand for readjustment or adaptation. The mother who is suddenly told that her only son died in battle suffers a terrible mental shock. If years later it turns out that the news was false and the son unexpectedly walks into her room alive and well, she experiences extreme joy. The specific results of the two events, sorrow and joy, are completely different, in fact opposite to each other, yet their stressor effect—the nonspecific demand to readjust herself to an entirely new situation—may be the same.[2]

Certainly "new situations"—environmental change and novelty—runs as a common thread through many of the items listed in table 7–2. Another such thread is lack of environmental "clarity," i.e., uncertainty as to one's position, of what is to happen, or the appropriateness of one's responses. Obviously, uncertainty and change are closely related and a combination of the two has been shown over and over again to constitute a potent inducer of stress responses. For example, in experiments designed to study stress responses, the investigators must keep in mind that plasma cortisol will inevitably be elevated during the subject's first session, even when it is a benign interview. This elevation can be minimized by providing the subject in advance with as complete information as possible about the experiment.

As important as are psychosocial stimuli per se, and the characteristics of novelty, change, and uncertainty, the presence of another ingredient seems to be critical for determining the magnitude of the stress response—the individual's degree of involvement in the social

---

*Based on the viewpoint that "stress is the nonspecific response of the body to any demand made upon it" Selye had advocated use of the term "distress" to denote damaging or unpleasant stress, but this suggestion has not really caught on.

environment, and how much he is trying to cope with the situation. Indeed, John Mason and Joseph V. Brady, two of the major workers in the field of stress responses and psychosomatic disease, believe that the degree of adrenal cortical activity serves "as a general index of interaction or involvement of the animal with the physical and social environment."[3] In the same vein, Mason has emphasized that increased adrenocortical activity is not related to any specific affective state such as anxiety but "appears to reflect a relatively undifferentiated state of emotional arousal or involvement, perhaps in anticipation of activity or coping."[4]

This view nicely states present thinking concerning the double function of the physiological responses to psychosocial stimuli; these responses prepare the organism for increased physical activity (the fight-or-flight paradigm) but also for the mental processes required for immediate coping with an altered social environment and for the learning of new responses.

The idea that mental processes are influenced by the neuroendocrine responses to psychosocial stress has always been a dominant theme in our view of the role of epinephrine and the sympathetic nervous system. We know that, in positive feedback fashion, increased arousal enhances epinephrine secretion which, in turn, further increases the state of arousal. We know also that the presence of an increased blood level of epinephrine is associated with better performance of a variety of tasks, particularly those which are repetitive or monotonous.

The really new insights came when trying to ascertain just what adaptive effects the pituitary-adrenal system might exert on brain function and coping. Several animal studies had shown that cortisol could strongly influence electrical activity in the brain and is preferentially taken up by nerve cells in those areas of the brain having to do with memory and motivation. It was irresistible to hypothesize that activation of the pituitary-adrenal system associated with psychosocial stimuli might facilitate learning of the behaviors appropriate for coping with the situations that had elicited the hormonal response. This hypothesis is now being intensively studied in many laboratories and although the details still remain unclear, a general outline is emerging (at least for rats). I'll describe just a few of these fascinating experiments.[5]

Perhaps the first direct evidence that the pituitary-adrenal system is involved in behavior was obtained about twenty-five years ago in studies of the learning of an avoidance response by rats. The animals were placed in a box divided into two compartments by a barrier, which had to be crossed in order for the animal to avoid or terminate a shock announced by a buzzer. The learning period of such a response is characterized by a marked increase in pituitary-adrenal secretions (stress response). Animals whose pituitaries had been surgically removed were found to have great difficulty learning this "active avoidance" response, a defect completely eliminated by the injection into them of ACTH. In addition, this pituitary hormone had a profound effect on the "extinction" of active avoidance responses, the time it takes for the animal to stop crossing the barrier when the cue (the buzzer) is presented but no longer followed by the shock. Extinction is normally associated, just as is the original learning of the response, with increased activity of the pituitary-adrenal system, and animals lacking a pituitary were found to extinguish learned active avoidance responses very rapidly. In contrast, ACTH injections greatly delayed the rate of extinction. Thus, animals lacking ACTH learned slowly and "forgot" or "unlearned" quickly.

Since physiologists have always assumed that the only action of ACTH in the body is to stimulate the secretion of cortisol (or corticosterone in the rat), it was logical for them to hypothesize that the effects ascribed to ACTH in these experiments were really due to the glucocorticoid. However, much to their surprise, they found that ACTH still produced these effects on learning and memory in animals from whom the adrenal cortex had been removed. Moreover, administration of corticosterone rather than ACTH did not enhance learning and actually speeded, rather than delayed, extinction. Clearly, the actions of ACTH on learning and memory are not due to its stimulation of the adrenal cortex but seem to be direct actions on the brain. (Just how ACTH and cortisol, which normally both rise together in response to psychosocial stress, interact to influence the rate of extinction in intact organisms is still unclear.) The actual way in which ACTH facilitates learning and prolongs memory retention (this is what slow extinction implies) seems to be by improving the animal's attention, perhaps by increasing the motivational value of external cues.

This same approach has been applied to other hormones known

to increase during psychosocial stimuli. The most striking finding has been that vasopressin also has effects on memory retention. Unlike the situation for ACTH, animals lacking vasopressin have little difficulty learning a conditioned avoidance response but their ability to remember the response for even four hours is markedly impaired. Surprises like this are one of the joys of research, for here is a hormone which has been assumed to have a single function—the regulation of urinary water excretion—but which now turns out to be intimately involved in memory retention of the behaviors required for coping with psychosocial stimuli.

For obvious reasons, the study of these types of effects in human beings is difficult, but what data do exist indicate a close correspondence with the rat results. For example, injections of ACTH into people improve visual memory (but not verbal, a finding which suggests a considerable degree of specificity and complexity to these hormonal influences), prolongs the EEG pattern typical of increased alertness, and improves performance of a repetitive task. Perhaps most exciting is the finding, not subject to study in rats, that the administration of ACTH decreases the anxiety of subjects during the learning of new material.

In summary, to quote one of the pioneers in this field:

> It appears that ACTH and vasopressin . . . are involved in the registration, consolidation, and retrieval of information that the organism uses in selecting the most appropriate response to environmental change.[6]

In addition to these effects on learning and memory, the hormones of the pituitary-adrenal system and the adrenal medulla are being studied for still other possible effects on brain function, particularly on emotions. For many years, scientists had attempted to determine whether increased plasma concentrations of epinephrine induce not only nonspecific arousal but specific emotions as well. Almost all the evidence indicates that it does not. Epinephrine seems to intensify whatever emotions a social situation elicits, but does not itself play a role in determining just which emotions that will be (happiness, sadness, aggressiveness, etc.). The story for the pituitary-adrenal system is much less clear. Most interest has centered on the role ACTH and the adrenocorticoids might play in enhancing agressive behavior, but we simply know too little at the moment to draw any conclusions.

The Interaction of Personality and Social Environment

A raw list such as that shown in table 7–2 can be quite misleading since it implies a simple cause and effect relationship between a psychosocial stimulus and a physiological response. The fact is, of course, that psychosocial stimuli do not trigger responses in the straightforward quantitative way that a low temperature induces shivering or a low oxygen environment increases breathing. Rather, the magnitude of our physiological response to a psychosocial stimulus depends on our perception, both conscious and unconscious, of its significance to us, on our past conditioning and personality, and on the setting in which it occurs. These are, of course, not discrete entities, but are closely interwoven.

It is a truism that what is stressful to individual A may not bother individual B at all (and might not bother A either if it were to occur in a different setting). Winston Churchill wrote in his memoirs that, after being notified that he had just been appointed Prime Minister, he went to bed and slept soundly for the first time in years. Stress for Mr. Churchill was being out of power, whereas most of us would have been exceedingly stressed by having to bear the responsibility for our country's fate during war. This has certainly been documented for much lesser degrees of responsibility. For example, adrenocorticoid secretion by pilots of two-man jet aircraft crews is much larger than that of the passive radiomen. The secretion of these adrenal hormones was also higher for officers than for enlisted men during a time of anticipated Viet Cong attack in Vietnam.

A good general overview of the interaction of social environment and individual characteristics like personality has been given by Stewart Kiritz and Rudolf H. Moos.

> Social stimuli do not act directly on the individual. Rather, it is his perception of the social environment, as mediated by personality variables, role and status relationships, and his behavior within the environment, which affects him directly, and which in turn affects his personality and behavior.
>
> There are two main ways in which individual and social environmental variables can interact, leading to different physiological responses.
>
> (1) Given the same social environment, two individuals may perceive different levels of the same dimension. For example, a paranoid person might . . . perceive little support in an office seen as very supportive by his less suspicious coworkers . . .

Given similar perceptions, two individuals may still differ in their . . . responses to these perceptions. Person A and person B, for example, work in an office which both perceive as offering little support. Person A has a loving wife and children, many friends, and a history of interpersonal successes. Person B is recently divorced and has long regarded himself as an interpersonal failure. It is likely that A and B would differ in their . . . responses to the office environment and in their resources for coping with or defending against the emotions aroused.

In practice it is often difficult or impossible to distinguish the operation of an individual's perceptions of a situation from his defenses or coping strategies.[7]

These defenses, particularly denial, are extremely important in determining the magnitude of the stress response to any given situation. One of the most famous illustrations of this is a study of 17-hydroxycorticosteroid excretion in women with breast tumors awaiting biopsy which would reveal whether the tumor was benign or cancerous. These women were extensively interviewed and their "ego defenses" were categorized. Those who used one of the patterns classified as "stoicism-fatalism," "prayer and faith," and "denial with rationalization" experienced relatively little increase in their secretion of adrenocortical hormones, in contrast to those women who had fewer defenses.

Mason has drawn the conclusion from many such studies that we have paid too much attention to "situational criteria of 'stress' and [to] mean group values, with a relative lack of systematic evaluation of the important and often marked individual differences between subjects in their emotional and defensive reactions to a given situation."[8]

I have stressed this point because it has great significance for our subsequent discussion of the evidence for psychosocial stress being a risk factor for various diseases, and I shall deal with more environment-personality interactions in that context.

Habituation and Adaptation

These two phenomena also are important in any analysis of stress and disease. As we shall see, many stress-disease theories have as their fundamental assumption the idea that the usual physiological responses to stress, if induced over and over again for long periods of time, lead to disease. The problem is that the vast majority of information concerning the nature of physiological stress responses and the social environments which elicit them in people are based on acute (short-term) studies, and predictions concerning long-term responses to these situations are quite tenuous.

One reason is habituation, the reduction in response which occurs with continuous or repeated exposure to a particular stimulus. That habituation of physiological responses to stressful stimuli occurs has been documented in a very large number of different situations for both people and animals. This is precisely what one would expect as the uncertainty and novelty of the stimulus wears off and as one's ability to shut it out or cope with it increases.

But one cannot always assume that habituation will occur. Indeed, precisely the opposite event may happen, a type of acclimatization or adaptation which is manifested as a more rapidly occurring and larger response to the stimulus. For example, mice exposed to a chronic housing situation which prevents formation of a stable dominance-subordinance hierarchy and enhances interanimal encounters develop an increased activity of the adrenal medullary enzyme which catalyzes the synthesis of epinephrine, leading to a chronic hyperresponsiveness of this hormonal system to subsequent stresses.

The Effects of Stress in Early Infancy

Almost all experiences of infancy involve some handling by a parent or some other larger and supremely powerful figure. Even the tenderest handling must at times be the occasion of emotional stress. . . . In the ordinary world the infant must grow under the changing pressures and sudden challenges of an inconstant environment. One may well wonder how the stressful experiences of infancy affect the behavior and physiology of the adult organism later on.[9]

Dr. Levine proceeded to investigate this question and his findings and those of others in the field offer an excellent illustration of the "critical periods" concept. The basic design of his experiments was quite simple; one group of infant rats was subjected to a variety of stresses and degrees of handling, whereas a second group was left in the nest throughout infancy and never handled by the investigators at all. At first, the manipulated infants were subjected to mild daily electric shocks but it was ultimately found that simply picking up the animals and handling them very gently was enough to bring out the striking differences, both behavioral and physiological, between them and the unhandled group when they were tested as adults.

When placed in unfamiliar surroundings, the previously nonmanipulated rats usually crowded in a corner of the box or crept timidly about, defecating and urinating frequently, signs physiological psychologists interpret as increased "emotionality" and stress. In contrast, the manipulated rats tended to explore the area much more freely and to urinate and defecate much less. Not surprisingly, they learned to run a maze for reward more readily than the unmanipulated group.

Their hormonal responses also differed. First of all, the pituitary-adrenal system could be activated by stressful stimuli at an earlier age in the manipulated animals and secondly, during adult life, it responded more rapidly. Thus, the critical-periods development of adaptive responses to stress in both the behavioral and physiological realms seems to depend on the presence of some minimal level of stress during infancy.* If these results can be extrapolated at all to human beings (which is suggested by some observations of children raised in orphanages or other institutions), it is a further reminder that stress should not be viewed as an unmitigated evil. Just as we saw in the previous sections, some level of stress response to psychosocial stimuli is not only normal but is highly adaptive. The real question concerns not stress per se, but its quality and quantity as well as our perception of it.

Psychosocial Stress and Disease

Given these basic ideas about normal responses to psychosocial stress, we now turn to their possible pathophysiological implications and to the field of psychosomatic medicine. This last term, which is often misinterpreted to mean that "the disease is all in your head," might better be replaced by the more cumbersome title, "psychological factors in the causation of disease." The diseases subsumed under this heading are not in the person's "head," but represent true physical and chemical changes, damage to organs

---

*There is, at least at first thought, a problem in logic in these experiments, as illustrated by Dr. Levine's own original expectations. He had presumed that the unhandled rats would be the "normal" ones (since it is surely not a normal part of a rat's development to be picked up by a human being, handled, or electrically shocked) and that the manipulated infants would show signs of emotional disorder when they reached adulthood. When the findings turned out to be exactly opposite, Dr. Levine took the position, which makes good sense, that animals raised in the laboratory with its controlled temperature, humidity, light etc., the limited space within the cage for exploration or being carried by the mother, are really understressed compared to the normal situation in nature.

and tissues which results in illness and death. Based on the recognition that all diseases have multiple causes, the field of psychosomatic medicine asks the question: Are there physical diseases (hypertension, coronary artery disease, cancer, gastric ulcers, etc.) in which psychological factors help generate the observable anatomic and chemical changes in the body that are typical for the diseases? The evidence to be described in subsequent sections strongly suggests that there are, indeed, such diseases, and so the next question is: What are the intervening physiological links between the stress and the malfunction or disease?

One possible chain of events is usually visualized as illustrated in figure 7–2. This concept holds that the anatomical and chemical changes characteristic of the disease are due to a long-term excessive generalized stress response triggered by chronic continuous or intermittent stress. The known effects of increased sympathetic activity and very large amounts of cortisol make this concept so plausible that many people often treat its validity as a foregone conclusion. Before pointing out the problems and assumptions in this theory, let me use several examples to show just how seductive it is.

Let's look at coronary heart disease, asking the question: How might one explain the development of this disease in terms of the

Fig. 7–2.   Hypothesized pathway from stress to disease.

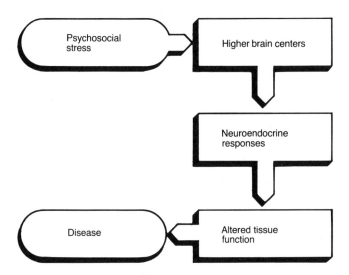

known effects of increased sympathetic nervous system activity? Figure 7–3 provides a guide for this description. First, we have already seen that increased sympathetic activity mobilizes fatty acids from fat stores, and this leads ultimately to enhanced synthesis of cholesterol by the liver and an increased plasma cholesterol. Second, increased sympathetic activity speeds the heart and increases the force of contraction, both of which increase the amount of blood pumped per unit time (the cardiac output). Third, it causes most small blood vessels to constrict, which impedes runoff of blood from the large arteries. This combination of increased cardiac output and decreased ease of runoff raises the arterial blood pressure, i.e., causes hypertension. Now we have two of the major known risk factors for atherosclerosis and coronary heart disease—increased blood cholesterol and hypertension. Add to these the increased coagulability of the blood caused by increased levels of epinephrine and you have the stage set for rapidly progressive narrowing of the coronary blood vessels by atherosclerotic deposits and clots. Moreover, in addition to the narrowing due to atherosclerosis, the coronary vessels might be further narrowed by a direct constrictor-producing effect of the sympathetic nerves supplying them (this is a hotly debated question among physiologists who study the coronary blood vessels, and it is still not clear whether the sympathetic nerves to these particular vessels ever do cause significant constriction).

Narrowing of the coronary vessels through atherosclerosis (and, possibly, direct constriction) is not the only way in which increased sympathetic activity could predispose to an outright heart attack. The heart does not actually suffer damage from atherosclerotic narrowing of the coronary vessels until its blood supply becomes inadequate to supply its metabolic requirements, i.e., to supply enough oxygen and nutrients to permit normal contraction by the heart muscle. Increased sympathetic activity can upset the balance between supply and demand not only by reducing the former (through vessel narrowing) but by enhancing the latter, i.e., elevating the work of the heart, which it does in two ways. First, a direct action on the heart muscle to increase force of contraction raises the requirement for oxygen; second, by increasing arterial blood pressure (as described above), it forces the heart muscle to pump against a higher pressure, and this increased work also requires more oxygen.

The combination of narrowed vessels (reduced blood supply) and

Fig. 7–3. Pathways by which increased activity of the sympathetic nervous system could lead to fibrillation of the heart and death.

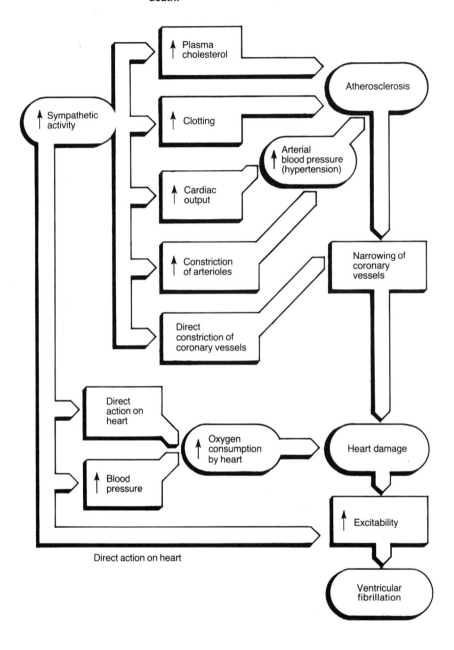

increased work (increased requirements for blood) is obviously ideal for the production of cardiac damage, temporary as in angina pectoris, or permanent as in a myocardial infarction (heart attack). One more action of the sympathetic nerves to the heart explains how the chances that a heart attack will be lethal can be enhanced. Damage, per se, causes the heart to be more excitable and to be susceptible to development of fatal ventricular fibrillation, and the sympathetic nerves act directly on the heart to raise excitability even more.

To summarize, this entire scenario is divisible into two components—a chronic phase characterized by slowly progressing atherosclerosis and an acute episode in which the effects of the sympathetic nerves on cardiac work triggers the actual heart attack and the effect on excitability makes it more likely to be lethal. Indeed, some have hypothesized that, if intense enough, increased sympathetic activity might induce ventricular fibrillation in a heart free of atherosclerosis.

Just because all this seems so logical is no reason to abandon our usual skepticism and not demand scientific proof that it really occurs. Do people who seem to be under chronic stress really have continuously hyperactive sympathetic nervous systems, or do they habituate? Even if some hyperactivity does persist, are the levels adequate to produce atherosclerosis or ventricular fibrillation? Remember that physiological studies of the effects of directly increasing sympathetic activity are almost all short-term, and we are not justified in drawing conclusions concerning the long-term effects from such data.

When we turn to cortisol, we encounter an equally seductive picture, this time not just applicable to hypertension and coronary heart disease but to almost every major disease. This is because very large amounts of cortisol are known to produce an extraordinary array of effects quite different from the physiological ones described earlier. But before tackling these so-called pharmacological effects, let us look at the physiological ones in the way we just looked at those of the sympathetic nervous system, asking the question: What diseases might we expect chronically elevated blood concentrations of cortisol to produce or worsen?

Certainly the most obvious disease is diabetes. As we have seen, cortisol raises the blood glucose concentration both by facilitating glucose formation (by the liver) and by blocking the sugar's entry into cells. There is no question that acute stress, whether physical or psychosocial, worsens the symptoms of diabetes, partly because of cortisol's effects and partly because several of the other hormones released during stress (epinephrine, glucagon, and growth hormone) also all tend to raise plasma glucose.

The second category of problems one would expect to be associated with an elevated plasma cortisol is that of protein breakdown. Cortisol's normal physiological effect is to facilitate the catabolism of protein, and mainly for this reason, any person subjected to severe physical stress, such as a major operation, will go, during that period, into negative nitrogen balance, i.e., will break down more protein than he simultaneously builds up.

Unlike the situation for the sympathetic nervous system, there is a great deal of information concerning the consequences of long-term marked elevations of plasma cortisol, not due to stress but to situations which, we have always presumed, produced cortisol levels in considerable excess of those achievable during chronic stress. Patients with excessively hyperactive adrenal cortexes (there are several causes of this disease, including adrenal tumors) represent one such situation, but the much more common occurrence is that of hormone administration for medical purposes. Both groups of patients manifest just what one might predict—a tendency toward diabetes, bone breakdown (the framework of bone is protein), muscle weakness, capillary fragility, poor growth in children, and other signs and symptoms of protein loss. (I must emphasize that not all patients receiving corticosteroids for medical purposes manifest all of these effects or the ones to be described subsequently, and to avoid them as much as possible, the physician keeps the dose as low as is consistent with the therapeutic purpose.)

In addition to these effects predictable from cortisol's physiology, such patients also manifest one or more effects collectively called pharmacological effects because they presumably occur only at levels of cortisol not seen in a normal person ("physiological"). The most all-encompassing is a profound reduction in the body's responses to foreign matter, i.e., in its immune responses to injury, infection, and transplants. To achieve just such an effect is the major reason that patients are given large amounts of steroids. The rationale for trying to block the body's immune responses in a person who is bearing a transplanted kidney is obvious, but why try to do so in other persons? The reason is that many diseases, including allergy and certain forms of arthritis, really represent the body's maladaptive response to relatively or completely harmless foreign substances. The symptoms of hay fever are due entirely to the body's overzealous and inappropriate attack launched against the otherwise innocuous ragweed pollen. Many other diseases represent the body's failure to recognize its own tissues and organs as "self," which leads to attempted self-destruction by way of the immune system. In all these situations large amounts of cortisol have been found to block many of the steps in the body's attack (for example, the production of antibodies) and so to minimize damage.

This is all fine and good, but there is a price to be paid. Any patient receiving (or producing on his own, because of abnormally hyperactive adrenal glands) pharmacological amounts of cortisol will show a decrease in resistance to both infection and cancer, since these disease groups are opposed by the same immune responses which the cortisol is inhibiting. Thus, increased incidences of infection and cancer must be added to diabetes and protein breakdown in our list of diseases caused by extremely large amounts of cortisol.

There are still others. Abnormally large ("pharmacological") amounts of cortisol decrease the resistance of the gastric mucosa to the damaging effects of the highly acid gastric secretions, the result being increased incidence of ulcers. They facilitate the development of hypertension and atherosclerosis (by unknown mechanisms). They cause personality changes, sometimes frank psychosis. They interfere with normal reproductive cycles in women, often resulting in sterility.

What a list! Its correspondence to the major causes of serious illness and death in industrialized countries makes it impossible not to speculate about the possible role of psychosocial stress, acting by means of increased cortisol, in all these diseases. However, we do not know whether the levels of cortisol which occur spontaneously in stress are large enough to produce these pharmacological effects nor do we have any really solid information about long-term patterns of blood cortisol (or any other hormone) in persons suffering from these diseases. Such studies are certainly deserving of a high priority in our attempts to track down the causes of our major "killer" diseases. Several of those already performed are certainly quite intriguing. For example, we shall see later that bereavement is one psychosocial situation strongly associated with an increased incidence of disease, and it has been reported that function of certain cells which mediate tissue rejection and cancer defenses is significantly depressed in persons mourning the loss of a spouse.

The same game we have played with the sympathetic nervous system and cortisol applies to the other neuroendocrine responses to stress. A logical case can be built for invoking a role for stress-induced increases in glucagon and growth hormone in the exacerbation of diabetes; for aldosterone and vasopressin, the hormones which cause retention of sodium and water, in hypertension; for disordered secretion of testosterone and estrogen in reproductive failure; for many hormones, such as ACTH, in behavioral and learning abnormalities. The list can be extended well beyond these possibilities, but the sticking point is always the same—there are simply too few hard facts concerning chronic dose-response relationships and actual hormonal measurements in persons suffering from these diseases to permit evaluation of these highly appealing speculations.

Before we leave this particular approach to psychosomatic medicine—one which postulates that the neuroendocrine components of the generalized stress response provides the intervening links between psychosocial stress and the actual physiological malfunctions—I'd like to point out a general theoretical criticism of the overall concept, one having to do with the question of specificity. If stress calls forth a relatively nonspecific physiological response, how can this account for the specific nature of the diseases which people actually develop? Why do some get hypertension and others cancer? Why do some get gastric ulcers and others heart attacks? Hans Selye, an adamant believer in the "general stress response" concept of psychosomatic disease,* has tried to explain specificity in terms of "conditioning factors" which can selectively enhance or inhibit one or the other stress effect. Such conditioning, he believes, may be internal (genetic predisposition, age, or sex) or external (dietary factors, for example). Moreover, since different stresses produce diverse specific effects, in addition to their nonspecific stress response, there is the opportunity for interaction between the two in selectively affecting the predisposed body area.

---

*A question which ought to be of considerable interest to historians or sociologists of science is why physiologists and clinicians have generally paid much less attention to Selye's views than have psychologists and the general public. At least one reason is that he has tended to blur the distinction between fact and theory in advocating the view that stress causes disease. He is quite certain, for example, that cortisol, in the amounts released during stress, exerts many, if not all, of the so-called pharmacological effects described earlier, despite the almost complete lack of evidence for or against this dose-response assumption.

More recently, another quite different explanation of specificity has emerged, one what deemphasizes the general stress response and focuses on discrete neuroendocrine links which are thought to be elicited preferentially because of learned or conditioned responses to stress. The theoretical base for this theory (and an entirely new concept of the control of bodily functions) was provided by the demonstration that "involuntary" neuroendocrine responses (such as the speeding up of the heart due to increased sympathetic activity, or increased secretion of insulin in response to elevated blood glucose) can be influenced by rewards or punishments, i.e., by operant conditioning. For example, rats could be "taught" to raise their blood pressure simply by rewarding them with food whenever their blood pressure spontaneously rose, as occurs over and over during the course of several hours. The rats, of course, were not conscious of the fact that their blood pressure had risen or that such a rise constituted the reason for the reward, but nonetheless, their blood pressure soon became permanently increased.

A high degree of specificity could be produced in these experiments. The rat could be conditioned to raise the blood flow in one ear but lower it in the other (responses presumably mediated by inhibiting or activating, respectively, the sympathetic nerves to the blood vessels of the two ears), raise or lower its urine flow (presumably by altering vasopressin secretion), and so on.

The original experimenters in this field believed they had demonstrated conclusively that such learning could not be an indirect result of the animals' simply relaxing or contracting their skeletal muscles, which, of course, are under voluntary control, but their experiments (utilizing complete drug-induced paralysis of all the animal's skeletal muscles during the learning period) have been very difficult to replicate. Nonetheless, whether the animal's (or person's) control over neuroendocrine function is direct or indirect, the fact is that some form of voluntary control is being exerted.

Researchers in this area (dubbed "biofeedback") have accumulated considerable data indicating that a large number of autonomic (sympathetic and parasympathetic nervous systems) and endocrine functions are, at least to some extent, subject to influence by operant conditioning. It is easy to imagine (but probably impossible to prove!) that a specific physiological response may have been "learned" because its occurrence was unknowingly rewarded, and so it occurs frequently, with possible consequences for disease induction. Whether or not such processes really contribute to the development of psychosomatic diseases, operant conditioning in the form of biofeedback offers a potential mode of therapy for persons suffering from a variety of diseases. For example, many physicians are experimenting with "teaching" hypertensive patients to reduce their blood pressure.

Now with all this discussion of possible mediating physiological links, we have become quite diverted from the central question of psychosomatic medicine which opened this section: Does psychosocial stress play a causal role in the development of physical diseases? The truth is that the validation of this hypothesis in no way depends upon elucidation of what the actual sequence of events might be between the psychosocial stress and the disease. If we know that persons seemingly under stress do, in fact, have consistently elevated activity of their sympathetic nervous systems, we might feel more comfortable with the hypothesis that such persons are more likely to develop coronary heart disease, but such evidence would not prove the hypothesis. By the same token, demonstration that chronically stressed persons do not have increased activity of the sympathetic nervous system would in no way disprove a stress-disease causal link but would only indicate that if such a link does exist, the sympathetic nervous system is not the intermediating variable forging it.

In a sense, then, I have tackled the question backward by describing potential mechanisms linking stress and disease before establishing that there is any link to be explained by a mechanism. What kinds of evidence, then, are required to establish a causal role for stress in disease, regardless of what the physiologic mechanisms might be? The answer, of course, is controlled laboratory animal experiments which attempt to produce physical disease by subjecting animals to psychosocial stress, epidemiological studies which try to associate stress and disease in human populations, and controlled human experiments in which an attempt is made to cure or prevent diseases by reducing the degree of stress to which persons are exposed.

Animal Experiments

There is absolutely no question that psychosocial stress, alone, can induce lethal diseases in experimental animals: hypertension, coronary heart disease, strokes, gastric ulcers, and kidney failure. Moreover, stress can greatly enhance the disease-producing potential of bacteria and viruses, including those that cause cancer in experimental animals. It is far beyond the scope of this chapter to describe all the studies upon which these statements are based, and I'll just pick out a few of the most important.[10]

A methodological problem that plagues this area of research is the difficulty of finding a meaningful form of psychosocial stress for the animals being studied, one which will not incorporate physical stresses as well. For example, one technique, which might be called the "triple threat," exposes animals to varying combinations of cage vibrations, flashing bright lights, and intermittent loud noises. This technique has been effective in eliciting the entire list of diseases given at the beginning of this section, and there is no question that the environmental stimuli used are stresses; however, separation of the physical stresses from any psychosocial ones in this technique is impossible, so that it really does not validate a role for purely psychosocial stress.

This same problem applies to several other techniques such as simply shocking animals intermittently. One way to minimize any effect of the shocks, per se, is to use classic Pavlovian conditioning methods. For example, at first a buzzer is sounded, followed by a shock to the animal; after a short conditioning period, the shock need not be delivered (except on a few occasions so as to maintain the conditioned associations), since the buzzer alone elicits the stress response. Pavlovian conditioning techniques like this have not been very useful in producing either sustained physiological responses or disease, because animals tend to habituate very rapidly to the situation.

Operant conditioning techniques are generally more effective than Pavlovian in minimizing habituation and in producing disease. They are usually of the shock avoidance type, in which, typically, a signal is delivered (a light or buzzer), following which the animal is shocked unless it presses a lever a certain number of times, upon which the signal is turned off, the lever reset, and the entire sequence repeated. The animal soon learns to make the appropriate response so that it receives very few shocks and it is assumed that any disease which develops more frequently in such animals, compared to controls, is the result of the psychological stress associated with this demanding task.

Shock avoidance techniques are presently being used to study the role of stress in the development of a variety of diseases in several species of animals. For example, monkeys fed an atherogenic diet were required over a period of twenty-five months (one hour/day, five days/week) to press a lever every thirty to fifty seconds to avoid a shock; compared to a control group fed the same diet but not exposed to the shock avoidance protocol, these animals developed higher plasma cholesterol concentrations and much more extensive coronary atherosclerosis.

A variant of the shock avoidance experiment, one which controls completely for any disease-producing effects of the shocks themselves, is the "yoked-partners" method. The most famous of these experiments, one which really caught the public's imagination, was performed many years ago by Joseph V. Brady and his colleagues, using monkeys who were paired so that when one received a shock, the other did also. One animal of the pair, the "executive" monkey, could prevent both of them from being shocked by pressing a lever approximately once every twenty seconds, as long as the red light marking the test period remained on. After a time, the executive monkeys developed severe gastrointestinal ulcers and died, whereas the yoked animals, who received precisely the same number of shocks but could do absolutely nothing to avoid them, survived with no discernible ill effects.

These results were consistent with a simplistic view of responsibility and stress, but the experiment turned out to be extremely difficult to replicate, and a more complex but satisfying explanation was not forthcoming until the work of Jay Weiss, of Rockefeller University, approximately ten years ago.[11] Weiss performed seemingly analogous experiments using rats, but obtained precisely the opposite results. The executive rats survived and the yoked passive rats were the ones to get ulcers and die. The diametrically opposed results, Weiss argued, reflect several critical differences in experimental design, and his explanation of how these operated has provided a solid theory for predicting just what makes a situation stressful and likely to cause disease. In Weiss' basic experiments, a warning signal sounded, and the "executive" rat, upon hearing it, could prevent himself and his yoked partner from being given an electric shock by touching a bar or turning a wheel; nothing the yoked "helpless" animal did could prevent the shock. The rats were subjected to one continual stress session lasting twenty-one hours, with the shocks scheduled to appear at the rate of one per minute (they actually occurred much less frequently because the executive rat prevented them). Under these conditions, the helpless rats developed approximately three times more extensive gastric ulceration than the executive rats. Other experiments were then performed using a similar basic design but different schedules of warning signals and delivery of shocks. Quantitative analysis of all these results led Weiss to formulate a general theory of how coping behavior affects gastric ulceration.

> The theory states that stress ulceration is a function of two variables: the number of coping attempts or responses an animal makes and the amount of appropriate or "relevant" feedback these coping attempts produce. When an animal is presented with a stressor stimulus, the animal will make coping attempts or responses. The first proposition is simply that the more responses one observes, the greater is the ulcerogenic stress. . . . If the responses, however, immediately produce appropriate feedback . . . ulcerogenic stress will not occur. . . . Perhaps the most important concept in this theory is that of feedback. . . . Relevant feedback occurs when a response produces stimuli that differ from the stressor.[12]

This definition of feedback is a psychologist's technical way of saying that the animal's response and the environmental change the rat is "trying" to achieve with this response are clearly related, that the rat "knows" it is accomplishing something (it is such anthropomorphic statements that Weiss' choice of words is trying to avoid, and the quotation marks denote the fact that the conditioning of an animal in no way depends on conscious "trying" or "knowing" of anything). Thus, the executive rats receive relevant feedback because their actions (pressing the bar or turning the wheel) consistently produce both absence of shocks and termination of the warning signal; in contrast, the helpless rats also make an appreciable number of coping attempts (they may press the bar or turn the wheel rapidly), but there is absolutely no consistent relationship between their actions and the presence or absence of shocks and the warning signal, the relevant feedback. The theory that feedback about the effectiveness of one's actions is a major factor in determining how stressful and disease-producing a situation is provides a pleasing analogy to other physiological control systems, the effectiveness of which also depends on continuous feedback. It is also one that, intuitively, we recognize as applicable to our own experience.

One immediate test of Weiss' two-factor (response rate and degree of relevant feedback) theory was its ability to explain Brady's earlier opposite results. It passed this test successfully. Brady's executive monkeys had had to respond at an extremely high rate (once every twenty seconds) to avoid shocks, and were given no external relevant feedback—the red light used in the experiment to alert the animal to start bar-pressing remained on throughout the test period, rather than being turned off by a certain number of bar presses; thus, the executive's rapid-fire responses did not change the external environment at all. At the same time, the yoked animals were making very few responses because the executive's high responding rate kept the number of shocks low.*

The results of operant conditioning experiments have not always been as striking as in the examples I have selected, but this is not surprising when, keeping in mind Weiss' concepts, one realizes how critical small changes in the enviornmental contingencies may be in eliciting stress responses and frank disease. Habituation also remains a serious problem in these experiments, and very few have been continued for long periods of time.

Despite the success that at least some shock avoidance experiments have had in documenting the role of stress in disease, the artificiality of the situation and its lack of real correspondence to the usual types of psychosocial stress normally experienced by animals make some scientists uneasy about generalizing too far from the results. Therefore, experiments which attempt to employ psychosocial stresses more representative of the types animals might encounter in their natural habitat are particuarly important.

Simple crowding of animals has been one extensively used technique, the pioneer studies being those of John B. Calhoun, working with rats. His crowded animals demonstrated increased mortality rates, especially among the young; decreased fertility rates; increased rates of spontaneous abortions, still births, congenital defects and death of the young soon after birth; neglect of the young by their mothers; extremely aggressive behavior within the colonies; total withdrawal of some animals from the community; sexual aberrations and other "psychotic" behaviors.

Many studies have confirmed these basic findings in a variety of laboratory rodent species, and have also strongly suggested that many of these same events may occur in free-living species in their

---

*There was another reason the yoked helpless monkeys made relatively few responses, one which really invalidated the entire experiment; in pretrials, animals found to be good bar pressers were assigned to the executive group, and poor bar pressers were placed in the "helpless" group.

natural habitats. Animals like the lemmings and meadow voles manifest marked swings in their populations, and when the population density reaches a peak, it is followed by a "crash" characterized by increased mortality, decreased fertility, and mass migrations. The lemmings are not seeking out cliffs from which to jump, but are simply moving out randomly in all directions (when one does this in a country like Norway, sooner or later, one encounters a cliff and the sea). Moreover, most of the lemmings die during the population crash not from drowning, but from overwhelming infections (from microbial organisms that normally inhabit them but give no trouble), and failure of the heart and kidneys.

All of these events have been produced in rodents in the laboratory by administering pharmacological doses of cortisol or epinephrine, and this, coupled with the fact that overcrowded animals (both in the laboratory and wild) manifest evidence of marked hyperactivity of these two neuroendocrine systems, has led to the following theory: As animals become more and more crowded, the number and intensity of their social interactions, particularly aggression, increase. This psychosocial stress so elevates plasma cortisol (and activity of the sympathetic nervous system) that the pharmacological effects become operative, resulting in decreased reproductive rate, increased mortality rate, and mass migration. These lead, in turn, to a marked population decrease. In negative feedback fashion, the reduced population density relieves the psychosocial stress, and the cycle of population buildup and crash begins all over again.

These experiments and observations have had a twofold effect on our view of stress and disease. First of all, they provide a powerful demonstration of how psychosocial stress may induce a wide variety of malfunctions. Second, and I believe even more important, they have provided a biological explanation for why animals carry within themselves a potentially destructive time bomb in the form of the pharmacological effects of cortisol and the disease-producing effects of extreme sympathetic nervous system activity. Prior to these studies, medical scientists simply viewed the pharmacological effects of cortisol either as laboratory curiosities or, in the case of the anti-inflammation effect, something to be made use of clinically. But now it is a realistic hypothesis that these effects really do occur in nature, and serve the purpose of regulating population size and density. (The profound decrease in secretion of sex hormones produced by stress in laboratory animals also makes sense in this context.) It also may spur evolution of the species since the male animals most affected in the laboratory are the subordinates. They have the highest levels of adrenocortical activity, and the greatest death rate. Assuming (and it is only an assumption!) that an animal's position in the dominance-subordinance hierarchy has some genetic basis, one can see that this phenomenon will change gene frequencies in the surviving population.

All this, of course, immediately raises the question of whether such a population control mechanism operates in human beings also (certainly not all mammalian species manifest it), a question to which I will return in a subsequent section.

Another "natural" psychosocial stress is exposure of animals to others of the same species who have been conditioned to be highly aggressive. For example, when subordinate adult male tree shrews were introduced into a cage with a trained fighter, the latter animal immediately attacked while the former submitted. The two animals were separated before any physical injury could occur but were allowed to remain in sight of each other. Within two to sixteen days, despite normal eating and drinking, the subordinate animal would die of kidney failure brought on by such profound activation of the sympathetic nerves to the blood vessels of the kidneys (a normal component of the fight-or-flight response) as to seriously impair blood supply to these organs.

One of the first studies to use as a stressor chronic disruption of social interactions without crowding was performed with dominant male Hamadryas baboons, each of whom had taken, as is the natural situation with these species, several females at an early age and remained with them. When a male was then separated from his females and young and another male placed in their cage in his full view he would become very agitated and remain so indefinitely. After several months, these dispossessed males manifested very high incidences of hypertension, coronary heart disease, and frank heart attacks.

The single most important "natural" animal model for studying the interaction of psychosocial stress and disease is the ingenious one developed by James P. Henry and his coworkers at the University of Southern California.[13] These investigators have studied mice in special "population cages" which greatly enhance social interactions and prevent stable territory formation, i.e., simply exaggerate the types of psychosocial stress that wild mice almost certainly encounter in their natural environment. To further exaggerate the interactions, the male mice used in the experiments were often isolated from the time of weaning until they were placed in the population cages with normally socialized females at approximately four months of age. The cages consist of a system of six boxes with narrow connecting tubes all forming a circle. Additional spokelike tubes connect each box to a seventh central feeding and watering place. Sixteen previously isolated males and sixteen females constitute one experimental colony.

Under such conditions, the males are quite aggressive and fail to establish a stable social hierarchy. The control animals for these experiments are mice either left in isolation for a lifetime, or more commonly, normally socialized animals who are housed simply in standard boxes, rather than in population cages. It must be emphasized that crowding is not a stimulus in these experiments; the population density is the same for the animals in the standard cages and those in the population cages. Nor is physical trauma a confounding variable, since almost all the aggressive behavior is symbolic.

Using this model, and several variants of it, Henry has demonstrated that the population-cage mice develop a striking array of diseases completely absent in the controls or occurring in much lesser degree and at an older age. They develop severe hypertension, characterized by the same progression over time of hormonal and neural changes suspected of occurring in people with hypertension. They develop atherosclerosis (on normal mouse diets!) with prominent involvement of the coronary arteries, and degeneration of the heart muscle. Their kidneys become scarred and develop the anatomic and functional features typical of kidney failure in people. The females develop a very high incidence of mammary tumors.

This last finding is typical of a growing body of studies on experimental animals which indicate that psychosocial stress has profound effects on immune defense mechanisms and susceptibility to the diseases they defend us against. Shock avoidance experiments like those described earlier have resulted in increased susceptibility of the animals to many different viruses, bacteria, and parasites. Simply housing mice together rather than alone does the same, as does stressing mice by exposing them (in protected cages) to a hungry cat. The development of tumors, both benign and cancerous, can also be increased by stresses as innocuous as brief daily handling and mild electric shocks. Moreover, this is observed even when the stresses are administered only during the first days of life, the tumor cells or tumor-producing viruses being injected during adulthood. (Remember my warning about concluding from Levine's experiments that early handling is an unmixed blessing.)

Probably the most striking study of stress and tumor-development is that performed in 1975 using mice carrying a virus which produces mammary tumors in 80 to 100 percent of female mice eight to eighteen months after birth under standard laboratory housing conditions. Simply placing the animals in new facilities which eliminated drafts, minimized thermal fluctuations, reduced noise, and eliminated the transfer of odors from cage to cage reduced the incidence of tumors at 400 days of age from 32 percent to 7 percent. When handling of the mice by laboratory personnel was also reduced as much as possible, the incidence fell to zero percent!

All these findings are consistent with other abundant evidence that psychosocial stresses such as avoidance conditioning, "triple threat," or crowding can inhibit antibody formation, diminish the number of circulating T-lymphocytes (the immune cells which attack cancer cells), and prolong the survival of tissue transplants. Some of these responses to stress could be prevented by prior removal of the adrenal glands from the animals but others could not. Prior damage to the hypothalamus, the brain center so involved in emotional behavior and the integration of neuroendocrine responses, also abolished many of these responses, particularly those involving changes in antibody production. Clearly, we have a long way to go before the specific physiologic mediators for the different responses are identified, but there should no longer be any doubt that, in experimental animals, the immune system can be strongly influenced by psychosocial stress.

The final group of animal experiments I'd like to mention is that pertaining to ventricular fibrillation, the leading cause of fatality among patients with coronary heart disease. In the United States, ventricular fibrillation is responsible for an estimated 500,000 deaths per year. What makes this lethal event so important to understand is that prolonged survival is the rule if acute resuscitation is successful. To quote two of the investigators in this field, Bernard Lown and Richard L. Verrier:

> [Ventricular fibrillation] seems to represent an electrical accident rather than the culmination of extensive, irreversible structural damage to the heart. Indeed, in most cases of sudden death, pathological

studies have failed to uncover acute lesions either in the coronary arteries or in the [heart muscle]. How, then, is the heart catapulted into such disorganized electrical activity?[14]

As we have seen, the stress hypothesis indicts increased activity of the sympathetic nervous system acting upon a heart already electrically unstable because of reduced coronary blood flow, and this is the basic hypothesis investigated in animal models.

The first evidence that the nerves to the heart are essential for the development of ventricular fibrillation during acute reduction of coronary blood flow was the finding that denervation of the heart prevented most of the deaths associated with the occlusion of a major coronary artery in dogs.

That psychosocial stimuli alone could induce ventricular fibrillation was shown in monkeys with or without preexisting heart muscle damage, using a yoked-partner avoidance technique analagous to that of Weiss. Acute damage to the heart and ventricular fibrillation could be elicited in animals which were helpless to anticipate and avoid an electrical shock, but no such response occurred when the animals had control over the administration of the shock (even though a greater total number of shocks was delivered) and were receiving relevant feedback establishing the existence of this control.

The most extensive quantitative studies of the role of psychological factors in ventricular fibrillation are those of Drs. Lown and Verrier.[15] By means of electric wires previously implanted in their dogs' hearts, they were able to pass electric current painlessly into the heart and measure exactly how much current it took to produce the very first evidence of an abnormal rhythm. They then exposed the dogs to two different environments for short periods of time on three successive days: a cage in which the animal was not disturbed and another in which the animal received a single painful electric shock (not to the heart!) at the end of each day's period. Then, on days four and five, the animals were tested in the two different environments for how much current in the heart wire it took to produce an abnormal heart rhythm. The animals clearly exhibited evidence of stress at being in the environment in which they had previously received shocks; they were restless, salivated frequently and excessively, and exhibited muscle tremors and a high heart rate. The important finding was that, in this stressful environment, it took only one-third as much current to produce an abnormal rhythm as when the dogs were in the nonaversive cage. Moreover, if instead of passing current into the heart, a major coronary artery was occluded (by a balloon previously implanted in the artery) the dogs developed diverse abnormalities of rhythm while in the aversive environment, and these completely disappeared when they were placed in the nonaversive cage. Finally, in still other experiments, using the shock avoidance model, all behaviorally induced changes in cardiac excitability could be abolished by treatment of the dogs with drugs that block the actions of the sympathetic nerves on the heart. All of these studies leave no doubt that in experimental animals, psychological stresses can predispose to ventricular fibrillation, mediated by increased sympathetic neural activity to the heart.

Epidemiological Studies

An extremely large number of epidemiological studies has been performed looking for associations between psychosocial variables and increased incidences of mortality rates from different diseases. They may be divided broadly into two categories: (1) studies of disease rates in populations presumed to differ in their degrees of stressfulness; (2) intrapopulation studies of specific psychosocial variables.

Interpopulation Comparisons

The classic example of this type of comparison is that between Japan and the United States with regard to coronary heart disease.[16] Japan has the lowest rate of coronary heart disease of any industrialized nation, only one-eighth that of the United States. As I have already pointed out, a study of Japanese-Americans has documented that little, if any, of this difference is ascribable to genetic differences. During the ten-year period covered by this prospective study of 3,800 men living in the San Francisco Bay area, those who had adopted Western ways suffered a much higher rate of coronary heart disease than did those who had continued to live a traditional Japanese life-style.

Because many of the more acculturated men had not adopted a Western diet, it was possible to factor out the influence of diets on this increased incidence of heart disease, and doing so produced very little change in the relative numbers. Neither did controlling for smoking, plasma cholesterol, blood pressure, relative weight, or plasma glucose. The variables that did correlate very strongly with the increased incidence were American cultural upbringing and the degree to which the men had become disassociated from their ethnic group. American cultural upbringing alone raised the rate two and one-half times and the addition of cultural dissociation raised the rate to five times higher than that of the most traditional men.

Sociologists have for years pointed out that the traditional Japanese culture has built-in buffers to stress that are not found in the United States. Traditional Japanese have considerable stability in their lives. They live in closely knit groups whose members are highly supportive of each other. Their future occupations are determined when they are young, and most jobs carry virtual tenure. They have strict customs to guide action in most situations. There is much more emphasis on the group than on the individual, which greatly reduces the pressure for competition. These are only a few of the features of traditional Japanese life which minimize social, personal, and occupational pressures, protect the individual from unfamiliar situations and excessive choices, and provide continuous feedback to him that his actions are appropriate and are leading to desirable and anticipated consequences.

Many of these same features apply to other societies and subgroups which have a low incidence of coronary heart disease. For example, when studied in 1966, the exclusively Italian-American population of Roseto, Pennsylvania, had an extremely low death rate from coronary heart disease, about one-half that of their neighboring communities, despite a diet rich in animal fat and an average weight excess of twenty pounds per person, compared with the American average.[17] Sociologists and anthropologists who have studied this community report a remarkable degree of cohesiveness, gregariousness, and mutual support, along with clearly defined male and female roles. Apparently, upon arrival from Italy, the emigrants reinforced those elements of their traditional culture which gave them security and served to insulate them from hostile surrounding communities. The result was that this community became more homogenous and traditional than the parent village of Roseto, Italy! As the culture of Roseto moves inevitably toward the usual American pattern, will the incidence of coronary heart disease increase? If it does, the stress hypothesis will have received strong support.

Another American group which has been intensively studied because of its supposedly peaceful, highly structured life is Benedictine monks. During the early 1960s, American Benedictine monasteries were inhabited by two different groups of monks who ate the same high-fat American diet at the same tables but otherwise had very different life-styles. The Benedictine brothers spent much of their time in prayer and meditation, whereas the Benedictine priests worked at an intense level in the outside world, running churches, schools, and the like. The incidence of heart attacks in the priests was approximately two and one-half times that of the brothers.[18] Of course, this study runs into the self-selection problem I have pointed out so many times; a high percentage of the priests had extreme Type A personalities (defined later in this chapter), which predisposed them to the stresses of the considerable work pressure they experienced.

The largest mass of whole-population data attempting to relate a disease to psychosocial factors is in the realm of hypertension. The reasons such studies have been so numerous is that blood pressure is very easy to measure and hypertension would seem to be the "obvious" disease inducible by stress, via increased activity of the sympathetic nervous system. All these population studies have been reviewed by James Henry and John Cassel,[19] who believe that they provide a strong case for indicting psychosocial factors. The basic argument is as follows.

The general population of the United States and most other Westernized nations shows a clear-cut steady rise in blood pressure with age. In contrast, there are at least forty cultural groups throughout the world (including some of every race and from every continent) whose blood pressures are low and do not change with age (these are essentially the same populations which have very low incidences of coronary heart disease and strokes). Analysis of the psychosocial characteristics of these groups led to the following conclusion:

> A man living in a stable society and well-equipped by his cultural background to deal with the familiar world around him will not show a rise in blood pressure with age. This thesis holds whether he is a modern technocrat who became a fighter pilot early in life or a Stone Age Bushman who is a skilled hunter-gatherer living in the Kalahari Desert.[20]

One problem with this type of approach is the post hoc nature of the analysis; it is usually possible to find evidence of either social stress or stability once one knows whether the group in question belongs to the hypertensive or normotensive category. In at least one case involving six tribes, where separate "blind" scorings were made of the social environment with particular regard to degree of acculturation, the association with hypertension was not very impressive.[21]

A far greater problem than this methodological one is the confounding of the analysis by dietary salt (sodium chloride). A very large number of the low-pressure populations ingest very little salt. Here we have a very striking parallel to dietary fat and coronary heart disease. On a worldwide basis, there is a strong association between salt intake and blood pressure. Indeed, there is not a single population whose members habitually ingest less than 1 to 2 g salt per day which exhibits a high incidence of hypertension. Moreover (and here the salt-hypertension association has it over the cholesterol-heart disease one), drastic reduction of salt intake will lower the blood pressure of the great majority of hypertensive persons, at least to some degree. In the light of all these facts, many authorities ascribe the relatively low blood pressures of most of these forty-odd groups to their low salt intake rather than their psychosocial characteristics.[22] Cassel and Henry do not deny that salt almost certainly plays some role but they argue that there are enough exceptions to establish that it cannot be the whole explanation. For example, Buddhist farmers in Thailand in 1960 were eating 20 g of salt per day, yet maintained normal blood pressures throughout their lives.

The salt problem also plagues studies of persons from these low-blood pressure cultures who migrate to other areas. The Zulu, for example, in their usual rural tribal setting have low blood pressures which do not increase with age; those who migrate to large urban centers soon begin to manifest increased blood pressures, but is this due to the undoubted stress of this new life or to the well-documented marked increase in their salt consumption? Or to weight gain? Obesity unquestionably plays an important causal role in the development of hypertension, although the mechanism by which it exerts this effect is unknown. Both in retrospective and prospective studies, obesity emerges as a clear-cut risk factor, particularly in young people, for whom it may be the only known predictor for the later development of hypertension. Most important, controlled human studies have proven that simple weight reduction is highly effective in lowering the blood pressure of even modestly overweight hypertensive persons. Now, we know that most persons who migrate from rural societies to Westernized cities not only increase their salt intake but gain weight, due both to diminished physical activity and to increased food intake. How much does this weight gain contribute to their increased likelihood of developing hypertension?* Obesity could also account for the fact that in Westernized countries the incidence of hypertension increases as socioeconomic class decreases, for the incidence of obesity follows the same pattern.

American blacks offer a particularly vivid and important example of how difficult it is to untwist all these variables. Hypertension is extremely prevalent among this population, and is a major factor contributing to their shorter life expectancy. The number of young and middle-aged blacks suffering from this disease ranges from three to twelve times higher than that of whites, and there are more fatalities at a younger age. Yet we know that most Africans in their native tribal setting have low blood pressures which change little with age. One hypothesis to explain this phenomenon is that blacks have become adapted to the low-salt environment of Africa, and that one feature of this adaptation is a tendency to retain salt when it is available. Therefore, the plentiful salt ingestion of American blacks brings about a greater degree of hypertension than would an equivalent salt intake in whites. This hypothesis is certainly a reasonable one, but there is virtually no solid evidence documenting that blacks hold on to ingested salt more than whites.

A competing (but not mutually exclusive) hypothesis is that American blacks develop so much hypertension because of severe psychosocial stress both in the ghettos of the North and their disintegrated societies of the rural South.

Yet a third view is that there is nothing unique about blacks as regards susceptibility to hypertension, that a higher proportion of blacks belongs to the lower socioeconomic classes, which have higher incidences of hypertension in all Westernized countries. Whatever the explanation for this association with socioeconomic class—stress, obesity, or poor medical care, to name a few possibilities—it affects whites and blacks equally according to this view.

----

*One investigator has suggested an interesting *deus ex machina* for this dilemma. He argues that stress might predispose to hypertension indirectly (rather than by directly increasing sympathetic nervous system activity) by causing persons to eat more, thereby both ingesting more salt and gaining weight. (A. Ostfeld, cited in J. L. Marx, "Stress: Role in Hypertension Debated," *Science* 198 [1977]:907.)

Life Change and Illness. If the preeminent psychosocial stress is change, and if psychosocial stress plays a causal role in disease, then there ought to be an observable epidemiological association between the amount of recent change in people's lives and the amount of illness they suffer. This simple but reasonable logic led Thomas Holmes, Richard Rahe, and their colleagues to look for such an association, originally for American naval shipboard personnel.[23] Their positive findings and the relative ease of performing such studies (at least on a retrospective basis) has led to a huge number of life-change studies on an international basis and with an extraordinary number of different groups.[24] A significant positive association has been found in the great majority of these studies, and yet, for good reasons, the conclusion that life changes are an important risk factor for disease remains unconvincing. Elaboration of some of these reasons provides us with an excellent opportunity for reviewing a few basic concepts in statistics and epidemiology.

First, let us review the basic approach of this type of research and some of its findings. Holmes and Rahe defined as "change" any life event which requires socially or psychologically adaptive responses on the part of the individual. In their formulation, all that matters is the intensity and length of time necessary to accomodate to the life event, not the desirability of the event, for pleasant changes, too, challenge the individual's coping mechanisms. In order to quantitate forty-three commonly occurring life events, they had an average sample of the adult Seattle population rate the events as to relative degrees of necessary adjustment, using marriage as the standard, assigning it a score of fifty. The Scale of Life Change Events (or Social Readjustment Rating Scale) constructed from this endeavor is shown in table 7–3. This checklist or ones comparable to it but constructed for use by particular groups, such as college students, is used by most investigators in the field; each subject simply marks the events which pertain to his or her experience, usually covering the previous six to twenty-four months in retrospective studies, and a simple score can be calculated for that person simply by adding up all the life change units (LCUs).

Typical of these studies is an early retrospective one by Rahe, in which more than 2,000 naval personnel reported both their life changes and histories of illness during the previous ten years. The

TABLE 7–3 Holmes-Rahe Life Change Events for Seattle Adults

	LCU values
Family	
Death of spouse	100
Divorce	73
Marital separation	65
Death of close family member	63
Marriage	50
Marital reconciliation	45
Major change in health of family	44
Pregnancy	40
Addition of new family member	39
Major change in arguments with wife	35
Son or daughter leaving home	29
In-law troubles	29
Wife starting or ending work	26
Major change in family get-togethers	15
Personal	
Detention in jail	63
Major personal injury or illness	53
Sexual difficulties	39
Death of a close friend	37
Outstanding personal achievement	28
Start or end of formal schooling	26
Major change in living conditions	25
Major revision of personal habits	24
Changing to a new school	20
Change in residence	20
Major change in recreation	19
Major change in church activities	19
Major change in sleeping habits	16
Major change in eating habits	15
Vacation	13
Christmas	12
Minor violations of the law	11
Work	
Being fired from work	47
Retirement from work	45
Major business adjustment	39
Changing to different line of work	36
Major change in work responsibilities	29
Trouble with boss	23
Major change in working conditions	20
Financial	
Major change in financial state	38
Mortgage or loan over $10,000	31
Mortgage foreclosure	30
Mortgage or loan less than $10,000	17

Source: R. H. Rahe, "Subjects' Recent Life Changes and Their Near-Future Illness Reports." *Annals of Clinical Research* 4 (1972):250–65.

numbers of LCUs for each year was then related to the number of illness episodes for the subsequent year. In general, those who reported fewer than 150 LCUs for a given year had little illness the next year, 50 percent of those with scores between 150 and 300 reported some illness, and 70 percent of those with scores greater than 300 suffered illness, often in multiple episodes.

A typical prospective study by these same investigators employed 2,500 naval personnel, who recorded life events for the six months prior to subsequent six-month shipboard tours of duty. Those in the lowest 25 percent for life-events score suffered 1.4 illnesses as recorded in the shipboard medical records, whereas those with the top 25 percent LCU scores suffered 2.1 illnesses, this difference being statistically significant.

To summarize the voluminous literature in this field, in both retrospective and prospective studies, modest but statistically significant associations have been found between life change and the occurrence or onset of a remarkable number of diseases—heart attacks, accidents (including athletic injuries), tuberculosis, various forms of cancer, diabetes, psychiatric disorders, to name just a few—with little obvious specificity in the associations. Why, then, the debate as to the importance of this association?

The most extensive critique of life-change studies is that of Judith G. Rabkin and Elmer L. Struening, epidemiologists in the New York State Department of Mental Hygiene. The first issue they take is a statistical one. Remember how, in chapter 2, I emphasized that the test of statistical significance, the P value, provides information concerning how likely the difference between groups is to be a true population difference but that it says nothing about how important the difference is? The P values are almost always less than 0.05 in life-change studies (in large part because so many subjects are used), indicating that real differences are being observed, but how important are they? When we want to answer this question we use the reflexion coefficient, which tells us how much the differences in one variable (the life-change score) can account for differences in another (illness episodes). In most life-change studies, correlation coefficients are not even calculated, and when they are present they are usually very low, typically below 0.30. Such values suggest that life events account for less than 9 percent of all differences in illness among the subjects (remember that one takes the square of the correlation coefficient to obtain such estimates). In Rahe's naval data, for example, the correlation coefficients were consistently around 0.12, indicating that less that 2 percent ($0.12 \times 0.12 = 0.014$ or 1.4 percent) of the differences in illness episodes among the men were ascribable to differences in life events. As Rabkin and Struening conclude, "in practical terms, then, life event scores have not been shown to be predictors of the probability of future illnesses."[25]

The second criticism strikes even more deeply, indeed at the very question of whether the significant association ($P < 0.05$) observed in almost all of these is real, at all, or an artifact due to methological errors. The great majority of life-change studies are retrospective and are usually flawed by lack of adequate comparison groups. As C. David Jenkins, an epidemiologist at Boston University, has pointed out:

> Use of patients as their own controls—comparing life changes recalled from the six months before acute illness with those recalled from earlier periods of the patients' lives—allows the possibility that the usually greater number of life changes reported for the most recent period occurs because recent memory is more complete than distant memory.[26]

Moreover, as Joseph Connally, a British psychiatrist and himself a life-change researcher, has vividly stated:

> The interview with a man wired to a monitor in a Coronary Care Unit and well aware of his dangerous situation is very different from that with an airline employee, able to break up a day's work to talk with a visiting physician. The interviewer may feel that he has conducted as rigorous a search for predesignated, coarse, memorable events happening to . . . people in both groups, [but] this will assuage the unease of none but the more generous of his critics.[27]

Life-change studies are also particularly prone to other sources of "retrospective contamination." For one thing, sick people may feel the need to exaggerate past events to justify present illness. For another, cause and effect may be reversed in studies covering a short period, that is, the initial undetected stages of a disease may lead the individual to make life changes. This is most obvious in the case of emotional disorders, but applies to physical disorders as well. Thirdly, the crisis of serious illness may sensitize people to attach more importance to earlier life events. Finally, there is suggestive evidence that life changes may not bring on an illness, but rather may lead people who may have been sick for some time to seek out medical assistance, that is, stress may trigger not illness but use of a medical facility.

All these methodological problems may explain why associations between life changes and disease tend to be stronger and more consistent in retrospective studies than in the few prospective ones reported (and even the latter may not be free of some of these sources of bias if their time span is fairly short), some of which have yielded negative results. For example, a prospective study of 6,579 Swedish workers 41 to 61 years of age found no association between life-change scores and heart attacks for the ensuing twelve to fifteen months. (There were associations, however, with several other diseases.)

All in all, Dr. Jenkins' assessment of life changes and coronary heart disease seems to me to apply to virtually all other diseases as well.

> The totality of findings thus far generated regarding a possible association between increased rate of life changes and the timing of myocardial infarction are provocative but remain unconvincing because of the inconsistencies among them. Furthermore, the studies that are stronger methodologically are the cases with negative results. . . . The best way to perform a definitive test of this hypothesis is through further prospective study.[28]

My descriptions so far have dealt with the association between the sum total of all life changes and the occurrence of disease. Several studies have singled out specific particularly stressful changes and tried to associate them with disease. For example, men whose jobs had been abolished were shown to develop, over the next months while out of work, marked increases in their incidence of hypertension and arthritis (the latter up to a ten-fold increase), which were reversed shortly after they found new satisfactory jobs. Even more striking are the data concerning death rates for persons who have recently lost a mate. During the first six months after loss of their wives, 213 out of 4,486 widowers of 55 years of age or older died (mainly from heart attacks), a death rate 40 percent greater than that expected for married men of the same age. (Only about one-quarter of the husbands' deaths were from the same disease that caused their wives' deaths, making it very unlikely that environmental factors to which both had been exposed prior to the wives' demise were responsible for both mates' deaths.)

What seems to be the critical component of this "bereavement phenomenon" is whether the surviving mate "gives up." In one study, fourteen women (ages 20 to 50) whose husbands were known to be dying of cancer were intensively interviewed so that they could be broadly classified into two groups according to the strength of their psychological defense mechanisms and the likelihood of their "giving up" after their husbands' deaths; incredibly, the nine who were predicted to "give up" all became ill within six months whereas the five predicted to "carry on" remained well, a perfect score for the predictors.

Other Psychosocial Variables. Change is not the only psychosocial factor which has been associated with increased incidence of or mortality from a disease, and I'll just briefly mention a few of these others.[29]

Mortality rates in the United States for all causes of death are consistently higher for single, divorced, or widowed individuals of both sexes and all races. These differences are greatest for the younger age groups and more apparent in males. In some cases, the married-unmarried discrepancy is quite remarkable. For example, the death rate from coronary heart disease of divorced white males, ages 35 to 44, is two and one-half times greater than that of married men of the same race and age; the ratio is 1.84 for widowers and 1.47 for single men. No consistent differences in plasma cholesterol, blood pressure, or smoking have been found to account for these differences. The fact that death rates for all diseases are affected makes it very likely that psychosocial factors play an important role in the phenomenon, for it is difficult to imagine other environmental factors which would exert such across-the-board effects.

Dissatisfactions with life have also been associated with disease, particularly coronary heart disease. A large prospective study showed that problems and conflicts concerning money, family, work, co-workers, and supervisors, all were associated with the subsequent development of angina pectoris (but, interestingly, not with frank heart attacks) at a rate two and one-half times that for men reporting no problems in these areas. Similar findings emerged from a prospective study of twins in Sweden.

An association between work pressure and cardiovascular disease has also been found in several studies, including industrial workers on a conveyor line system, telephone operators working in a large exchange and under pressure to complete a large number of transactions per unit time, invoicing clerks being paid price-wages and so working at a very fast rate, and air traffic controllers. The very high incidence of hypertension and peptic ulcers in this last group certainly suggests a synergism between work pressure and responsibility, for these men work under extreme time pressure and with the constant responsibility for hundreds of lives.

Another psychosocial factor dear to the hearts of stress researchers is status incongruity, said to exist when there are discrepancies in the different aspects of an individual's social status—his education, income, occupation, quality of housing, and so on. Status incongruity also applies to discrepancies between individuals within a family (wife's level of education versus husband's income), and across generations (father's income versus son's income). Such inconsistencies are presumed to breed tensions, conflicts, and dissatisfactions, and a large number of studies, both retrospective and prospective, have found associations between status incongruity and the incidence of various diseases, particularly coronary heart disease.

Crowding. Does crowding produce in human beings responses similar to those earlier described for some mammalian species? The inhabitants of cities the world over tend to have higher incidences of many diseases, particularly coronary heart disease and cancer, but this could, of course, be explained by a host of socioeconomic variables other than population density, and by physical risk factors as well. Therefore, by far the most important of all human "crowding" studies is that of Galle and his associates for different areas of the city of Chicago, since they took many of these other variables into account.[30] They looked for five types of social pathology modeled after Calhoun's work with rats: age-adjusted mortality rate; fertility rate; the percentage of 18-year-olds or younger on public assistance (a measure of parental care); the percentage of males brought to court on juvenile delinquency charges (a measure of aggressive behavior); admissions to mental hospitals. All five correlated positively with density (persons/acre); this means that all but fertility rate, which should have correlated negatively, were in the direction predicted by Calhoun's work.

The next step was to control for (i.e., factor out) socioeconomic factors such as class, income, ethnic or racial status, and so on. When this was done, all the associations disappeared, but only when the measure of density was persons per acre. This is not surprising since it is not population density per se that should matter, but the intensity of psychosocial interactions resulting from crowding.

When these scientists used other more meaningful markers for true crowding, the results were quite different. Even after factoring out socioeconomic factors, there were strong positive associations between all five indicators of social pathology and either persons per room or rooms per family housing unit. If the inferences drawn from this study are correct, then human beings may, indeed, resemble rats in their response to chronic stressful crowding, except in the matter of fertility (and we have never lacked for evidence that high population densities do not reduce human reproductive rates).

Of course, we must not expect that such associations would be seen worldwide. Many cultures (such as the Japanese and Chinese) have developed powerful social and psychological techniques for coping with crowding. Indeed, at least one population—the !Kung—seem to crave it. Ostensibly one of the least crowded peoples on earth (one person per ten square miles), they in fact build their huts in such close contact and crowd in upon each to such a degree that the average space per person in their encampments is 188 square feet. Moreover, they spend a very large fraction of the total twenty-four hours in actual physical contact with other persons. This is particularly true of children.

"Personality" and Behavior Patterns. Associations with disease have been documented not just for "external" psychosocial stresses, but for emotions, personality types, and behavior patterns. For example, in a very large number of prospective studies (in this particular case retrospective studies are probably useless), coronary artery disease has been consistently associated with expressed feelings of anxiety, depression, general nervousness, and emotional drain as well as with sleep disturbances. In many of these studies, the elapsed time between the evaluation of emotional status and the onset of symptoms of coronary heart disease was long enough to make it unlikely that these feelings were really early manifestations of subclinical levels of the disease.

Psychiatrists and physicians have also tried to identify entire personality profiles which correlate with particular disease—a "hypertensive personality," "cancer personality," and so on. Perhaps the greatest success in these endeavors has been with cancer, the cancer-prone individual being characterized as one who is prone to feelings of "helplessness and hopelessness," uses excessive denial and repression of negative emotions, particularly anger, and is unable to cope successfully with a major emotional loss such as death of a loved one.[31] One of the earliest and most extensive studies to establish this association was that of Dr. M. Kissen, University of Glasgow, who studied workers (all of whom smoked) and concluded, on the basis of psychological interviews and questionnaires, that the more psychologically repressed the persons were, the fewer cigarettes it took to induce cancer.

The presence of feelings of hopelessness or of recent emotional loss is claimed to be a prominent feature of breast cancer, uterine cancer, and leukemia. For example, one investigator, Dr. William Greene, University of Rochester, believes his data indicate that nine out of ten cases of leukemia occur when a person feels "alone, helpless, and hopeless." Lawrence LeShan, a New York psychologist, feels that this phenomenon applies to persons coming down with virtually all forms of cancer. He has reported that 72 percent of more than 400 cancer patients he has had in psychotherapy had suffered the loss of a very important relationship during the period from eight years to a few months prior to the first symptoms of their cancers. This compares to only 10 percent of his control group of persons in psychotherapy for other reasons. Moreover, the great majority of these cancer victims had been suffering from "despair, futility, and isolation" for many years before their cancers emerged.

Now, impressive as many of these studies seem to be, they must be viewed with great caution because they are retrospective. All these personality characteristics (as well as the importance attached to an emotional loss) may be the result of having cancer, which obviously exerts a profound emotional impact upon its victims. Two major prospective studies are presently being performed but the results are not yet in.

The most productive (and provocative) of the attempts to associate personality characteristics with a disease is that championed by Drs. Meyer Friedman and Ray H. Rosenman for so-called Type A behavior and coronary heart disease.[32] These physicians at the Brunn Institute for Cardiovascular Research in San Francisco set out to answer the question: Is there a pattern or style of behavior that, like other risk factors, permits prospective identification of persons at higher risk of development of clinical coronary heart disease? Research from several countries seems to have answered this question in the affirmative.

The coronary-prone behavior pattern can be defined as an overt behavior syndrome or style of living characterized by excesses of competitiveness, striving for achievement, aggressiveness (sometimes stringently repressed), time urgency, acceleration of common activities, restlessness, hostility, hyperalertness, explosiveness of speech amplitude, tenseness of facial musculature, and feelings of struggle against the limitations of time, and the insensitivity of the environment. This torrent of life is usually, but not always, channeled into a vocation or profession with such dedication that Type A persons often neglect other aspects of their life, such as family and recreation. Not all aspects of this behavior pattern must be present simultaneously for a person to be classified as possessing it. *The pattern is not a personality trait or a stress reaction* [emphasis added], but rather the observable behavior that emerges when a person predisposed by his character structure is confronted by a "triggering situation." The converse of this behavior pattern, Type B, is marked by an absence of Type A characteristics.[33]

The italics added to this description are to emphasize that the Type A behavior pattern is defined neither by an inherited trait alone nor any single environmental influence; it is defined by the struggle that develops when an individual possessing this trait and confronted with several environmental influences decides to "do battle." It is not the same as stress, nor does it represent a distressed response; rather it is a style of behavior with which some persons habitually respond to environmental circumstances that arouse them. Friedman and Rosenman believe that this behavior pattern is now so widespread because the contemporary Western environment encourages its development. In this formulation, we may view work pressure and the other environmental triggers as the psychosocial stresses (stimuli) which elicit the behavior pattern and its accompanying physiological responses—an increased activity of the sympathetic nervous system, hypersecretion of cortisol, and the other components of the classic stress response, almost all of which have been documented to occur to a greater extent in Type A persons than in Type B in response to appropriate psychosocial stimuli (for example, problem-solving with severe time limitations).

Since 1970, more than twenty studies, both retrospective and prospective, have looked for an association between Type A behavior and coronary heart disease in a variety of populations, using either a structured interview or a computer-scored questionnaire to classify the subjects. All but a few have been successful in documenting a positive association, although the strength of the association varies considerably from study to study.[34] One of the most convincing is the Western Collaborative Group Study (WCGS), a double-blind prospective study which included at its outset a structured interview specifically designed to quantitate how Type A the participants were. After 4.5, 6.5, and 8.5 years of surveillance, the men judged to be Type A at the beginning of the period (either by interview or questionnaire) had suffered 1.7 to 4.5 times the rate of new coronary heart disease as men judged to be Type B.

Now, your immediate response to such findings should be: Do Type A men smoke more than Type B, eat more animal fat, get less exercise, and differ in other risk factors, any one of which could be the real explanation of their increased incidence of coronary heart disease? The WCGS study factored out the traditional risk factors (using the approach developed for use with the extensive Framingham data), and still found a strong association with Type A behavior, one which added appreciably and independently to the overall prediction of coronary risk (this is a very important finding since the traditional risk factors account for less than 50 percent of total risk prediction). It seems fair to conclude, at present, that the Type A behavior pattern is a significant risk factor for coronary heart disease; whether the explanation for this association is to be found in potentially damaging effects of hyperactive stress responses or simply represents some inherent difference in body chemistry having nothing to do with environmental influences still remains unknown. To me, the latter possibility seems unlikely, but it cannot be ruled out until we document more fully the effects on coronary incidence of altering the environment of Type A persons. This will be a very difficult task, much more so than evaluating the protective effects of altering dietary fat intake.

Measurement of Neuroendocrine Processes. This is a very different epidemiological approach to the relationship between psychosocial stress and disease. Instead of attempting to associate the disease with a psychosocial factor, the investigators look for evidence of enhanced stress responses, using one or more of the types of measurements described earlier in this chapter—plasma epinephrine, urinary corticosteroids, increased heart rate, and so on. There are still very few data of this type and hypertension has been the best-studied disease in this regard.

Since increased activity of the sympathetic nervous system is the major hypothesis for how stress could induce hypertension, most of the studies have concentrated on this system. To sum up a very large amount of data, heart rate and plasma catecholamines (epinephrine and norepinephrine) have been found to be significantly elevated, relative to the values of normotensive persons, in a considerable number of persons with hypertension, but by no means in all. This is particularly true for young patients and those with relatively mild hypertension, and it may well be that hypertension is commonly initiated by stress, acting through the sympathetic nervous system, but that some other factor takes over at a later stage.

Other studies have tested not for levels of sympathetic activity at rest but for the responsiveness of this system to an artificially imposed stressful stimulus—for example, submerging one's arm in ice water. The results of these studies, too, are consistent with hyperactivity of the sympathetic nervous system in subgroups of patients with hypertension.

Controlled Human Studies

For obvious reasons, controlled human experiments in the realm of psychosomatic medicine have been limited to trying to ameliorate disease by combating stress. A variety of behavioral and psychiatric techniques are being used to try to achieve this aim. One is biofeedback, which I mentioned earlier. However, this method really tells us nothing about what caused the disease in the first place; of course, the modest successes it has had in the treatment of hypertension and other diseases does strongly reinforce the general concept that disease processes are subject to alteration by neurally controlled pathways.

In striking contrast to the techniques of biofeedback, which are designed to elicit (or repress) highly specific responses, a host of new methods aims to produce a widespread integrated state of relaxation mediated by the central nervous system, in essence just the reverse of the fight-or-flight response. Those who are sold on the benefits of these techniques have inherently accepted the view that generalized stress responses contribute to a host of physical and mental disorders, and that by dampening these neuroendocrine responses, the individual's health and well-being are improved.

The most popularized of such techniques is that known as Transcendental Meditation (TM), in which the individual, using a systematic method that he has been taught, perceives a particular sound or thought, without really attempting to concentrate specifically on this cue. The initial studies of the basic physiological responses occurring during the actual period of meditation revealed changes consistent with decreased sympathetic nervous system activity; decrease in oxygen consumption, blood lactate concentration, respiration rate, and heart rate. Blood pressure did not go down, but there was a suggestion that the meditators already had a low basal blood pressure during the premeditation control period. Taken together with observed changes in the electroencephalogram, these effects were thought to characterize a "hypometabolic" or "restful" state different from sleep and opposite to the hypermetabolic aroused state associated with increased activity of the sympathetic nervous system.

Dr. Herbert Benson, a physiologist and clinician at Harvard Medical School, who performed many of these early studies, went on to demonstrate that these physiological changes were not unique to TM but could be induced by a variety of relaxation techniques, and he dubbed it the "relaxation response." It is still not clear whether this response truly does represent a diminution in sympathetic activity, for measurements of plasma epinephrine and norepinephrine during meditation do not differ significantly from those of persons simply sitting quietly but not practicing any relaxation technique. This is true for cortisol as well.

However, of far greater potential significance than any acute changes which may occur during the relaxation response are the possible long-term effects. A large number of studies have claimed that the practice of TM has long-term beneficial effects on many parameters of physical and mental health. Unfortunately, most of these studies are poorly controlled (for example, they rarely take into account the placebo effect), and it is presently impossible to evaluate the claims objectively or ascertain whether TM does anything different than simply relaxing for twenty minutes twice a day would. Dr. Benson, who feels he has documented that regular eliciting of the relaxation response significantly reduces the blood pressure of patients with hypertension (but by only a very small amount), acknowledges that establishing a preventive role of the relaxation response in hypertension will require large, expensive, and difficult investigations which may take years to complete.

The most controversial of the methods used in an attempt to influence disease by nonphysical means is psychotherapy. Its practitioners have often been quite hostile to the use of conventional medicine and surgical therapies and so have rightly incurred the wrath of most physicians and scientists, who accuse them of endangering their patients' lives. There are several groups, however, who practice psychotherapy along with traditional therapy. Some of their claimed results in the area of cancer treatment are quite impressive but the published data are too few to really permit any conclusion in this potentially important question. Finally, as Lewis Thomas has emphasized, it is strange that we have usually shrugged off the well-documented placebo effect in so many diseases (including cancer) as something that interferes with our research. The fact is that it exists and we should be devoting an immense amount of attention to figuring out how it works.

Conclusion

The great mass of data from animal experiments and epidemiological studies, I believe, fully justify the following statement by Richard S. Lazarus, a psychologist at Berkeley:

> We are beyond the period of Koch and Pasteur in which illness was regarded as the result of an external agent, say a bacterium, and we now recognize that illness is the result of many factors, . . . including the vulnerability of the person. I think we also agree that vulnerability can be affected by . . . multiple psychological and social factors such as psychological stress, faulty coping, social isolation or alienation, or some combination of these. The disagreements among researchers seem to center largely on which of the many physiological and psychological factors and mechanisms are most important.
>
> When one asks about how psychological and social factors operate, some . . . favor a highly general model in which stress factors are said to increase *general susceptibility* to all illnesses, while others. . .suggest there are also *specific links* between stress factors and given diseases.[35]

Lazarus argues, convincingly to me, that the lack of consistency in the huge number of studies on the general question of stress, personality, and disease, and the relative weakness of the association even in the positive studies, stems mainly from the failure on the part of researchers to recognize that stress does not exist as an independent entity the way a bacterium does.

> Again and again, writers seem to be saying that stress as an agent is either out there in the social or physical environment, or within the person as an intrapsychic defect. . . . However, stress is a special kind of transaction, or relationship between a particular kind of . . . per-

son . . . and a particular kind of environment. . . . At the psychological level, . . . stress depends on the ways an individual appraises a transaction and copes with it.[36]

This fact comes out clearly, as I have described, in all studies of physiological stress responses, and obviously must apply to disease processes as well. A perfect example of failure to take it into account is provided by the studies we have reviewed on life changes and disease. Use of the Holmes-Rahe charts ignores completely the individual's perception of the change in his life and the coping mechanisms he can bring to bear upon it. Remember how remarkably the predictability of the disease-inducing ability of a stress improved when these factors were taken into account in the study of bereavement and giving up I described.

Lazarus believes that the usual kinds of epidemiological studies performed in this field have been useful but have gone as far as they can. The inclusion of large numbers of subjects and evaluation of isolated characteristics has served its purpose of establishing statistically significant associations and the general kinds of factors to look for. Now what is required, he argues, is to study fewer people much more intensively than is usually done, by measuring their physiological and psychological responses longitudinally, that is, in the many real-life situations that impinge upon them over time.

I share with him the view that such research will ultimately clarify those precise interactions between individuals and their psychosocial environment which lead to disease, as well as the physiological processes which form the connecting link. That there is some causal interaction has, I believe, already been proven beyond a reasonable doubt.

Part **IV** | Toxic Chemicals

Chapter 8 | The Body's Responses to Environmental Chemicals

Monsanto's advertisement, "Without chemicals, life itself would be impossible" is a pernicious truism. Its implication is that, because many chemicals, like the nutrients, are essential for life, chemicals in general must be pretty good things to have around. Of course, this is nonsense, for many chemicals in the environment are highly toxic to human beings and other living organisms.

There are several categories into which these toxic environmental chemicals conveniently fall.

1. *Nutrient chemicals in excess.* As we have seen in the previous chapters, many nutrients may exert toxic effects when too much is ingested. This is true of the fat-soluble vitamins, most of the trace metals (iron, zinc, copper, etc.), glutamate (popularly known as MSG), nitrates, and many others.

2. *Naturally occurring bacterial, fungal, and plant toxins.* We are all aware of the deadly effects of certain mushrooms, but there are other extremely dangerous and far more prevalent toxins of plant or bacterial origin. Two of the most important are aflatoxin, a product of certain fungi, and cycasin, produced by the cycad nuts used to prepare flour in Guam and Japan. Both of these chemicals are potent carcinogens and unquestionably are leading causes of cancer in those parts of the world where their ingestion is common. The aflatoxins were discovered in the 1960s when 100,000 turkeys died after eating fungal-infected peanut meal, and contaminated peanuts remain the most common source of

aflatoxins in the human diet wherever peanuts are harvested when they have a high moisture content, and no precautions, such as rapid drying, are taken against mold formation. Other plants containing carcinogens are the bracken fern (suspected of being the cause of the high incidence of stomach cancer in Japan), the betel nut (a cause of mouth cancer in those areas of Asia where it is chewed), and, of course, tobacco.

3. *Naturally occurring nonnutritive inorganic elements.* As we have seen, many inorganic elements such as iron and zinc are essential nutrients, but many more—lead, cadmium, mercury, etc.—have no known biological function, and are toxic when present in large enough amounts. Biological organisms have evolved in the presence of these elements, and it is reasonable to suppose that they have evolved protective mechanisms against the amounts usually present in their surrounding environment. The problem now is that man has, for his own purposes, generated high local concentrations of these materials, often in forms more toxic than those occurring naturally. These then become dangerous not only to the workmen who participate in their mining, processing, and incorporation into products, but to the general population through inadvertent exposure.

4. *Synthetic chemicals.* This is far and away the largest category of chemical hazards we face. It includes an immense number of pesticides, fertilizers, herbicides, food additives, fuel additives, household chemicals, industrial chemicals, and drugs, all of which are "foreign" in the sense that they are not normally found in nature. They all find their way inevitably into the body, either because they are purposely administered as drugs (medical or "recreational"), or simply because they are in the air, water, and food we use.

We no longer even know how many there are. Over two million have been synthesized at one time or other, and the Environmental Protection Agency estimates that approximately 60,000 are presently in everyday use, with the number growing by 500 to 1,000 every year. Obviously, evaluation of risk for all commonly used synthetic chemicals is a massive project, one which can never be completely finished.

Barry Commoner's so-called third law of ecology, "Nature knows best," may well apply to every one of these chemicals: "any man-made change in a natural system is likely to be detrimental to that system."[1] This dictum, applied to synthetic chemicals, was justified by analogizing the chemical to the product of a genetic mutation. As we have seen, when a gene mutates, the altered DNA molecule may code for a previously nonexistent protein, which in turn may catalyze the production of a substance previously unknown to that organism. Since most mutations are known to be harmful, by analogy it is likely that most synthetic chemicals will also carry some risk. Indeed, Commoner has hypothesized that the ultimate test of toxicity may already have been performed for some of these chemicals in the dim past, that given the immense time during which evolution occurred and the flexibility of the genetic apparatus, it is extremely likely that many of our present and future synthetic chemicals really were produced by some mutant organisms; if so, their subsequent disappearance from the natural world signifies that natural selection has already tested them and found them wanting.

Unfortunately, there is no single term that encompasses all four categories of toxic environmental chemicals. "Pollutant" is often used to denote the last three, that is, all but the nutritive chemicals, but it seems a bit strange to categorize chemicals taken for medicinal reasons or deliberately added to food as "pollutants." I will, for simplicity, simply refer to them all as environmental chemicals.

The present mushrooming concern over the health effects of environmental chemicals stems not only from the fact that our exposure to them, particularly the synthetic ones, is increasing exponentially, but from our recognition that many diseases hitherto regarded as spontaneous diseases of aging are, in fact, related to environmental causes, many of them chemicals. Our dangerous predicament was really brought home to us in the late 1960s with the rapid-fire announcement of three animal study results: DDT causes cancer; captan, a commonly used fungicide, causes mutations and birth defects; cyclamates, the most common nonnutritive sweetener in use at the time, causes bladder cancer, chromosome abnormalities, and birth defects. These agents had all been used for many years, without our being aware of their potential dangers. It was clear that previous methods of testing had been inadequate, had concentrated almost exclusively on acute toxicity, and had almost entirely ignored the much more relevant question of low-dose, long-term toxicity. How many agents already spread through the planet and present in most of our bodies were contributing to the development of cancer, cardiovascular diseases, alteration of our genetic pool, birth defects, chronic kidney disease, and the like?

Rapidly, our scientific approach to environmental chemicals altered. Scientists increased their research into how the body handles chemicals and responds to chemically induced damage. New laboratory tests for toxicity were developed, and epidemiologists began searching for clues. At the same time, government agencies already in existence (like the FDA) or soon to be created (like the Environmental Protection Agency) undertook more vigorously to regulate exposure to potentially toxic environmental chemicals.

This chapter will detail what we have learned concerning body-chemical interactions and the next will document, using several specific cases, the enormous difficulties encountered by regulatory agencies in applying these facts—toxicity results from animal studies and epidemiological findings—to the task of setting "acceptable levels of exposure."

Basic Approach

One can study the body's responses to nonnutritive environmental chemicals with the same approaches described in chapter 3 for nutrients, since for all chemicals, whether beneficial or toxic, the central focus is on those factors which determine the effective internal concentration of the chemical at its sites of action. Thus, the first task is to analyze the pathways for gains (inputs to the body) and losses (outputs from the body), since these determine what the total amount is in the body at any moment. Second, the factors which influence the chemical's distribution within the body must be analyzed, for as with nutrients, the total amount in the body is often less important than just where the chemical is and in what concentration. Finally, we must study the homeostatic control points in these pathways and here is where the focus might seem to differ from our previous discussions of nutrients. The homeostatic control of nutrient intake, output, and distribution is aimed at maintaining some optimal concentration of the nutrient at its major sites of action; in contrast, ideal homeostatic controls of nonnutritive environmental chemicals attempt to rid the body entirely of the chemical or at least to minimize the chemical's concentration at its site of toxicity. Really, the principles are the same if one simply imagines that the operating point of homeostatic control systems for toxic chemicals should, ideally, be zero. Just how closely this operating point is approached, and how rapidly, determines the success of the system. One more feature common to many homeostatic systems exists here as well—the capacity for long-term improvement in responsiveness, i.e., acclimatization.

In the descriptions to follow, I will be, in essence, constructing a checklist of questions to be asked about the body's handling of any given environmental chemical, using figure 8–1 as a guide. For the sake of continuity, I will frequently use DDT as an example, not to infer that DDT is an unusually great environmental hazard, but simply because it is quite typical of many organic pollutants and because we know a good deal about what the body does to it. For purposes of orientation, here is a brief description of this pesticide and its suspected toxicity.

The insecticidal potency of DDT (dichloro-diphenyl-trichloro-ethane) was first discovered in 1939, in time to be used extensively in World War II. Its structure, based on the cyclic benzene ring, is quite typical of the huge number of chemicals synthesized by the petrochemical industry in the past thirty years and used for an incredible variety of purposes. By 1962, when Rachel Carson's book, *Silent Spring*, appeared, hundreds of millions of pounds of DDT had already been released around the world, and DDT had been universally credited both with saving 500 million lives (from malaria, typhus, and other infectious diseases carried by insects) and dramatically improving crop yields. Carson was the first to bring home to the public the facts that DDT was everywhere on the surface of earth and in the bodies of all living creatures, including man, that it took years to deteriorate, that its concentration was markedly increased at each step in food chains, and that it was an extremely poisonous substance to many animals other than insects, in particular to birds. Her discussion of toxicity marked a crucial transition in our way of looking at environmental chemicals, for it made people recognize that the real danger from DDT was not one of acute exposure and effects like the ones responsible for killing insects (it takes truly huge amounts of DDT to cause significant acute toxic effects in people), but rather of chronic effects such as cancer, resulting from continuous low-level exposure. Moreover, the potential targets were every living thing in the world.

Silent Spring therefore ushered in the contemporary consciousness concerning environmental chemicals and stimulated development of the methodology required to test for chronic effects. Where do we

Fig. 8–1. **Metabolic pathways for foreign chemicals.** (Redrawn from A. J. Vander, J. H. Sherman, and D. S. Luciano, *Human Physiology: The Mechanisms of Body Function*, 3d ed. [New York: McGraw-Hill, 1980].)

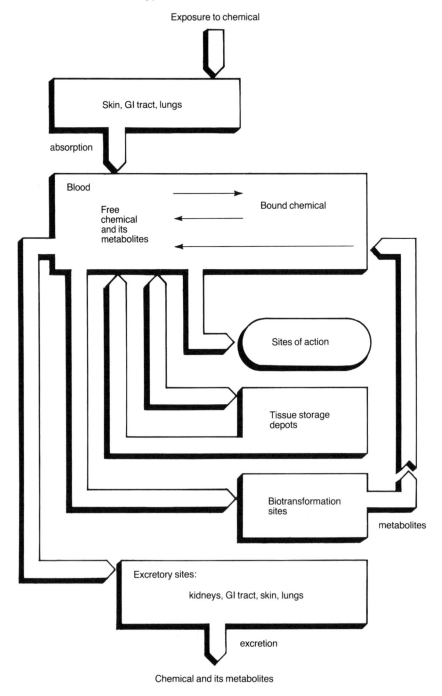

stand on DDT today?[2] Rachel Carson's charge that it interferes with reproduction in birds has been substantiated (although a class of chemicals discovered later, the PCBs, may be more responsible than DDT); the situation for mammals is less clear, and we are also still quite uncertain as to the effects of DDT on the plants and animals of the ocean. DDT has been proven unequivocally to cause several forms of cancer in mice; the doses used were, as is customary, very high relative to human exposure, and there is no proof that DDT causes cancer or other long-term adverse health effects in human beings. However, this lack of proof is not very conclusive, since the controlled human studies have been for relatively short periods of time and have employed very few subjects; moreover, epidemiological studies of such an ubiquitous substance are quite insensitive. In 1972 the Environmental Protection Agency banned the use of DDT, although exceptions have since been made. In contrast, the World Health Organization strongly supports the use of DDT, arguing that its withdrawal would give rise to catastrophic outbreaks of malaria in many parts of the world.

Now let us turn to the central theme of this chapter—the body's handling of environmental chemicals.

Entry to the Body

Possible sites of entry of environmental chemicals are the gastrointestinal tract (following ingestion), the respiratory tract (after inhalation), the skin, and the placenta—the site of chemical exchange between mother and fetus.

Gastrointestinal Tract

Just because a substance has been ingested doesn't mean it will actually be taken up (absorbed) by the blood supplying the gastrointestinal tract. Some environmental chemicals are unstable in the high acidity of the gastric contents, some combine with insoluble or otherwise unabsorbed material in the gut (the metals are prime examples), some are rapidly broken down either by gastrointestinal enzymes or by the bacteria which inhabit the tract. Any of these events preclude absorption of the chemical. In addition, even when the chemical remains intact and unbound, its inherent molecular structure may prevent complete absorption. In chapter 3, I talked about absorption of nutrients from the gastrointestinal tract without really going into the mechanisms by which such transport from the interior (lumen) of the tract to the blood vessels is achieved. Now we must look a little more deeply at these processes.

Transport mechanisms across any biological membrane can be categorized broadly as being diffusion or carrier-mediated. Diffusion is the movement of a substance from one location to another by means of the random continuous motion undergone by all molecules. The term "random" denotes the fact that a molecule moving in one direction may in the next instant be moving in a completely different direction, all directions being equally probable. Because these spontaneous molecular movements are random, if equal concentrations of the substance (i.e., equal numbers of molecules per unit volume of fluid in which they are dissolved) are present initially on two sides of a membrane permeable to the substance, the numbers of molecules passing through the membrane from each side will be equal; there will be a lot of shuttling back and forth but no net movement from one side to the other. In contrast, when the concentrations are different on the two sides of the membrane, there will occur a *net* movement from the initially more concentrated side to the less concentrated, simply because more molecules randomly strike the membrane and pass through it from the more crowded side. This explains what we all know intuitively—diffusion results in net movement of a substance from a region of higher concentration to one of lower concentration.

The actual rate at which such net movement proceeds depends upon the nature both of the moving molecule and the membrane through which it must pass. Biological membranes are highly selective barriers to diffusion, allowing some molecules to move through rapidly, others much more slowly, if at all. Size of the molecule is one determinant—the smaller the molecule, the more likely it is to move through—but the degree to which the molecule can dissolve in lipids is far more important. This is because the major constituent of biological membranes is lipid, and so a highly lipid-soluble molecule can dissolve in the membrane after striking it and move through to the other side. In contrast, lipid-insoluble substances cannot enter the lipid portions of the membrane and are restricted to the far less extensive network of water-filled channels interspersed between the lipids of the membrane (lipid-insoluble substances are highly water-soluble and vice versa, so I will use water-soluble and lipid-insoluble as synonyms).

What determines whether a molecule is mainly lipid-soluble or water-soluble? The major factor is its electrical characteristics or polarity. The more electrically charged (either negative or positive) a molecule is, the more polar it is said to be and the more easily it dissolves in water, because the water molecules themselves are very polar and exert an electrical force which breaks the bonds holding other polar molecules together. Likewise, completely nonpolar molecules, those with no electrical charge, easily dissolve in the extensive nonpolar regions of lipid molecules.

I've been using the term "charged" rather loosely here to include either of two characteristics: the molecule, as a whole, may possess more or less electrons than protons so that the entire entity is truly charged (such a molecule is known as an ion); or, the numbers of electrons may equal the number of protons but be distributed unevenly around the molecule, so that parts of the molecule tend to be negatively charged, parts positively charged. Examples of the two kinds of charged molecules are sodium ions (the symbol for which is Na^+ to denote that this is an ion bearing one net positive charge, i.e., one less electron than proton) and water molecules, respectively.

The significance of all this is that diffusion is an important means by which nonpolar (another synonym for lipid-soluble) molecules like DDT can cross biological membranes, but is generally of much less importance for polar molecules. I would not have inflicted this discussion on the reader if its relevance were limited to the gastrointestinal tract; in fact, we will make use of it over and over again in a variety of contexts.

What about polar molecules? Are they doomed not to be able to cross biological membranes or to cross only extremely slowly? No, such cannot be the case, and to realize this, you need only recognize that many nutrients are highly polar molecules. Evolution has supplied us with transport alternatives to diffusion in the form of protein "carriers" embedded in the lipid matrix of biological membranes. There are a variety of types of these membrane proteins and each type interacts more or less specifically with a given molecule (or family of molecules) to aid the latter's movement across the membrane. We know that the first step in this process requires chemical interaction between the protein carrier and the molecule to be transported, but just how the membrane traverse is achieved remains unknown (the term "carrier" is a holdover from a time when we believed that the protein somehow "carried" the molecule

| THE BODY'S RESPONSES TO ENVIRONMENTAL CHEMICALS

combined with it through the membrane; we now recognize this is probably untrue but the name has stuck).

To reiterate, the membrane itself plays very different roles in diffusional processes and carrier-mediated transport. In both cases, in order to move through the membrane, molecules must interact with the constituents of the membrane, but for diffusion, the interaction is quite nonspecific and almost any substance capable of dissolving readily in the lipid components can move through; in contrast, the interaction between membrane component (the protein "carrier") and transported molecule is more or less specific. If there is no membrane carrier whose structure accommodates a particular type of molecule, then no carrier-mediated transport can exist for that substance. As you would predict, evolution has supplied us with the appropriate carriers for all essential polar nutrients. The carriers present may differ considerably (both in number and type) from location to location in the body.

The specificity between carrier and transported substance may not be complete, and several closely related molecules may all be able to use the same carrier. This accounts for competition between them, i.e., the presence of a high concentration of one may decrease the rate of transport of the other. The number of carriers in any given cell membrane is finite, and if a carrier is occupied in aiding the transport of one molecule, it is not available for transport of another. This also means that the total number of molecules transportable per unit time is limited; no matter how many molecules are available to be transported, once the carriers are saturated they simply can't handle any more. Both these characteristics of competition and saturation, like that of specificity, distinguish carrier-mediated systems from diffusion.

We can now return to the question of gastrointestinal absorption and apply this information. A very large number of synthetic chemicals are nonpolar and, therefore, highly lipid-soluble. The gastrointestinal tract offers no barrier to them, and since following ingestion their concentrations in the lumen of the gastrointestinal tract are much higher than in the blood supplying the tract, absorption down this concentration gradient may approximate 100 percent. There is really nothing the body can do to prevent this.

For substances which are invariably nonpolar, no matter what the conditions, the story is that simple. However, many substances which belong to the category known as weak acids or bases can exist either in polar or nonpolar forms, depending upon the acidity of the solution in which they are dissolved. Look for example at aspirin, which exists in two forms given by the equation:

$$\text{Acetylsalicylate}^- + H^+ \rightleftarrows \text{Acetylsalicylic Acid}$$

| (an ion, highly polar and not soluble in lipid) | (nonpolar and highly lipid-soluble) |

The negative sign by acetylsalicylate denotes the fact that the entire molecule has an extra electron so is a negative ion. H^+ is a hydrogen ion, which has an extra positive charge (or, what amounts to the same thing, has lost an electron). The equation states that when the acetylsalicylate and hydrogen ion combine, the result is a neutral molecule of acetylsalicylic acid. The double arrows indicate that the reaction is reversible so that, if there are very few hydrogen ions around to combine with acetylsalicylate, that species will predominate; in contrast, when the solution contains many hydrogen ions (i.e., is very acid—the acidity of a solution is merely a measure of how many free hydrogen ions are present in it), the acetylsalicylate will almost all be converted to acetylsalicylic acid.

What has all this to do with absorption from the gastrointestinal tract? You know that the lining of the stomach secretes lots of hydrogen ions into the lumen so that the gastric contents are very acid. This means that almost all the aspirin you ingest will end up as the nonpolar, and therefore highly absorbable, acetylsalicylic acid in the stomach. (Despite what the ads tell you, buffering the aspirin does not facilitate absorption of aspirin but actually has the opposite effect.)

Aspirin offers, therefore, an example of how weak acids (those which exist as neutral molecules in acidic solutions) are absorbed by diffusion across the lining of the stomach. Now look at weak bases, typified by another drug, quinine (Q):

$$Q + H^+ \rightleftarrows QH^+$$

When quinine picks up a hydrogen ion, it is converted to a positively charged ion, one which is, of course, not soluble in lipid. Therefore, quinine will not be absorbed by diffusion from the acid stomach contents. But what happens in the small intestine? The liver and pancreas dump large quantities of alkali into the small intestine and this neutralizes the acid coming from the stomach. The quinine loses its hydrogen ion and once again becomes a nonpolar substance readily absorbable by diffusion from the small intestine.

So, whether it be from the stomach, in the case of weak acids, or the small intestine, in the case of weak bases, just about any foreign molecule belonging to these two classes ends up being absorbed simply by diffusion. Again, there is no way the body can prevent this.

All right, what about those molecules or ions which only exist in a highly polar form and so cannot be absorbed to any extent by diffusion? Does this automatically prevent them from getting into our blood after ingestion? No, it does not, for many of these substances end up being absorbed anyway, not by diffusion, but by carrier-mediated transport mechanisms. This may seem strange, for how could we have evolved carriers for synthetic molecules which the body never encountered during evolution? The answer is that these foreign molecules masquerade as nutrients. They usually bear a close resemblance to nutrients and because the gastrointestinal tract's carriers are often not extremely specific, the foreign molecule can hitch a ride on a carrier evolved to assure absorption of a nutrient. For example, the potent poison fluorouracil (uracil with a fluoride atom attached) is absorbed by the carrier which ordinarily absorbs the nutrient uracil.

The fact that the foreign chemical is actually competing with the nutrient for the carrier (with diffusion, there is no competition between molecules; each can get through the membrane independently of all others) offers our first instance of how an individual's diet may influence the toxicity of foreign molecules. The less of the nutrient available to compete for the carrier, the more likely it is that the foreign chemical will latch on to it and get absorbed. Conversely, a high intake of the nutrient can partially block absorption of the competing foreign chemical.

What I have said so far applies equally to organic molecules and the inorganic elements. The class of environmental chemicals most poorly absorbed from the gastrointestinal tract is the nonnutrient metals (mercury, cadmium, lead, etc.). They are not absorbed to any significant degree by diffusion and must depend on carrier-mediated mechanisms, frequently those which exist for the nutrient metals (zinc, copper, iron, calcium, etc.). That they are not absorbed too well should therefore, not be too surprising since we saw in chapter 3 that the same generalization applied to nutrient metals as well. Competition for transport is particularly important for the absorption of non-nutrient metals. They may compete with each other for transport but also with the nutrient metals. Thus, a diet rich in calcium profoundly lowers the intestinal absorption of lead. Conversely, a calcium-deficient diet is associated with a high rate of lead absorption. So is a diet low in iron. Interactions like these are just one more reason that one cannot make statements about what constitutes the optimal intake of a nutrient without reference to the rest of the environment; for persons exposed to large quantities of lead, this effect of a low iron diet to potentiate lead toxicity might outweigh all considerations of the possible benefits of a low-iron diet, whereas it is of no consequence at all in a lead-free environment.

Recent findings concerning metal absorption from the gastrointestinal tract have presented us with a nasty surprise and a warning that we must never assume that children are simply little adults so far as their metabolism of environmental chemicals is concerned. Infants and young children manifest much greater absorption of several nonnutrient metals than do adults, often more than tenfold more. This means that they are at far greater risk from ingested metal pollutants than are adults.

In summary, the gastrointestinal tract is not an effective barrier to the absorption of most environmental chemicals. The only class of substances which constitutes a relative exception to this generalization is the metals. There is really no homeostatic defense against absorption of lipid-soluble environmental chemicals. There is against substances whose absorption is dependent upon carrier-mediated transport but it is simply a passive one—carrier-mediated systems have only a finite transport capacity which sets a limit on the amount of chemical which can be absorbed regardless of how much is present. Finally, infants and young children may differ greatly from adults in their ability to absorb environmental chemicals from the gastrointestinal tract. A question intimately related to that of the infant's capacity for absorbing environmental chemicals is just how easily these chemicals get into their major source of nourishment— milk. The only safe generalization at present is that all environmental chemicals present in the mother's (or cow's) blood will get into her milk but in varying quantities. For example, the concentration of

DDT in an American mother's milk is one and one-half times greater than in her blood.*

Skin

The absorption of environmental chemicals through intact skin is a very simple phenomenon. Carrier molecules are not involved (the outer layers of skin cells are dead) and so diffusion is the only pathway available. The result is that only highly lipid-soluble substances are able to penetrate intact skin. Since so many environmental chemicals fit this description, the skin should not be neglected as a potential entry point. DDT deposited on the skin during spraying, and estrogen in cosmetics are examples. Of course, chemicals for which the skin itself is the target site for damage do their dirty work without having to move through the skin and gain entry to the body.

Respiratory Tract

The lining of the airways are fairly thick and offer a relatively tight barrier to the entry of environmental chemicals (again, as just described for skin, many chemicals exert their actions directly on the lung lining [the carcinogens in tobacco smoke, for example] and so, to do damage, need not cross). In contrast, the tiny air sacs in which these airways terminate and across which oxygen and carbon dioxide exchange with the blood are extremely permeable to most chemicals. Even metals penetrate them fairly easily, much more than they do the gastrointestinal tract. For this reason airborne atoms of metals generally pose a greater hazard to the entire body than does the same quantity of ingested metal.

There is a second reason, in addition to greater entry, that an air pollutant, particularly an organic one, may exert a greater effect than an identical amount of ingested material. Almost all of the blood leaving the stomach and small intestine flows first into the liver before returning to the heart to be pumped to the rest of the body. Therefore, the liver gets first crack at any ingested chemical absorbed into the blood, and as we shall see, the liver is the major organ for metabolizing many environmental chemicals. This means that the amount of intact chemical escaping the liver and reaching

---

*This represents a hefty ingestion of DDT for the infant relative to the usual adult intake. DDT in breast milk is 80 micrograms per liter (μg/L); multiplied by 0.64 L/day (the intake of a 4 kg infant) gives a total of 48 μg DDT/day or 12 μg/kg body weight/day. Compare this to the average adult intake of 1 μg/kg body weight/day.

the rest of the body may be smaller than the amount absorbed by the gastrointestinal tract. In contrast, anything gaining entry to the lung capillaries from the air sacs gets distributed to the entire body without any initial processing by the liver. Of course, the fact that blood from the gastrointestinal tract goes directly to the liver means that chemicals whose site of toxicity is the liver itself may cause much more damage when ingested than when inspired, since they reach the liver in higher concentration in the former case.

What I have said about chemicals being able to penetrate the terminal air sacs (called alveoli) is also true of microorganisms. Moreover, the airways themselves are susceptible to injury by both chemicals and microorganisms. It is not surprising, therefore, that we have evolved important defense mechanisms for preventing such agents from moving very far down the airways. These defenses operate mainly upon particulate materials (very likely because the major sources of danger during our evolution were microbes, not nonparticulate gases), and so are particularly effective against air pollutants which, as is quite common, are breathed in as components of particles.

The nose is the first line of defense. The largest inhaled particles are filtered out by the hairs at the front of the nose. Then as air flows through the nose, it is diverted by the bones of the nasal passageway into multiple turbulent streams which cause many of the large particles escaping the initial barrier of hairs to contact the mucus-lined walls. The particles stick to the mucus which is continuously propelled by cilia, the tiny hairlike structures on the surface of the lining cells, to the back of the nose, and thence into the throat, where it is swallowed and its adhering particles thus prevented from reaching the airways beyond the throat.

Many particles are too small to be trapped by the nasal defenses and these remain in the air passing through the larynx and entering the airway system leading to the alveoli. Along its entire length, but ending just above the alveoli, is a coating of mucus resting on cilia, just as in the nasal passages. Many of the particles adhere to this mucus and are carried by the cilia-propelled mucus escalator up to the throat and swallowed. In addition, the cough reflex, called into play by particularly irritating particles, helps expel entrapped materials.

One last defense remains against those particles, usually the very small ones, that do reach the alveoli. Scattered among the extremely thin cells of the alveoli across which gases exchange (and pollutants may move) are scavenger cells called macrophages, which can engulf particles and catabolize them with strong digestive enzymes.

Placenta

Very few areas in the field of toxicology are as urgently needing of study as the movement of environmental chemicals across the placenta from maternal to fetal blood. This is, of course, the site of nourishment for the fetus, but it is also the site at which any environmental chemicals which have gained entry to the mother's body can enter the developing fetus, so at risk as its various organs undergo their critical periods of development.

The major reasons for great concern at present are the figures for birth defects, and the fact that pregnant women are exposed to a large number of chemicals. Approximately 2 percent of live-born infants suffer from major birth defects, but this number certainly underestimates the incidence of birth defects. At least 20 percent of all pregnancies terminate in spontaneous abortion, and most of these are likely to be due to fetal abnormalities. Moreover, we have no idea at all of the incidence of more subtle forms of birth defects such as behavioral alterations or increased susceptibility to cancer later in life. The recent experience with DES has proven that the latter possibility is not mere theory, and a growing number of studies in laboratory animals and people is also documenting the existence of behavioral abnormalities particularly with regard to drugs given during labor and delivery.

Recent studies have documented that 82 percent of all pregnant women received prescribed medication during pregnancy, 65 percent took self-prescribed drugs (excluding alcohol and tobacco), 57 percent smoked, 85 percent used alcohol, and 95 percent received some form of medication during labor and delivery.[3] Add this voluntary exposure to the huge number of environmental chemicals which gain entry to the pregnant woman's body via food, air, and water, and you have the setting for potential disaster if the placenta permits their passage.* And it does. Despite our considerable ignorance, an overall generalization, one similar to that made for breast milk, is possible. Almost all environmental chemicals which can

---

*Moreover, evidence is slowly accumulating that exposure of the mother or father to teratogens before their offspring are conceived also causes an increased incidence of birth defects in the offspring (G. B. Kolata, "Teratogens Acting through Males," *Science* 202 (1978):733).

make it into the mother's blood stream will pass, to lesser or greater extent, into the fetus. Lipid-soluble substances have little difficulty, for the placenta is, in large part, designed for effective diffusion; for example, the concentration of DDT in fetal blood is almost half as high as in maternal blood. Polar substances generally have a much more difficult time, unless, as is sometimes the case, they can hitch a ride on one of the carriers present to transport organic nutrients and ions into the fetus. Often we simply don't know how a substance enters. Lead, for example, against all theoretical predictions, moves across the placenta fairly readily.

Internal Distribution

Once an environmental chemical has gained entry to the blood across the gastrointestinal tract, respiratory tract, skin, or placenta, it can be eliminated either by excretion or metabolism (i.e., changes in its molecular structure). However, between entry and elimination, the ability of the chemical to exert its actions may be greatly diminished by internal factors which lower its concentration either in the blood or at the site of action itself.

A first line of defense is the plasma proteins, particularly albumin. Many environmental chemicals have a strong attraction for plasma proteins, to which they bind reversibly. A chemical bound in this manner is still, of course, circulating in the blood but it is unable to get out of the blood at its sites of action and exert effects. Only the free (unbound) chemical can do so. This means that binding to plasma proteins reduces the intensity of action of a given total dose of the chemical.

Binding to plasma protein is a double-edged sword, for although it keeps the free blood concentration lower than would otherwise be the case, it prolongs the duration over which the free chemical persists in the blood. This is because the organs responsible for eliminating the chemical from the body—mainly the liver and kidneys—also operate mainly on the free chemical in the blood, so that protein binding hinders their getting hold of the chemical. Of course, since the binding is reversible, the bound protein is in equilibrium with the free, and as the free chemical is eliminated, some of the bound chemical is released from the protein, and so can be excreted in turn. Thus, binding to plasma protein does not completely prevent elimination but does prolong it.

So we see that partial binding of a chemical to plasma albumin produces a trade-off—peak intensity of the chemical's action after entry is reduced but the duration over which some chemical persists in the blood is prolonged. Which of these opposing phenomena turns out to be most important depends on the amount of chemical entering and its dose-response at its sites of actions. Binding might completely eliminate the action of a chemical which is effective only at very high free concentration; in contrast, it might potentiate the action of a chemical which is effective at very low concentrations but only if present for long periods of time (for example, some cancer "promoters," as we shall see).

Binding to plasma proteins is not the only way of altering the fraction of any given total amount of chemical which remains free in the blood. For many chemicals, there occurs a similar and quantitatively even more important type of binding to certain intracellular proteins and to the protein meshwork of bones. The latter provides a potentially very large storehouse for a variety of environmental chemicals, both organic and metallic. In bone there is no specialized storage protein; the chemical simply binds to the same bone protein which normally binds calcium salts. This nonspecificity also characterizes much intracellular binding to protein but in at least one case, there seems to be a true intracellular storage protein, specific for cadmium and other metals. This protein (known as metallothionein) also binds several essential metal nutrients (zinc, for example) and it may have evolved to prevent toxicity from overdoses of these nutrients. Its importance lies in the fact that its synthesis is highly inducible; thus, if the amount of cadmium in the body starts to rise because of increasing exposure, the metal somehow triggers the DNA-mRNA-protein-synthesizing machinery to start turning out more metallothionein, which can then lock up the metal.

Binding to proteins is not the only way the body "stores" environmental chemicals. The body's fat cells are far and away the most important storage site for lipid-soluble chemicals. Each fat cell consists of a narrow band of cytoplasm containing all the cell's organelles—nucleus, mitochondria, etc.—surrounding a homogeneous interior pool of fat molecules. Lipid-soluble environmental chemicals don't have to "bind" to this fat, they merely dissolve in it!* Therefore

---

*The fetus seems to have an additional storage site for lipid-soluble environmental chemicals reaching it across the placenta. The vernix caseosa, a greasy coating over the skin, has been found to contain extremely high concentrations of lipid-soluble environmental chemicals such as DDT, and it is shed soon after birth.

the relative solubilities of the molecule in water and lipid determine, respectively, its relative concentrations in blood (which in mainly water) and fat cells. DDT, for example, being much more soluble in lipid than in water, has an average blood concentration in Americans of 50 ppb (parts per billion) in blood and 10,000 ppb in fat (1 ppb is equal to 1 microgram [μg] of chemical per kilogram of blood fat cells, kidney, seawater, or any other material; 1 ppm is 1 μg/g of fluid or tissue).

As is the case with binding to plasma protein, the binding of chemicals to bone protein and intracellular proteins, as well as the storage of lipid-soluble chemicals in fat cells, is reversible. The bound or lipid-storage forms are in equilibrium with the free chemical in blood and so are released whenever this free concentration falls. Therefore, these processes, like the binding to plasma protein, reduce the intensity of action of any given total amount of the chemical, but increase the length of time that some chemical, no matter how low in concentration, persists in the blood. For example, if exposure to environmental DDT were to fall to zero tomorrow, most of us would still have some DDT coming out of our fat to be metabolized and excreted for months or even years.

Two other phenomena are attributable to the sheer magnitude of storage of environmental chemicals: toxicity from sudden release, and multiplication in the food chain. The latter stems simply from the fact that, at each step in the food chain, the concentration of the chemical in the body of the plant or animal ingested is higher (because of storage) than that in the preceding stage. For example, the concentration of DDT (in parts per million, i.e., μg DDT/g whole body weight) in plankton, minnow, and green heron are, respectively, 0.04, 0.94, and 3.50.

Rapid release from storage occurs mainly in two circumstances, the first being weight loss. During fasting or weight loss due to disease, the body's fat stores are progressively mobilized, and as the fat molecules are released from the shrinking fat cells into the blood, so are the chemicals dissolved in them. Blood DDT concentrations in people may more than double at this time, and this provides an interesting example of how vague statements like "fasting is good because it 'cleans out the system' " may be illogical; yes, fasting does potentiate the excretion of DDT from the body but only because it considerably increases the plasma concentration of DDT. Only if it were less dangerous to have a higher plasma concentration of DDT for short periods of time than a lower concentration for a longer time would intermittent fasting be protective against the toxic effects of DDT. This is certainly not the case for the acute lethal effects of large quantities of DDT as demonstrated vividly by the huge number of fish which died in the Mississippi a few years ago; the fish had accumulated large amounts of DDT in their fat during the summer, and then this DDT poured out of the fat cells during the winter as the fish mobilized the fat for energy. The potential danger of DDT to human beings is not, however, this pesticide's acute effects but rather chronic effects such as carcinogenesis.

While we are on the subject of weight loss and DDT, let me emphasize one more implication of chemical accumulation in fat, this one essential for proper interpretation of epidemiological data. Several years ago, a highly publicized retrospective study reported that persons dying from cancer had singificantly higher concentrations of DDT in their fat than did a control group of the same age, socioeconomic status, and place of residence, who had died in automobile accidents. The inference: DDT may be a causal factor in carcinogenesis. This inference, of course, was based on the assumption that the cancer patients had more DDT in their bodies (whether because of increased ingestion or decreased elimination), but this assumption was wrong. The scientists had used DDT *concentrations* in fat as a marker for total body DDT, but this is valid only if the two groups had possessed identical quantities of fat. This sounds complicated but is not at all. Imagine dissolving the same quantities of DDT in one quart of lipid and one-half quart of lipid; the *concentration* of DDT would be twice as high in the one-half quart than in the one quart. This was essentially the case in this study; patients generally die of cancer slowly, losing large amounts of weight, much of which is fat, in the process; as the volume of fat in the body shrank, the DDT left behind in the remaining fat simply became more concentrated. Thus, it is far more likely that the presence of cancer caused the elevated DDT concentrations in fat rather than vice versa.

The other circumstance associated with rapid release of a chemical from storage, particularly from bone, is acute exposure to a second chemical which competes with the first for the binding sites. An example learned the hard way concerns the antimalarial drugs—primaquine and atabrine. Both bind strongly to bone, and some persons previously receiving primaquine for long periods of time suffered toxic effects from rapidly rising blood concentrations of this chemical when they were abruptly switched to atabrine. The latter drug had simply displaced large amounts of primaquine from bone binding sites.

So far I have been describing only those internal factors—binding to or dissolving in storage molecules—which influence how much of the total body content of a chemical will actually be free in the plasma. Now we can shift our focus to the next anatomic level of importance, from the blood to the tissue or organ which constitutes the site of action of the chemical. The point is that, at any given blood level of free chemical, not all tissues and organs can be penetrated to the same degree by that chemical. One very important reason is that the chemical must leave the blood vessel by diffusion in order to gain access to cells, and the capillaries (the small blood vessels across which such diffusion occurs) in the different parts of the body differ in the ease with which they permit diffusion. The liver capillaries, for example, are extremely "leaky" so that almost any chemical can gain access to liver cells (this is in keeping with the liver's functions in chemical metabolism). In contrast, the capillaries in the brain and the gonads (ovaries and testes) are very "tight," and this provides these areas with a large degree of immunity from influence by environmental chemicals. This offers an example of how one's concept of "good" vis-à-vis the body's barriers and responses to environmental chemicals depends on the context; it is fine that potentially toxic chemicals have a hard time getting at the brain, but the other side of the coin is that it is difficult to get therapeutic drugs into the brain to combat infections and other diseases.

Excretion of Environmental Chemicals

There are three major routes for the excretion of environmental chemicals: the respiratory tract, kidneys, and gastrointestinal tract. Loss via the respiratory tract is pretty much limited to environmental chemicals which are quite volatile, i.e., can vaporize easily, like acetone or alcohol. In contrast, the kidneys and gastrointestinal tract excrete a wide spectrum of environmental chemicals.

Kidneys

To really understand the role the kidneys play in excreting environmental chemicals, one must become familiar with a little basic kidney (renal) physiology (fig. 8–2). Each kidney is composed of approximately one million similar functional units called nephrons. Each of the nephrons begins as a blind-ended hollow capsule in intimate contact with a nest of capillaries (the glomerulus). The pressure of the blood in the capillaries is much higher than that of the fluid in the hollow capsule, and so filtration of fluid occurs from the blood into the capsule, and this is the initial event in urine formation. We have just added a third type of transport to diffusion and carrier-mediated movement; in *filtration*, driven by a pressure difference, bulk-fluid flow occurs in a single oriented direction, in marked contrast to the random movements of individual molecules characteristic of diffusion, the energy for which comes not from an external pressure but from the internal energy of the molecules.

The small pores through which this glomerular filtration occurs are too small to permit plasma proteins to pass, but everything else in the plasma can. Thus, the filtered fluid is basically protein-free plasma, and an average person filters 180 liters of this fluid each day!

Fig. 8–2. **The three basic components of renal function.** (Redrawn from A. J. Vander, J. H. Sherman, and D. S. Luciano, *Human Physiology: The Mechanisms of Body Function*, 3d ed. [New York: McGraw-Hill, 1980].)

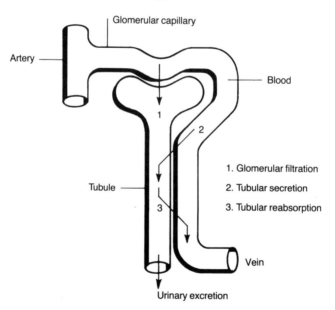

Glomerular capillary

Artery

Blood

1

2

1. Glomerular filtration

2. Tubular secretion

3. Tubular reabsorption

Tubule

3

Vein

Urinary excretion

The second part of the nephron is the tubule, an elongated small tube lined with a single layer of cells, which runs from the hollow capsule to merge ultimately with the tubules of other nephrons and drain its urine into the plumbing system ending in the bladder. Along their entire lengths, the tubules are adjacent to capillaries (not the glomerular capillaries but a different set into which blood from the glomerular capillaries ultimately drains), and this permits exchanges of materials between the blood vessels and tubules in both directions. When a substance moves from tubule to blood vessel the process is called reabsorption. Reabsorption permits a molecule, filtered upstream at the glomerulus, to be reclaimed by the blood and so not to appear in the final urine.

You could have predicted the existence of reabsorption once you were informed that 180 liters of protein-free plasma filter each day. You know you don't urinate 180 liters of water each day, and the reason is that about 99 percent of the filtered water is reabsorbed, only the remaining 1 percent being left behind in the tubules to appear in the final urine. Many other substances undergo reabsorption, to greater or lesser degrees than water. For example, large amounts of glucose are filtered through the glomerulus each day, but none of it appears in the urine of normal persons because it is all reabsorbed back into the blood (diabetics lose glucose in their urine because the amounts filtered may be so huge as to exceed the tubules' capacity to reabsorb this sugar). In contrast, only about 50 percent of the filtered urea (you'll recall that this is the nitrogenous end product of amino acid catabolism) is reabsorbed.

The fact that different percentages of water, glucose, and urea are reabsorbed underscores how different the mechanisms for reabsorption are from filtration, in which everything (excluding the proteins) moves together. Reabsorption does not occur by filtration (beyond the glomerulus there is little pressure difference between the tubule and its surrounding blood vessels), but rather by our old friends, diffusion and carrier-mediated transport. The principles here are precisely the same as those described for gastrointestinal absorption. Highly lipid-soluble substances can more readily cross the tubule and so the existence of a concentration gradient will automatically drive net diffusion in the direction of reabsorption; polar substances, in contrast, generally require interaction with more or less specific membrane carriers for their reabsorption.

Perhaps surprisingly, net movement of a molecule can occur

across the tubules in the direction opposite to reabsorption, i.e., from blood vessel into tubule. This is called secretion and it obviously offers another route (glomerular filtration being the first) by which a substance can gain entry to the tubule and appear in the urine. This route can be very important quantitatively, since only about 20 percent of the plasma flowing into the glomeruli filters into the tubules; the rest passes into the blood vessels adjacent to the rest of the tubules' length, and the remaining 80 percent of the plasma's molecules could theoretically be secreted into the tubules, either by diffusion or carrier-mediated transport mechanisms.

To summarize, the kidney handles any particular substance by a combination of glomerular filtration, reabsorption, and secretion. The first and third processes facilitate the excretion of the substance whereas the second opposes excretion. Filtration is a common pathway for all plasma substances except proteins (and everything else bound to these proteins), whereas reabsorption and secretion are discrete processes. Whether a substance will undergo them depends on its molecular structure (particularly its lipid solubility), the presence of a concentration difference for it (to drive diffusion), the existence of membrane carriers for it, and the orientation of these carriers in the cells lining the tubules (one kind of orientation causes reabsorption, whereas the opposite will cause secretion).

We can now apply this basic information to the renal handling of environmental chemicals. To be excreted, environmental chemicals must gain entry to the tubules by glomerular filtration or secretion across the tubule. All chemicals in the plasma not bound to proteins automatically and quite nonspecifically undergo glomerular filtration, so that this mode of entry constitutes an extremely important pathway. We can now see why the binding of an environmental chemical to plasma proteins slows its excretion; filtration of the bound chemical simply does not occur. The importance of glomerular filtration also explains why patients suffering from a disease-induced reduction in the number of functioning glomeruli are likely to excrete most environmental chemicals quite slowly and therefore, to experience higher blood concentrations of these chemicals than normal persons do for any given level of exposure.

In contrast to glomerular filtration, which applies to all chemicals not bound to plasma proteins, secretion is a route of excretion for only a few types of environmental chemicals, mainly those for which membrane carriers oriented in the secretory direction exist.

As is the case for the gastrointestinal tract, these carriers are, for the most part, carriers of normally occurring plasma constituents, and can be utilized by structurally similar foreign chemicals because the carriers may not be terribly specific. Penicillin is a good example of a foreign chemical which utilizes a secretory carrier-mediated system, in this case one which normally handles endogenous organic acids (fig. 8–3). Quinine uses the system which normally secretes endogenous organic bases. It should be obvious that foreign substances which undergo secretion tend to be cleared from the body quite rapidly and so are less likely to accumulate. (Early in World War II, supplies of penicillin were quite low and in order to keep the penicillin in the body longer, a drug capable of blocking penicillin's secretion, by competing with it for the carrier, was sought and found.)

Just as is true for normally occurring bodily chemicals, neither its glomerular filtration nor secretion assures an environmental chemical's excretion. Reabsorption, i.e., movement of the substance from tubule back into the blood, may cancel these processes partially or

Fig. 8–3.   **Diagrammatic representation of the kidney's handling of penicillin (filtration and secretion) and DDT (filtration and reabsorption).** (Redrawn from A. J. Vander, J. H. Sherman, and D. S. Luciano, *Human Physiology: The Mechanisms of Body Function*, 3d ed. [New York: McGraw-Hill, 1980].)

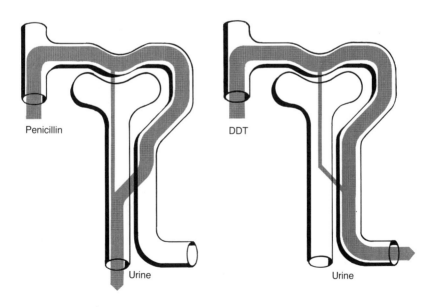

Penicillin

DDT

Urine

Urine

completely. In some cases, reabsorption may occur via carrier-mediated systems, when the environmental chemical resembles the endogenous molecules usually reabsorbed by these systems, but far more important is the nonspecific reabsorption, by diffusion, undergone by all lipid-soluble environmental chemicals. Recall that net diffusion of a lipid-soluble substance across a biological membrane will occur whenever there is a concentration difference for that substance across the membrane. The crucial point is that such diffusion gradients always exist for lipid-soluble environmental chemicals from tubule to blood. Let us see why, using DDT as an example.

The fluid filtered through the glomeruli contains free DDT (DDT not bound to protein) in the same concentration as exists in plasma (remember that everything in plasma, except the proteins, filters together with water). Therefore, in the very first part of the tubule, no concentration difference exists for DDT between tubular fluid and blood. But now, as the filtered fluid moves along the tubule, water reabsorption occurs, and this removal of pure water concentrates everything left behind in the remaining water (just think of how a salt solution in a glass becomes more and more concentrated as pure water is lost, in this case by evaporation). This includes, of course, DDT, so that now the concentration of DDT in the tubule rises above that in the plasma, and this concentration difference drives the reabsorption of DDT by diffusion (see fig. 8–3).

To realize the potential magnitude of this process, just recall that approximatley 99 percent of the filtered water is reabsorbed. Since the tubule is so permeable to the highly lipid-soluble DDT, the reabsorption of this pesticide lags only slightly behind that of water, so that almost all of the filtered DDT is also reabsorbed, extremely little being left behind to be excreted in the final urine. This is why the kidneys are so ineffective in ridding the body of DDT and other highly lipid-soluble environmental chemicals in their original forms. One practical application of this information is that drinking large quantities of water enhances the excretion of many lipid-soluble chemicals because the less water reabsorbed, the less chemical.

Gastrointestinal Tract

We have seen that gastrointestinal absorption may be incomplete for some ingested environmental chemicals, the unabsorbed fraction simply moving the length of the tract and appearing in the feces. I remind you of this only to emphasize that incomplete absorption of ingested chemical is not what is meant by excretion via the gastrointestinal tract. One does not refer to this as excretion (i.e., loss from the body), because the chemical never really made it into the body in the first place (as long as an ingested substance remains in the lumen of the gastrointestinal tract, it is not counted as a gain to the body). For a substance truly to be excreted (lost) from the body via the gastrointestinal tract, it must move from the blood or cells lining the tract into the lumen of the tract, i.e., in the direction opposite to absorption, and be lost in the feces.

The major source of such loss is the bile, the fluid produced by the liver cells and conducted by the biliary duct from the liver to the lumen of the gastrointestinal tract. Other glands, notably the salivary glands, pancreas, and glands within the tract itself, secrete fluids into the lumen, but the bile is by far the most important so far as environmental chemicals are concerned.

Again, however, there is a counteracting process. The bile enters the very first part of the small intestine just below the junction of stomach and intestine, and so its contained chemicals must travel the length of the intestine in order to escape in the feces. This means that the intestine has a shot at absorbing the chemicals and returning them once again to the blood, cancelling the liver's action in removing them from the blood in the first place. As should be predictable, the lipid-soluble environmental chemicals are particularly subject to this sequence, since they readily move both from blood across liver cells into the bile and across the intestinal wall back into the blood.

So now we have seen two distinct seemingly useless cycles, one in the kidneys (filtration or secretion counteracted by reabsorption) and the other in the digestive system (secretion into the bile counteracted by absorption of the biliary constituents from the intestinal tract). These cycles are particularly prominent for lipid-soluble substances and account for the poor excretion of these substances in their original forms. We shall see in the next section that the body has a way out of this predicament, namely, altering these "original forms."

Biotransformation

The body possesses enzymes capable of altering, or biotransforming, the molecular structure of a wide spectrum of organic environmental molecules. Often the resulting molecule, termed a metabolite, does not possess the biological activity of the original parent molecule so that biotransformation is said to have "detoxified" the environmental chemical. However, this is not always the case and, in fact, the metabolite may be even more biologically active than the original molecule. So biotransformation, alone, cannot be counted on to nullify toxicity. Nevertheless, biotransformation is the single most important bodily defense against environmental chemicals, because even when it does not detoxify a chemical, it prepares the chemical for excretion; this is the common denominator of virtually all biotransformation reactions in the body.

These reactions are mediated by enzymes located in any of several tissues and organs, including the liver. The liver is the site where by far the greatest number of biotransformation reactions occur. This makes sense for several reasons. First, the liver is the primary processing plant for almost everything—nutrients and environmental chemicals alike—entering the body by ingestion and absorption across the gastrointestinal tract. I have already emphasized how the flow of blood from gastrointestinal tract to liver assures that the liver gets first crack at most absorbed substances before they can be distributed to the rest of the body. However, I don't want to exaggerate the importance of this fact, since usually only a fraction of the total quantity of an absorbed chemical undergoes biotransformation during this first trip through the liver, so that a reduced but often still considerable amount of intact chemical does make it to the rest of the body; of course, blood keeps returning to the liver over and over again so that the remainder of the molecules can be transformed on these return visits. This is also the fate of chemicals entering the body via the skin and lungs.

The second reason for the liver being a logical site for the majority of biotransformations is that it can secrete many of the metabolites formed during the reactions directly into the bile via which they reach the intestine and can be excreted in the feces. However, I do not wish to leave the impression that the bile is the major recipient of the metabolites; most of them, following their formation, are released by the liver cells not into the bile but into the blood, in which they circulate to the rest of the body and are excreted by the kidneys (of course, this circulation also exposes all the body's organs and tissues to the metabolites, a fact the significance of which I shall deal with later).

It also makes good adaptive sense to have biotransforming enzymes in sites other than the liver. Those in the skin, gastrointestinal tract, and respiratory tract get an opportunity to metabolize a contacted chemical before it ever gets a chance to be taken into the blood. Similarly, those in the placenta provide a last opportunity to metabolize an environmental chemical before it can enter the fetus.

The enzymes which transform foreign molecules were first discovered in the context of their metabolism of drugs, and so they were termed drug-metabolizing enzymes. This name is too restricted, however, for the enzymes act upon many types of chemicals other than drugs. The other commonly used name, microsomal enzyme system (MES), is derived from the location of the enzymes within cells. They are embedded in the membranes of the endoplasmic reticulum, the function of which is to synthesize them and then serve as the actual site for them to perform their transformations. When liver cells are homogenized and centrifuged, these membranes break up and form tiny vesicles (membrane-bound spheres) known as microsomes—thus the name MES. The enzymes retain their function in these laboratory preparations, and so microsomes have provided an extremely valuable tool for studying the biotransformation enzymes *in vitro* (this latter phrase signifies a test-tube experiment, one performed on cells, tissues, or organs removed from a complex organism, or on intact simpler forms of life such as bacteria).

Biochemically oriented scientists have had a field day working out the numerous enzymes of the MES and the variety of reactions they catalyze, but out of this complexity has emerged a single unifying generalization: The essential effect of these reactions is to convert lipid-soluble organic compounds into water-soluble (lipid-insoluble) ones. This is what I was referring to in the previous section when I said the body had a way out of the predicament posed by the fact that lipid-soluble substances are so difficult to excrete since they are readily reabsorbed by the kidney tubules. The MES alters the molecule's structure in such a way that the metabolite becomes much less lipid-soluble than the parent molecule and so, following its filtration at the glomeruli (lipid-solubility has little bearing on filterability at the glomerulus), it is no longer able simply to diffuse across the tubule back into the blood and so will remain in the tubule to be excreted in the urine (unless, of course, as is not usually the case, it can hitch a ride on a reabsorptive carrier-mediated pathway). Thus, the liver transformations permit the kidneys to serve their rightful role as the major excretors of foreign molecules. For analogous reasons, transformed chemicals secreted into the bile are much more likely not to be absorbed by the intestine but to be excreted in the feces.

How does one make an organic molecule less lipid-soluble? It really isn't very hard—adding or removing one or more oxygen atoms, hydrogen atoms, hydroxyl (OH) ions, or water molecules will usually do the trick, since any of these transformations tends to cause a clustering of electrical charge in certain regions of the molecule, in contrast to the uniform charge distribution which is the major determinant of lipid-solubility. This increased polarity is often achieved not in a single step but in a sequence of reactions. Frequently, the final step is not just a subtle fiddling with a few atoms but the wholesale addition to the molecule of a charged natural constituent of the body such as the glucose derivative, glucuronic acid, or the tripeptide (a molecule consisting of three amino acids), glutathione. Such additions are called conjugation reactions and are highly effective in making the new molecules formed in the process insoluble in lipid.

Because so many of the transformations involve oxygen and the transfer of electrons, it is not surprising that the key enzyme in the MES is a protein similar to hemoglobin and the mitochondrial enzymes involved in the cell's utilization of oxygen and provision of energy. Termed cytochrome P-450, it is really not a single enzyme but exists in different forms within a single cell, the different forms acting upon different molecules. The multiple forms of cytochrome P-450 are not the only source of diversity in the MES, which includes many other enzymes (such as the one which catalyzes the addition of glucuronide), and these, too, exist in multiple forms which operate on different molecules. Finally, even a single enzyme in the MES is usually able to act upon more than one chemical.

The result of all this diversity is that the MES, taken as a whole, is relatively nonspecific. It will metabolize an incredible variety of lipid-soluble substances covering almost the entire spectrum of foreign organic molecules. How did such a system evolve? By now, you ought to be able to answer this question with ease. The MES did not evolve to metabolize foreign organic molecules (to which our distant ancestors were never exposed), but rather to metabolize naturally occurring bodily compounds, preparing them for excretion. The normal endogenous substances the MES is known to metabolize include steroid hormones, the fat-soluble vitamins, thyroid hormone, bilirubin (the breakdown product of hemoglobin catabolism), cholesterol, and fatty acids. Thus, the MES is really a component of the homeostatic control systems regulating the amounts of these useful substances (only the waste product, bilirubin, of those mentioned doesn't deserve the label "useful"), and it operates on the foreign chemicals as well simply because they have molecular characteristics similar to those of the endogenous substances.

Induction of the MES

Now for the feature of the MES that completes its qualifications for the single most important component of our defenses against environmental chemicals—it is a highly inducible system! Upon prolonged or repeated exposure to a particular environmental chemical, the DNA-RNA-protein-synthesizing machinery responsible for manufacturing the enzymes of the MES is stimulated, and the result is more of the enzymes, which leads to a faster rate of metabolism of the inducing chemical at any given blood concentration of the chemical.

Clearly, we have here a system which *actively* resists any rise in the blood concentration of DDT; it is a form of acclimatization, as defined in chapter 1, since it represents an improvement, over time, in the body's resistance to DDT. I stressed the word "actively" because this is really the first time (except for the earlier example of the metal-binding protein, metallothionein) that we have seen the body doing anything more than passively responding to increasing amounts of foreign chemicals. Yes, the gastrointestinal tract has a limit to its ability to absorb those foreign chemicals which use carriers, and this offers protection against larger amounts of the chemical; but the presence of the chemical doesn't cause the gut to make fewer carriers and so improve the protection. Yes, the kidneys filter more of a chemical when its blood concentration is elevated, simply because they can't help doing so; but the high blood concentration doesn't cause the kidneys to increase the volume of plasma they filter so as to get rid of the chemical faster. Yes, the higher the blood DDT gets, the more moves into fat cells, thereby helping to minimize the blood concentration, but only because this is an inevitable consequence of increased concentration causing an increased rate of diffusion; the increased DDT doesn't drive an increase in the number of fat cells or their capacity to establish a higher internal DDT concentration for any given blood concentration.

In contrast to these examples, a high concentration of DDT does cause the liver to make more enzyme molecules (or activate more of the ones already present) so that DDT is metabolized more rapidly than it otherwise would be at the same blood concentration. This induction usually requires repeated or prolonged exposure to the chemical, and once achieved, the enhanced MES activity is long-lasting; indeed, it usually persists for several weeks after the disappearance of the inducing chemical.

Table 8–1 gives just a sampling of the more than 200 chemicals and chemical families known to induce the MES and, in turn, acted upon by the MES. Notice how many commonly used drugs and ubiquitous environmental pollutants appear on this list. Ethanol, for example, is a potent inducer, and this accounts, in large part, for the well-known tolerance to ethanol developed by heavy drinkers; because induction increases the rate of metabolism of ethanol, the alcoholic must drink progressively more and more to achieve a given blood level of ethanol. (Enzyme induction is not, however, the explanation of the tolerance developed to narcotic drugs such as morphine; that type of tolerance reflects changes in the brain cells upon which the narcotic acts, not changes in the metabolism of the narcotic.)

Table 8–1 leads us to another very important generalization. Because of the relative nonspecificity of the MES, induction of in-

TABLE 8–1   Some Foreign Chemicals Which Stimulate Induction of the MES in Man

Nicotine
Ethanol ("alcohol")
Meprobamate (a commonly used tranquilizer)
Many barbiturates
Many food preservatives
Many dyes used as coloring agents
DDT and other halogenated hydrocarbons
Urea-containing herbicides
Many volatile oils
Polycyclic aromatic hydrocarbons (such as benzapyrene in cigarette smoke)
Polychlorinated biphenyl (PCBs)

Source: A. H. Conney and J. J. Burns, "Metabolic Interactions among Environmental Chemicals and Drugs," *Science* 172 (1972):576–86.

creased MES function by one chemical almost invariably causes an enhanced metabolism not just of the inducing chemical but of others acted upon by the same enzymes. This phenomenon is what first led accidentally to the discovery that the MES is inducible. The length of time rats slept after receiving various doses of hexobarbital was being routinely measured, as an indication of the blood levels of this sleeping medicine achieved with these doses, when the scientists observed that, over a few days, the hexobarbital seemed to have become much less potent; the rats were barely going to sleep at all at doses that had previously been quite effective. In searching for the possible cause, they found that the rat cages had been sprayed with the insecticide, chlordane, a few days prior to these striking changes. Ultimately it was shown that the chlordane had induced the liver enzymes which metabolize hexobarbital (as well as chlordane) so that the rats' livers were already "revved-up" when the hexobarbital was given, the result being a very rapid transformation and excretion of the drug.

One must not gain the impression that complete nonspecificity exists in the MES and that the chlordane caused all the enzymes of the MES to be induced and all the chemicals of table 8–1 to be metabolized more rapidly. Scientists are slowly working out just which other chemicals have their metabolism most affected by any given inducer, but such details go way beyond the scope of this book. What is critical for our purposes is to recognize that one foreign chemical can have, via the MES, a profound stimulatory effect on the metabolism, and therefore the actions, of others. This is one of the major reasons that it is very difficult to make quantitative predictions concerning the toxicity (or benefit, if the chemical in question is a medicinal drug) of a foreign chemical in the real world, in which so many other chemicals are also present, from controlled experiments using that chemical alone, even when human beings are the subjects.

There are many examples of this type of interaction, and description of a few involving the barbiturates, a family studied extensively because of its wide clinical use, may clarify the basic principles just described.

1. Persons treated with phenobarbital have lower concentrations of DDT in their blood than do control untreated persons, because the drug induces the enzymes which metabolize the insecticide.

2. The enzymes induced by phenobarbital also metabolize the anticoagulant drugs used commonly to treat patients suspected of being subject to excessive blood clotting. If the patient is receiving phenobarbital as well as the anticoagulant, a considerably larger dose of the latter is required for effective therapy. If the phenobarbital is then withdrawn, this dose of anticoagulant may achieve such a high blood concentration as the inducing effect of the barbiturate is lost, that clotting may be completely blocked, with resulting hemorrhage.*

3. In the first two examples, the barbiturate was the inducing agent. This one reverses the situation. Persons who chronically ingest ethanol in large amounts are quite resistant to the effects of barbiturates (when they are sober) because the ethanol induces the enzymes which metabolize barbiturates. (However, once the alcoholic has destroyed his liver, this, of course, no longer applies.)

4. This example makes a very different point. An alcoholic (or a normal person) who imbibes a single large dose of ethanol is extremely sensitive (not resistant) to a simultaneous dose of barbiturates. Here, induction is not involved at all, for there has been no time for it to occur. Rather, we are seeing the competition of two drugs for the same enzyme. The ethanol combines with most of the metabolizing enzymes' sites, and prevents the barbiturate from being metabolized. The blood level of the barbiturate may go so high that, in combination with the depressant effects of ethanol on the brain, it may kill the person. I have given little attention to this type of competitive interaction because the one involving induction is of far greater general importance to the problem of long-term toxicity of environmental chemicals.

Inhibition of the MES

Because of the central importance of the MES in our defenses against environmental chemicals, anything which inhibits this system (or interferes with its inducibility) can be quite dangerous. Such an inhibitor will increase the potency of a large number of other chemicals simply by diminishing their rates of biotransforma-

---

*A similar relationship holds for DDT and the anticoagulant, warfarin, used commonly as a raticide. Wild rats have clearly become more resistant to warfarin, and among the hypotheses suggested to explain this resistance is the possibility that DDT, present in high concentrations in rats, may be inducing the MES and, thereby, speeding the metabolism of warfarin.

tion and thereby causing higher blood concentrations of these other chemicals for any given level of exposure.

Unfortunately, the capacity to inhibit the MES is a characteristic of many environmental agents. These include organophosphorous insecticides, many metals such as lead, certain pesticide synergists (used specifically to enhance the potency of DDT and other MES-metabolized pesticides), carbon monoxide, carbon tetrachloride, and morphine.

Environmental chemicals are not the only factor capable of inhibiting the MES. Perhaps the most important one of all is malnutrition, particularly protein deficiency. This explains why DDT and many other pesticides are so much more toxic in laboratory animals maintained on subnormal protein intakes; total body DDT in these animals is many times greater than in control animals fed the same amount of DDT with normal amounts of protein. The possible implications of this for human beings is obvious, particularly since DDT is presently used most extensively in developing countries, and these are precisely the places in which protein deficiency is most prevalent. Whether this synergism is actually able to raise DDT levels high enough in people to produce toxic effects is simply not known.

Protein has been the best studied dietary factor affecting the MES, but it is by no means the only one. Indeed, it now appears that the basal activity and inducibility of the MES is subject to influence by many nutrients. Diets deficient, for example, in polyunsaturated fatty acids prevent full inducibility of the MES by barbiturates in rats. Diets relatively low in vitamin C have a similar blocking effect on the induction response of DDT. This latter defect was observed even though the vitamin C intake was in excess of the amounts required to prevent scurvy and, indeed, were higher than the present RDA for vitamin C. The role of nutrition in the metabolism of environmental chemicals clearly is an extremely important research area, one which beautifully illustrates how the concept of "optimal" intakes must always be in terms of a specific environment.

There is one more extremely important situation characterized by low activity of the MES. In newborn and very young animals (including people), the MES simply has not yet matured fully. This means that the young may be more susceptible than adults to certain environmental chemicals. This has been clearly demonstrated for DDT and several other MES-metabolized substances.

Toxicity of MES-formed Metabolites

The logical inference which one might draw from what has been described so far is that MES induction is an unmitigated benefit in our defense against environmental pollutants. Surely it seems a good thing to metabolize pollutants more rapidly so that they can be excreted, and by the same token, it seems good protection for the induction triggered by any particular pollutant to speed the biotransformation of others as well. It would also seem a bad thing for the system to be inhibited. Most of the time this is all true, but unhappily not always. For two reasons, induction of the MES by foreign chemicals can have maladaptive consequences as well as the obvious beneficial ones. Moreover, under certain conditions, inhibition of the MES might turn out to be a blessing. The bases for these generalizations have already been mentioned in passing: (1) the metabolites of some environmental chemicals are far more toxic than the parent compounds; (2) the enzyme induction may result in excessively rapid metabolism of the endogenous (naturally occurring) bodily substances which share the same metabolic pathways.

More than fifty chemicals have been proven to yield metabolites, upon biotransformation, which are considerably more toxic than the parent molecules from which they were generated, and this will unquestionably turn out to be the case for many other still untested chemicals. Indeed, many chemicals, like carbon tetrachloride, are completely nontoxic until they are metabolized by the liver. As luck would have it, this creation of toxic molecules from relatively harmless ones applies to the class of environmental chemicals we most fear—carcinogens! The majority of environmental chemicals proven to cause cancer are completely or relatively harmless until the MES in the liver (or other tissue) converts them to their carcinogenic form, usually a highly reactive type of molecule known as an epoxide.

This phenomenon has been most extensively studied for the class of chemicals called polycyclic aromatic hydrocarbons, which includes benzapyrene, other components of cigarette smoke, chemicals in polluted city air, and charcoal-broiled or smoked foods, to name just a few. The MES enzyme which acts upon these molecules to produce epoxides at an early stage in their biotransformation is called aryl hydrocarbon hydroxylase (AHH), a name worth remembering because of its profound importance in the production of active carcinogens. This enzyme is found not only in the liver but in the lungs, gastrointestinal tract, the kidneys, the skin, white blood cells, and the placenta, so that carcinogens can be produced in high concentrations not only in the liver but in other organs as well, where they act immediately. It is highly inducible by cigarette smoke, and so smokers have much higher activity in their lungs (and other sites) than do nonsmokers (in human placentas, for example, this enzyme is highly active in smokers but almost undetectable in nonsmokers). Environmental chemicals other than polycyclic aromatic hydrocarbons can also induce it, the PCBs for example.

Once this is all realized, the logic concerning the beneficial nature of biotransformation enzymes and their inducibility (or inhibitability) gets reversed. It is a disaster that benzapyrene is biotransformed by the MES, because the result is production of a carcinogen; better to have the molecule be more slowly excreted than to have it converted to a metabolite which gets out of the body faster but may cause cancer before doing so. It is also a disaster that benzapyrene induces the MES (to be more specific, the AHH component of the MES), because that results in an even higher blood concentration of the potent carcinogenic form. The fact that PCBs also induce the AHH component of the MES no longer can be viewed as one pollutant (PCB) inducing protection against another (benzapyrene) but just the opposite. Finally, inhibition of AHH, for example by mild protein deficiency, might be protective against cancer development in a heavy smoker, and the relatively low activity of AHH in the fetus might also be protective if the mother were a smoker (of course, as we have seen, the placenta has a highly inducible AHH and so can supply the fetus with plenty of benzapyrene epoxide; moreover, the AHH system is only relatively immature in the fetus but it is still present). This only emphasizes what a danger the placental AHH may be to the fetus whose mother smokes or is exposed, as we all are, to environmental chemicals capable of generating carcinogens.

The fact that biotransformation by AHH is required for the production of many carcinogens makes it very likely that much of the genetic difference in cancer susceptibility between people can be accounted for by differences in the activity or inducibility of their AHH. Studies (using white blood cells, the AHH inducibility of which correlates well with that of lung and other tissues) have revealed that normal persons differ markedly in the extent of AHH inducibility, 53 percent being classified as low inducibility, 37 percent intermediate, and 10 percent high.[4] Very importantly, these proportions were strikingly different in patients who had lung cancer; only 4 percent were in the low category with 66 percent intermediate and 30 percent high. The overall data suggest that persons with intermediate and high inducibility of AHH have, respectively, sixteen and thirty-six times higher risk for developing lung cancer than those with low inducibility. We may well be on the way to understanding why some persons can smoke very heavily yet never get lung cancer, whereas some relatively light smokers do.

Another mysterious aspect of carcinogenesis which may well be explainable by epoxide formation is the organ-specificity of the cancers produced by environmental carcinogens. Why does one chemical cause cancer in the lungs, another in the kidney, and so on? There are unquestionably multiple explanations, but at least one is that the MESs of different organs have different specificities and activities, so that the carcinogenic form may be produced to a much greater extent in one than in the others.

Because biotransformation of a compound frequently involves multiple steps, the interaction of the beneficial and dangerous aspects of the overall metabolism may be quite complex. For example, aflatoxin (the fungal product mentioned earlier) can produce cancer only after the MES converts it to its epoxide form. On this basis you might predict, logically, that induction of the MES, say by phenobarbital, would increase the ability of a given dose of aflatoxin to produce cancers in experimental animals. Yet, when the experiment was done, the result was precisely the opposite. Pretreatment with phenobarbital actually reduced aflatoxin's carcinogenic potency. This is because the epoxide of aflatoxin is produced at an early step in the metabolism of aflatoxin, and subsequent reactions inactivate the epoxide; it is likely that the phenobarbital has a greater inducing effect on the enzymes acting beyond epoxide formation than on those yielding epoxide. The net effect is that, even though the epoxide is formed more rapidly after phenobarbital-induction, it is inactivated even more rapidly so that its blood concentration ends up being lower after induction than before. Clearly, predictions concerning the influence of one pollutant or drug (the inducer) on the toxicity of another require a high level of knowledge (generally lacking at present for most chemicals) concerning just which enzymes are induced and just how toxic all the metabolites in the biotransformation sequences are.

To make matters more complex, species differences in the relative effects on the multiple steps can actually result in opposite effects in various species. Thus, pretreatment of mice with phenobarbital increases the liver-damaging effect of acetaminophen (a drug requiring metabolism before it can be toxic), whereas in hamsters, pretreatment with the barbiturate decreases acetaminophen's toxicity. Apparently, in mice, phenobarbital induces mainly the MES enzyme catalyzing the formation of the toxic metabolite; it induces this enzyme in hamsters to a much lesser degree and, more important, markedly induces the enzyme which hooks glucuronide on to the toxic metabolite, thereby creating a harmless molecule.

This should also make it clear that attempts to provide some kind of pharmacological across-the-board protection against environmental pollutants, by developing a drug whose only action would be to induce MES, is out of the question. Even if a drug could be found which enhanced only a conjugation step like glucuronide addition (this step seems never to increase a chemical's toxicity), it would run afoul of the next problem to be described.

Effects on Endogenous Molecules

The second reason that the inducibility of the MES system by environmental pollutants may be, in some cases, a mixed blessing is that, once induced, the enzymes might so accelerate metabolism of one or more of the naturally occurring bodily chemicals which share the system that a serious deficiency of that chemical arises. That this type of interaction can definitely occur in human beings has been documented for several drugs, notably for phenobarbital and the anticonvulsant phenytoin. These drugs, both of which are potent inducers of the MES, are frequently given in combination, and may so accelerate the metabolism of vitamin D via the MES that overt rickets occurs.

Interestingly, there may be ways in which the ability of drugs to enhance the metabolism of endogenous substances could be made use of deliberately. Bilirubin, the breakdown product of hemoglobin, has toxic effects on the brains of infants, and it is not uncommon, due to a variety of causes, for this chemical to be dangerously elevated after birth. This high concentration can be markedly reduced by giving the mother a fairly small dose of phenobarbital for a few days prior to expected delivery; the drug crosses the placenta and induces the bilirubin-metabolizing enzymes of the fetus' MES, enzymes usually quite immature at birth. Unfortunately, there are potential dangers to this therapy, which must be carefully studied before its widespread use is contemplated.

To return to the induction by environmental chemicals, of disease-producing excessive metabolism of endogenous substances, perhaps the best publicized case involving an environmental pollutant, rather than a drug, concerns the effects of DDT on reproduction of predatory birds. PCBs seem to do similar things and may well be even more responsible than DDT for the profound decreases that have occurred during the past three decades in the populations of falcons, bald eagles, ospreys, pelicans, and other flesh-eating birds. These decreases are due to a failure to reproduce normally, itself reflecting at least three problems: delayed breeding or failure to lay eggs altogether, thinning of egg shells so that breakage becomes a problem, and a high mortality of embryos and fledglings. Several lines of evidence have demonstrated that the high levels of DDT and PCBs in their bodies (a predictable finding considering the position of these birds at the top of a food chain characterized by a high degree of pesticide accumulation at each step) were responsible. Multiple sites of action seem to be involved, but the delayed breeding and failure to lay eggs are accounted for, in large part, by a marked lowering in the plasma concentration of the key hormone— estrogen—involved in these processes. Just as in humans, this hormone is normally metabolized by the liver's MES and the high rate of MES activity induced by the pesticide and the PCBs caused such rapid metabolism of the estrogen that a deficiency of the hormone resulted.* That this sequence of events is not limited to birds is strongly suggested by the premature pupping that has been occurring in sea lions living in certain locations. Those mothers having premature pups have much higher concentrations of DDT and PCBs in their bodies than those delivering at the right time.

What about human beings? Are the levels of DDT in our blood high enough to induce the MES, and if so, is it induced enough to interfere significantly with our normal metabolism? Data from controlled animal experiments suggest that the answer to the first may be yes, since the minimum exposure to DDT required for induction of the MES (as estimated by increased metabolism of test doses of

*Estrogen and DDT interact in a variety of ways so that we still don't have a completely clear picture; for example, DDT itself has estrogenlike activity.

phenobarbital) in laboratory rats produces a fat cell concentration of 10 to 15 ppm, a value found commonly in the general human population. Of course, the extrapolation to human beings may not be valid, and so we must turn to human studies. Unfortunately, because the MES is influenced by so many factors and because DDT is in all of us, it is almsot impossible to find a proper control group for epidemiological study of the general population. Therefore, we must depend heavily on data obtained from DDT-exposed workers whose plasma concentrations are so high (twenty to thirty times that of the general population) that failure to find evidence of induction in them would pretty conclusively rule out the likelihood of induction by the levels of DDT occurring in the rest of us. (That our society permits workers to be exposed to large amounts of chemicals of unknown toxicity is an unintended boon to toxicological research but an ethical disgrace.)

The first question posed above was tested by administering a chemical (phenylbutazone) known to be metabolized by the MES and measuring, by repeated blood sampling, how long it took for 50 percent of the chemical to be metabolized; this time was significantly less (25 percent) in DDT-exposed workers than in control persons, indicating enhanced activity of the MES. To see whether normally occurring substances were also being metabolized more rapidly, the twenty-four-hour urinary excretion of 6β-hydroxycortisol, one of the metabolites of the hormone cortisol, was measured. DDT-exposed workers excreted significantly more (40 percent) of this metabolite than did control persons, these data suggesting that their MES is metabolizing cortisol more rapidly than normal. Yet, when the actual plasma cortisol concentrations were measured in DDT-exposed workers (in a completely separate study), they were found to be normal. How can the plasma concentration of the hormone be normal even though its rate of metabolism is increased? There is an exquisitely sensitive negative feedback control system regulating plasma cortisol (see chap. 1); if the plasma concentration were to start down because of increased metabolism, this would be detected and trigger an increased secretion of cortisol to keep pace with the increased metabolism, so that plasma concentration would be restored toward normal and maintained there. In other words, there is a safety reserve to all important biological functions so that interference with the system at one point can be more or less compensated by homeostatically triggered alteration at another point.

Other studies (but, at least to me, surprisingly few, considering the potential importance of the relationship) have been done trying to get at whether DDT has disease-producing effects on the metabolism of hormones and other endogenous chemicals in human beings, but the results have been, like those described above, inconclusive. I'd like to mention just one more to reemphasize some problems of interpretation encountered when doing human research, particularly in this area. Because of the information on birds and sea lions and because the sex hormones are so important for maintenance of pregnancy, one of the most pressing toxicological questions regarding DDT is whether it might be causing premature births in humans. In one study of the offspring of normal women (not DDT workers), the concentration of DDT (actually of DDE, a metabolite of DDT which is still highly lipid-soluble and very poorly excreted, and so can be used as a marker of chronic DDT exposure and accumulation) in the whole blood of newborns was measured. There was a striking correlation of DDT concentration with prematurity, and overall, the mean DDT level in premature infants was almost sixfold greater than in normal-term infants. Certainly one possible inference from these data is that high levels of DDT *caused* the premature births, but this may not be a valid inference. Implicit in it is the presumption that when the fetuses subsequently to be born at full term were the same age as those born prematurely, they had lower blood concentrations of DDT. Yet this may not be the case at all; rather, several weeks prior to their birth, i.e., when they were the age at which premature infants delivered, they, too, might have had very high blood DDT concentrations, which then fell during the additional *in-utero* weeks not enjoyed by the prematurely born infants. There are two good reasons why such a decrease would occur during the last weeks of normal pregnancy: (1) the fetus lays down a good deal of fat during this time so that DDT should move from blood into fat (remember the episode of DDT being higher in patients dying of cancer?); (2) the MES increases in maturity so that increased metabolism, followed by excretion (the fetal kidneys are working at this time, the formed urine draining into the fluid surrounding the fetus) would lower blood DDT concentration. Thus, rather than a high blood DDT causing prematurity, the last few weeks of pregnancy might lower blood DDT. Unfortunately, the DDT levels in the mothers were not measured, and this measurement would have been helpful in distinguishing between the two alternatives (as in the sea lion study). The problem clearly deserves intensive study.

Transformations Not Mediated by the MES

I have devoted so much space to MES-mediated metabolic transformations because of their great importance and the large number of environmental chemicals subject to them. However, there are other biologically important metabolic pathways for environmental chemicals, some acting only upon a single chemical, others on an entire family. For example, the reaction:

$$\text{Nitrates} \rightarrow \text{Nitrites} \rightarrow \text{Nitrosamines}$$

has nothing to do with the MES; it, too, results in the production of potent carcinogens (the nitrosamines). Thus, toxicologists cannot simply assume that the MES is the major pathway for every environmental chemical, but must search diligently for other routes and evaluate the consequences of the transformations.

The Gut Bacteria

The actions of the bacteria which inhabit the lower portions of the intestinal tract are another important determinant of the toxicity of environmental pollutants (and the efficacy of therapeutic drugs). The consequences of bacterially mediated molecular alterations cover a broad spectrum. First, the bacteria may transform a potentially harmful chemical into a harmless one; unfortunately they may also do the opposite. For example, the form in which cycasin (the plant product mentioned earlier) is ingested is quite harmless, but the gut bacteria split off a portion of the cycasin molecule, converting it into its toxic form.

Second, the bacteria may not alter the toxicity of the molecule but rather simply cause it to be more absorbable. For example, cyclamate is highly polar and is poorly absorbed, but the gut bacteria metabolize it to a more lipid-soluble form which is absorbable. This type of action is also quite commonly exerted upon the chemicals that gain entry to the intestine not by ingestion but in the bile; the synthetic estrogenlike substance stilbesterol, for example, is transformed by the liver's MES to the lipid-insoluble stilbesterol glucuronide and secreted into the bile, but once it reaches the intestine, the gut bacteria chop off the glucuronide, thereby permitting the lipid-soluble stilbesterol to be absorbed and returned to the blood.

Conclusion

If, by now, you are bemoaning the complexity of the body's handling of environmental chemicals, I have achieved my purpose, for then you are in a position to appreciate why there may be enormous differences in the action of an environmental chemical between persons, between species, and for the same person in different environments and physiological states. First, each of the pathways so important for determining how high a blood concentration will be achieved by a given amount of environmental chemical and, beyond that, how effective that blood concentration will be in exerting effects on the chemical's target tissues and organs is potentially a source of built-in (genetic) variability between persons and across species. There seems little doubt that the greatest degree of genetic variability exists in the biotransformation pathways. Secondly, how effectively all these pathways operate depends not only upon the genetic potential but upon the simultaneous influence, both inhibitory and stimulatory, of the host of environmental chemicals which impinge upon us, by the choice of foods we have made, the kinds and numbers of bacteria in our gut, and whether we happen to be pregnant, have diseased kidneys, are under stress, and so on.

There are many implications to be drawn from the existence of such complexity and sources of variability, but for me, two stand out, both relating to the central question of human toxicology, the quantitation of risk. First, the toxicologic evaluation of a chemical must include as complete an understanding as possible of the ways in which the body handles the chemical. This type of information often seems dull and irrelevant to the general public, not nearly as exciting as the latest demonstration that chemical X (in large doses) has been shown to cause cancer in mice; yet the finding that chemical X is converted into its epoxide form in human beings, and more, that the rate of conversion is fifty times greater in people than in mice, may be of equal or greater significance in deciding whether the levels of chemical X in a factory or the general environment are likely to be causing cancer in people. The finding that a low-calcium diet increases lead absorption has profound implications for poor urban children, many of whom are both calcium deprived and exposed to considerable amounts of lead; any evaluation of the potential hazard offered by lead must take into account this relationship.

The second implication concerns extrapolation from the results of animal experiments to the human situation. There are many well-documented species differences in the handling of foreign chemicals, particularly with regard to the biotransformation reactions, and these account for most known species differences in chemical toxicity. In other words, the difference in the ability of DDT to produce bladder tumors in different species of experimental animal is almost certainly due not to any intrinsic differences in the bladder cells but to differences in how much DDT gets to the bladders and in what forms. The really important point, accepted by most scientists, is that the differences in absorption, excretion, metabolism, and so forth, are generally quantitative, not qualitative. The "unity of biology" generally (but not always) assures that, for example, the MES reactions are almost all present in all mammals, and that only their rates of operation differ from species to species. This means that a chemical capable of causing brain damage in rats will almost certainly, at some dose, do so in humans. Similarly for cancer, kidney disease, birth defects, and so on. The dose (adjusted for body weight) required may be more or less, but it is extremely likely that some dose will do it. Moreover, even if, as can never really be the case, the rat's or guinea pig's gastrointestinal tract, lungs, kidneys, liver, and placenta behaved inherently in a manner quantitatively just like that of human beings, the dose-responses for chemical toxicity in the people would still inevitably be different from those determined on the experimental animals simply because the animal experiments could never possibly duplicate the many other environmental conditions (presence of other chemicals, dietary differences, etc.) which play upon the pathways, altering their inherent rates (thus, the word "inherent" has no real meaning in this context).

Knowing all this, how willing are you to believe in the "innocence" of an environmental pollutant based on the failure to observe, in experimental animals, a toxic effect at doses equivalent to those to which we are exposed? Conversely, how willing are you to shrug off evidence of toxicity in experimental animals because the doses used seem unrealistically large? The next chapter will provide you with more concepts essential for coming to grips with these questions.

Chapter 9 | Saccharin, Cancer, and the Delaney Amendment

The central mission of the governmental agencies* responsible for protecting us from toxic chemicals is the setting of safety standards, maximum acceptable levels of toxic chemicals permitted in food, air, and water. There are really two quite distinct processes involved in the setting of "acceptable risk," as should be obvious from the term itself.[1] The first step—the estimation of risk—is an empirical scientific activity; the second—deciding how much risk shall be deemed acceptable—is a value-laden political activity. Thus, it is quite possible, indeed the rule, to have two standards—one (the higher of the two) for workers and the other for the general population—for the same chemical; clearly the risk for any given amount of the chemical is the same whether it is breathed in the air out on the street or in the factory, but what is deemed acceptable differs for the two situations.

What is acceptable and what isn't is often determined by a risk-

---

*There are four major federal regulatory agencies: (1) the Occupational Safety and Health Administration (OSHA), which sets standards for the workplace; (2) the Environmental Protection Agency (EPA), which has the extensive authority to regulate chemical levels in the general environment; (3) the Food and Drug Administration (FDA), which has authority over chemicals in food, cosmetics, and drugs; (4) the Consumer Product Safety Commission, which has responsibility for over 10,000 consumer products, excluding those (like food additives, pesticides, and tobacco) covered by other jurisdictions. They operate in relative independence from one another, each under the mandates and constraints of the different pieces of legislation which govern them. Recently, they have attempted to improve coordination through the creation of an Interagency Regulatory Liaison Group (IRLG).

benefit, or cost-benefit, analysis. In theory the process is straightforward, but in practice it is fraught with difficulty. The basic idea is simply to weigh pluses and minuses. The first step—the purely scientific one—is to garner the evidence from epidemiology and animal studies and to calculate quantitative estimates of risk to humans from given concentrations of chemical. In the case of cancer, this would be expressed as the number of cases of cancer expected each year from different concentrations of the chemical in food, air, or water. The same procedure is performed for calculation of the benefits, both health and economic, which accrue from use of the substance. Then the magnitudes of the risks and benefits are weighed against each other. If the benefits conferred by a particular chemical are trivial or achievable by other safe substances, then the most appropriate regulatory response is an outright ban, even if the substances carry only a small risk. But such a clear-cut balance is the exception rather than the rule, and so a compromise is reached—the establishment of an "acceptable level," one which does not eliminate all risk but which is thought to reduce risk to a value substantially lower than benefits.

This second step—the actual setting of the acceptable level—requires the making of a host of value judgments. For example, what is the dollar equivalent of a human life? Or, how do you balance risk and benefits when, as is usual, those reaping the benefit are not the same persons taking the risk (coal miners versus the owners of the coal mines and all of us who use coal)? The list of such value judgments is endless.

Clearly, then, even if the scientific estimates of risk and benefit were quite precise, we would still have great problems in standard setting. But these problems, stemming from the need to make value judgments, are enormously increased by the simple fact that the scientific estimates, particularly for low-dose long-term exposure, are rarely precise. Scientists can usually say with considerable confidence that a chemical will, at some dose, cause cancer or some other disease, but they can rarely say exactly how much chemical will cause how much disease. At its best, estimates of risks are educated guesses, which, as we shall see, may be wrong by a factor of hundreds or thousands.

Thus, there are two sources of controversy in the setting of safety standards: the uncertainty of the scientific data upon which they are based and the differing value judgments which determine the use of this scientific data. But these scientific and nonscientific spheres are obviously not independent; for example, those who oppose a safety standard on the basis of value judgments often focus their case on the inadequacy of the supporting scientific data. I use the word "case" advisedly, for regulatory decisions are generally made on the basis of adversary proceedings.

A recent example of this is provided by the present dispute over OSHA's proposed new standard for occupational exposure to benzene. Stimulated by a study which revealed that the mortality rate from leukemia (a cancer of the white blood cells) for workers exposed to benzene in two Goodyear plants from 1940 to 1949 was seven times greater than that for unexposed workers, OSHA decided to lower the workplace standard from 10 parts per million (the 1971 standard) to 1 ppm. OSHA estimated that the cost to industry of complying with the new standard would be $500 million, but OSHA deliberately did not take this into consideration in making its decision. More than any other agency, it has resisted making quantitative estimates of risk or performing risk-benefit analyses, arguing that such attempts at quantitation are not scientifically sound. Rather OSHA simply set the lowest standard possible consistent with being able to manufacture benzene at all. Industry took OSHA to court, and in October, 1978, the Fifth Circuit Court of Appeals in New Orleans ruled against OSHA, arguing that the statute governing OSHA requires a quantitative risk-benefit analysis and that OSHA must make "rough but educated estimates" of the extent of risk and weigh this estimate against the $500 million cost of complying. OSHA took the case to the Supreme Court, arguing (in a brief filed by the Secretary of Labor) that "the Court of Appeals overestimated the precision available in scientific studies of risk from exposure to carcinogens. . . . The Secretary believes that it is not possible to conclude, with any precision, how many cases of cancer could be avoided by reducing exposure from 10 ppm to 1 ppm."[2] The Supreme Court upheld the Court of Appeals holding that OSHA must make some estimate of how much risk would be reduced by the new standard.

This case also highlights another prominent feature of the regulatory process.

> The entire level-setting process occurs in a regulatory morass involving several Federal agencies and a dozen laws (each of which is to some extent vague, inconsistent, or contradictory), state and local

agencies, the courts, Congress, business interests, environmentalists, independent testing laboratories, the National Academy of Sciences, hospitals and universities, a legion of lobbyists, and a growing number of health functionaries on virtually all levels of government. The result is pandemonium.

Lawyers play key roles in level setting because the process is not so much an ongoing clash of opposing scientific truths as one between conflicting social and economic priorities. Regulatory agencies have a real fear of being sued by industry, according to Dr. Sidney Wolfe, a physician who was on the staff of the National Institutes of Health before joining Ralph Nader's Health Research Group in Washington. "In order to keep the agency out of court, they act only when they have the most open-and-shut case," he claims. "When we go into a hearing, we not only see lawyers from industry, but Wall Street analysts, too. There's big money at stake."[3]

The result?

Officials of the Environmental Protection Agency (EPA) and the Occupational Safety and Health Administration (OSHA), the main actors, are often reluctant to take the first step in restricting exposure to toxic substance because they know what happens next; outside pressure is applied, both directly and through Congress, followed inevitably by a lawsuit, which may expose deficiencies in the original law [creating the agency and stipulating its mandate]. Familiarity with this chain of events suggests that a safe approach is to do nothing at all.

The consequences of such an attitude are two-fold. First, regulatory agencies typically do not act until pressure is exerted by outside citizen groups. . . . Unions or public interest groups have been the initiators of OSHA, EPA, or FDA action in 22 of the 26 instances through 1976 when the agencies regulated carcinogens. This record suggests that EPA and OSHA have been taking a passive role, acting as judges and not prosecutors in environmental protection.

Second, when [a regulatory agency] begins to regulate a toxic substance, the length of time spent deciding exactly what to do is immense. . . the average time for rule-making by EPA is now approaching four years.[4]

This sets the stage for the subject of this chapter—an analysis of the validity of the scientific assessment of risk for carcinogens. Saccharin will serve as our example, for the recent controversy over this chemical reflects, at least in part, the public's misunderstanding of how such assessments are made. People have been led to believe that the ban on saccharin was based on a misuse of animal experiments and an ignoring of epidemiological studies. Indeed, the ridicule and anger that this perception has generated threatens to undermine all attempts to regulate carcinogens. After all, if scientists are providing data which are completely irrelevant then any ban or safe level established by regulatory agencies on the basis of these data are worthless.

I shall try to show that, in fact, the experiments used to incriminate saccharin (and other carcinogens) are valid, and that the real problem in the scientific realm of standard setting is not irrelevant experiments but our inability to derive dependable estimates of human risk from them. Once this is recognized, then the policy decisions to be based on these estimates can be considered in terms of this real scientific problem, not a phony distracting one. For it is not the saccharin ban itself, but the regulatory policy which led to its ban, that is presently on trial, and the verdict will have profound consequences for the future regulation of all environmental carcinogens.

The Delaney Amendment

For purposes of regulation, the law classifies nonnatural constituents of food into three categories:

1. *Contaminants*, like DDT and PCBs, which get into food because they are used in agriculture or are present in the environment and simply find their way inevitably into food chains. This category also includes naturally occurring toxins such as aflatoxin.

2. *Direct ingredients*, substances added to food during manufacture or processing to achieve a particular function such as preservation or coloring. Popularly known as "food additives" (although the legal definition of this term is much more restricted), these substances are usually intended to remain in the final product.

3. *Indirect ingredients*, substances intentionally used in food processing or packaging, but not intended to be in the final product. An example is chemicals which leach out of packaging materials and enter the food.

There are thousands of all these substances in our food today, and the number continues to grow as chemical use in and out of the food industry expands. Moreover, our appreciation of just how many contaminants and indirect ingredients really do appear in food has been changed dramatically by the great improvements made recently in chemical detection methods. (We can now measure chemicals in parts per trillion.)

The basic law which protects us against toxic effects from all these chemicals (and naturally occurring food ingredients as well) is the Federal Food, Drug, and Cosmetic Act of 1938, amended so many times since then that the present situation concerning the standards and classifications applicable to given substances is immensely confusing. For purposes of orientation, however, let me mention just a few points. One particular section of the act (section 406) regulates contaminants, and it authorizes the FDA to set "tolerance levels," i.e., acceptable levels of toxins permitted in foods. A different section (409) regulates the other two categories. It requires food additives and indirect ingredients to be tested for safety by the manufacturer, who then submits the test results to the FDA in the petition for approval of the chemical. The law does not define "safety," but the FDA generally interprets it to mean that, with "reasonable certainty," no harm would result from use of the ingredient. This "general safety clause" takes only risk and not benefit into account; however, it does not expressly forbid the consideration of benefit, and the FDA more and more bases its decisions on risk-benefit analysis.

There are several important exceptions to section 409. For one thing, "food additive" does not legally include food ingredients "generally *recognized as safe*" (GRAS) or chemicals already approved before 1958, the date of passage of the Food Additives Amendment. Thus, thousands of substances which are popularly called food additives are exempt from FDA regulation. The vast majority of these substances have never been tested for anything but the crudest acute toxicity, since only such tests were commonly used up to the time the GRAS list was drawn up. A GRAS designation is not absolute, however, for a substance which ultimately comes under suspicion can have its GRAS status revoked (as occurred with saccharin) and then be regulated.

The second important exception to section 409 concerns the Delaney Amendment, added to the act in 1958. It specifies that

> no additive shall be deemed to be safe if it is found to induce cancer when ingested by man or animal, or if it is found, after tests which are appropriate for the evaluation of the safety of food additives, to induce cancer in man or animal.

What makes the Delaney proviso so different from the rest of section 409 is that it defines "safe" in absolutely rigid terms. There is no agonizing over "reasonable certainty," how carcinogenic the substance is, how much is actually added to the food, and so on. If well-done tests show it to be carcinogenic in animals at any dose, then it must go.

The scope of the Delaney Amendment is much less than popularly supposed. It does not, for example, apply to air or water. It does not apply to food contaminants or the substances on the GRAS list. It does not apply to animal drugs unless the drug can be shown to appear as a residue in food (or the carcass after slaughter). Moreover, the Delaney Amendment has no equivalent in the legislation governing the regulatory agencies other than the FDA.

Thus, for only one class of environmental chemicals—food additives—and one type of toxicity—carcinogenesis—has the government set the legal tolerance for a chemical at zero. The Delaney Amendment has been invoked by the FDA only six times (and resulted in a ban only twice), the last time being in 1977 when the FDA announced, with great reluctance, a ban on the use of saccharin (actually the FDA Commissioner, Donald Kennedy, appointed some time after the announcement, later explained that quite apart from the Delaney Amendment, the general safety requirements of food law would have required the ban). This announcement emphasized that the FDA had no choice in the matter despite the fact that the Canadian rat study upon which it was based utilized a dose of saccharin, the human equivalent of 800 cans of diet soda per day. The announcement also stated that saccharin had been in use for more than eighty years and had never been found to harm people. Many believe this announcement was deliberately worded to trigger a storm of protest which would force reevaluation of the entire issue, for the implications of the saccharin case go far beyond the specific case of saccharin and directly to the heart of the limits of toxicology in the evaluation of carcinogenic risks to human beings.

The common denominator of arguments against the Delaney Amendment is that, in two ways, it is overly rigid. First, it excludes any quantitative considerations of risk; second, it excludes both health and nonhealth benefits of the additive in question. In other words, it excludes any quantitative risk-benefit evaluations. Even if the amounts of the additive in food are so small that the risk of cancer, based on extrapolation from the best scientific data possible, is presumed to be nil (or close to it), and even if the use of these small amounts might add greatly to health or well-being, the additive cannot be used. The opponents of the Delaney Amendment acknowledge that quantitative risk estimation is not an exact science, but they believe that educated guesses are both possible and essential, or else we doom ourselves to banning a very large number of highly useful chemicals. They also argue that consistency is badly needed in the regulation of environmental chemicals and that singling out food additives for special treatment is unwarranted; to achieve consistency by moving in the opposite direction—setting zero tolerances for all environmental chemicals—is, they feel, totally impossible since our present methods of detection are so good that virtually everything can, or soon will, be detectable in food, air, or water.

Finally, the opponents of the Delaney Amendment, while acknowledging that the regulatory process is extremely complex and subject to influence by lobbying, argue that, given the central importance of value judgments in setting acceptable risks, the political and judicial arenas are precisely where the battles should be fought, that arbitrary governmental decisions are no more desirable here than in any other area of life. Related to this is their feeling that outright bans deny people their right to make educated voluntary choices.

The supporters of the Delaney Amendment reply that rigidity is precisely what is required for the regulation of food additives. They argue that there is no scientific way to estimate, with any confidence, the quantitative risk to humans, and that no scientific advances have altered the statement of the Department of Health, Education and Welfare in support of the Delaney Amendment during its original consideration by Congress:

> Our advocacy of the anticancer proviso . . . is based on the simple fact that no one knows how to set a safe tolerance for substances in human foods when those substances are known to cause cancer when added to the diet of animals.[5]

Benefits, too, are extremely difficult to quantitate, argue the supporters of the Delaney Amendment, and may be of a completely different nature than the risks; moreover, even when an implicated additive is clearly beneficial, we ought to be able to find safe alternatives to serve the same purpose. Their basic conclusion, then, is that since quantitative risk-benefit analysis is impossible, the prudent course of action, at least for food additives, is to be totally rigid, because, for a variety of reasons, food additives deserve particularly careful regulation. Exposure to additives is pervasive and prolonged so that the danger from miscalculation of risks is mammoth; consumers expect special care to be taken with food, and exposure cannot really be confined to voluntary users; in contrast to that for food contaminants, exposure to food additives is simple to control—just stop adding the substance to food.

Inherent in their view is a deep distrust of the FDA's ability to regulate carcinogens on any other basis; they believe that, because of the regulatory morass described earlier and the undue influence of industrial lobbyists on the FDA, opening the door to debate over every carcinogen would result in no regulation at all, or the setting of acceptable levels which reflect industry's interests rather than health considerations. They point to cases like that of benzene as examples of the interminable delays and legal problems arising from the use of risk-benefit analysis.

Note that, as I have presented the arguments, the two sides do not differ on their view of the validity of animal experiments to implicate chemicals as carcinogens. They both accept that quantitative estimates of risk from such data cannot be exact. Their differences of view really involve value judgments as to what to do with such data, how much importance to assign to other factors such as benefit, and the efficacy of the usual regulatory process. Yet, one might gather from reading the mass media that the real argument against the Delaney Amendment is the idiocy of the animal studies used to invoke it. Unfortunately, this view is promulgated not only by the mass media, but by industry, and is sometimes tacitly hinted at by some scientists and, at least in the past, by the FDA itself.

Saccharin: History and Metabolism

Saccharin, which contains no nutrients of any kind and no calories, is one of the sweetest substances known, approximately 500 times sweeter than sugar. It is manufactured in two different ways, the R-F process (Remsen-Fahlberg, after the original synthesizers) and the more recent Maumee process. Both methods yield the water-soluble sodium salt of saccharin and impurities that are subsequently consumed along with the saccharin, but the impurities differ; that which has attracted most attention is OTS (orthotoluenesulfonamide), which is not found in the Maumee product. (The saccharin preparations used in animal experiments have been the R-F product, except for the 1977 Canadian study cited earlier; for *in vitro* tests, both preparations as well as highly purified saccharin have been used.)

After ingestion, saccharin is very rapidly absorbed from the gastrointestinal tract (the mechanism is unclear), very little appearing in the feces. There is relatively little storage of saccharin in the body, although, depending on the amount and spacing of doses, some does accumulate in several organs and tissues, particularly the bladder (the site of the cancers produced by saccharin in rats). Saccharin moves across the placenta easily and, following an infusion of saccharin in pregnant monkeys, the fetal blood levels were greater than maternal, because saccharin was eliminated more slowly from the fetus than from the mother.

The urine is the major route for saccharin excretion, only a few percent being secreted into the bile, most of which is then reclaimed by absorption. Because the great majority of carcinogens require biotransformation to more reactive metabolites before they can actually initiate cancers, it is surprising that saccharin seems not to be metabolized by experimental animals or human beings, even when given in very large amounts over very long periods of time. The metabolism of a tiny fraction of saccharin (less than 1 percent) has been reported in a few studies, but not in most, and never in people.

Saccharin appears, therefore, in the urine as intact saccharin, not as a metabolite. Its large degree of binding to plasma protein hinders its filtration at the glomeruli but it also undergoes tubular secretion. Tubular reabsorption is either not present or proceeds at a low rate relative to the combined rates of saccharin filtration and secretion. The result is that saccharin is excreted quite readily, 43 percent of the amount contained in a single bottle of diet soda coming out in six hours and 96 percent in twenty-four hours.

Saccharin has been used in the United States as a substitute for sugar since 1907 when it was added to canned goods. However, it was not until after World War II that it began to be used widely, almost always in combination with another nonnutritive sweetener, cyclamate. Then, in 1969–70, a ban on cyclamates, because of carcinogenicity in animal studies, left saccharin as the only nonnutritive sweetener on the FDA's GRAS list.

Since then, the use of saccharin has skyrocketed. In 1976 approximately three million kg of saccharin were used in the United States,

45 percent in soft drinks, 18 percent as a tabletop sweetener, 14 percent in other foods, and the rest in an incredible variety of products—dietetic foods, wine, tobacco, pharmaceuticals, dentifrices, cosmetics, cattle feeds, and many others. The total value of foods and beverages in which saccharin is used comes to $2 billion annually; saccharin is clearly big business.

The average yearly per capita consumption of saccharin is estimated at 10 to 11 g (a bottle of diet pop contains 0.15 g), and 25 to 40 percent of the population uses it to some degree. Both of these figures are still rising quite rapidly, mainly because of increased use of diet drinks. Although it is popularly held that teenagers are the major consumers, this is not true; on a body weight basis, the greatest users are now women in the childbearing years (20 to 39 years of age) and male children from birth to 9 years of age (keep this in mind when we discuss the animal experiments).

The use of saccharin continues unabated because the FDA ban was rescinded. The 1972 announcement predictably provoked protest not only from industry (as represented by the Calorie Control Council), but from prestigious medical societies. The American Diabetic Association argued that saccharin was essential for the treatment of diabetic persons, the American Dental Association predicted a marked increase in dental caries because of substitution of sugar for the banned saccharin, and the American Cancer Society felt that saccharin's risk for humans was so small that it was dwarfed by saccharin's great medical benefits, vis-à-vis therapy for diabetics and weight control for the general population. This view was also taken by many prominent individual scientists and physicians. The general public also left no question as to where it stood on the issue. Spurred on by the mass media's emphasis on the contrast between the rat data and human findings, and the enormity of the doses used in the rat study, they bombarded Congress with telegrams and letters; two nationwide public opinion polls reported opposition to the ban by a margin of five to one.

In April, 1977, the new Commissioner, Donald Kennedy, tried to calm the storm in two ways. First, he proposed that saccharin be made available as an over-the-counter nonprescription drug to persons with diabetes or other medically relevant reasons; second, he patiently explained that the Canadian study was not an isolated case, that the methodology used was not idiotic but standard practice, and that the human data were inadequate for inferring saccharin's safety for people. Very importantly, he questioned whether the supposed great medical benefits of saccharin really existed.

But the antiban sentiment, coupled now, as it inevitably must be, with a drive to eliminate or amend the Delaney Amendment, continued to gain strength, and the ultimate result was a decision by Congress in the fall of 1977 to postpone the FDA ban for eighteen months, during which time the National Academy of Sciences was to undertake a full review of scientific evidence concerning both the risks and benefits of saccharin. This report was subsequently issued (in two parts) in November, 1978, and March, 1979.[6] The committee members were unanimous on the scientific questions but disagreed on the policy to be inferred from the scientific facts. The animal experiments demonstrating saccharin's carcinogenicity were unequivocally declared valid and the high dose used totally justified. The committee's second conclusion was that the epidemiological studies to which one might turn for estimation of the risk to humans were not adequate for the purpose. Third, the purported benefits of saccharin were found to be not quantifiable simply because no one had ever really tried to document benefit scientifically. Thus, neither the risks nor benefits of saccharin could be presently quantified.

Now, let us study the basis for these scientific conclusions by the committee. We must begin with a brief summary of what is presently known concerning the mechanisms by which chemicals cause cancer.

Chemical Carcinogenesis

As I described in chapter 1, scientists estimate that approximately 80 to 90 percent of all human cancers are caused by environmental factors, of which, on the basis of present knowledge, chemicals are by far the most important. At least 1,000 chemicals have been shown to produce cancer in experimental animals, and this is probably only the tip of the iceberg. Indeed, one extremely unfortunate result of our recent intensive search for chemical carcinogens has been, paradoxically, to desensitize most of the general public, who greet the most recent carcinogen-of-the-week announcement, based on results of animal experiments, with jokes and a shrug of the shoulder: "So what? Everything will cause cancer if you give enough of it to a rat." This is simply not so! For example, of several hundreds of pesticides tested, in very large doses, less than 10 percent were found to cause cancer.[7]

Another common misconception is that almost all chemically induced cancers are due to man-made synthetic chemicals. However, epidemiological evidence makes it clear that this is not the case.[8] Tobacco alone accounts for an estimated 30 percent of all cancers in men and 7 percent in women. Dietary constituents (either inherent in the food, contaminants due to fungal growth [aflatoxins], or generated by the cooking technique used) may be even more important, some experts claiming that diet is a risk factor for 30 to 50 percent of all cancers. Estimates of the percentage of cancers contributed to by synthetic chemicals vary widely, from as low as 5 percent to as high as 40 percent, depending upon just which epidemiological statistics one wishes to give most credence to. One problem that greatly complicates such estimates is that more than one chemical source may be a risk factor for a particular form of cancer. For example, dietary fats are risk factors for several forms of cancer (notably breast and large intestine) but fat molecules are very unlikely, themselves, to be the direct inducers of cancer; more likely, as will be described later, they promote the growth of a cancer induced by some other chemical. The reverse is true for dietary fiber, the absence of which is a risk factor for cancer of the large intestine. This all means that both diet and synthetic chemicals could be risk factors for the same type of cancer, so that every percentage point assigned to diet doesn't necessarily mean one less left over for synthetic chemicals.

What is cancer and how do chemicals cause it? Cancer cells differ from normal cells in two major ways. They have lost the usual controls over their rate of division, and they are able not only to invade and displace normal tissues but to metastasize, to escape from the tumor mass and migrate via the blood or lymph to other parts of the body where they form satellite tumors. The first of these two abnormal characteristics can be demonstrated in several ways *in vitro*. When normal cells are cultured in the laboratory with continual transfer so that they do not become crowded, they divide a certain number of times and then stop (this experiment is one of the bulwarks of the theory that normal aging is a genetically programmed built-in process); in contrast, cancerous cells do not stop at the appointed number but keep on dividing. Moreover, when normal cells are allowed to contact each other, they generally stop dividing as soon as they have filled the surface with a single layer of cells; not so with malignant cells, which keep dividing, piling up in layer upon layer. This loss of normal "contact inhibition" reflects an abnormality of the cell surface, as does the propensity of cancer cells not to stick together normally but to metastasize.

Another way in which the outer membranes of cancer cells differ from those of normal cells is that embedded in them are proteins not found in any of the afflicted individual's other cells. The cancer cells are producing foreign proteins, and it is very likely that these are, at least in part, responsible for the cancer cell's abnormal relationships with its neighbors.

This finding of foreign protein molecules is only one of many types of evidence that have convinced most scientists that the key change induced by carcinogens is damage to the cell's DNA, most likely a mutation. This view is supported by the fact that the molecular structures of most known carcinogens (really of their metabolites, as described in chap. 8) are precisely those expected to be toxic to macromolecules. Moreover, it is hard to see how else the initial change induced by the carcinogen could be passed on, often after a delay of many years, from cell to cell. Just how the alteration of DNA results in the cells' loss of control of division is simply not known (there seem to be almost as many theories as investigators).

Of course, we know that not all mutations necessarily lead to cancer, but we do not know why certain ones do and others do not. The chemical carcinogen (or virus, radiation, or other environmental factor) which actually causes the mutation ultimately leading to cancer formation is called, appropriately, the initiator; all that is required is a very brief exposure to the initiator, and its effects are dose-dependent, additive, and, at some point, irreversible. The qualification, "at some point," denotes the fact that the cell's DNA repair enzymes (chap. 1) may be able to repair or eliminate the defect immediately after its appearance but not after some crucial point in the further development of the cancer has occurred; indeed, some scientists believe that faulty DNA repair may, itself, play a prominent facilitative role in the cancer's development. The protective function of DNA repair, at least in skin cancer, is illustrated by patients with the rare disease, xeroderma pigmentosa; these people have a genetic defect in the enzymes which repair the DNA damage induced by ultraviolet light, and they suffer from an extremely high incidence of skin cancer.

These concepts of carcinogenic initiation explain why this type of chemical toxicity must be looked at very differently from, say, a chemical which directly kills liver cells rather than causing carcino-genic transformation. First, cancer lethal to the entire body can result from alteration initially of a single cell, theoretically from interaction of one lone molecule of the carcinogenic chemical with one site on one DNA molecule of that cell (this so-called single-hit model of carcinogenesis is by no means accepted by all experts). The outright killing of a single liver cell would, by contrast, never even be noticed. Moreover, even if a very large fraction of the liver cells were killed, full recovery is to be expected because the cells can be replaced—the damage is reversible. A second exposure to the same dose of liver toxin five years later would have a similar (perhaps somewhat enhanced) effect but again recovery would occur if only a fraction of the liver cells were damaged or killed. Not so with car-cinogens; even five years later, the effect of the second dose would add to that of the first, increasing significantly the risk of develop-ing that form of cancer.

One thing these characteristics do not explain is why there is always a latent period between the initiation of the cancer and its emergence as a rapidly growing tumor. For example, after single injections of a large amount of benzapyrene to mice, tumors do not start appearing until sixty days later; the latent period can be short-ened to some extent by using larger doses, but cannot be eliminated. Actually, sixty days is very short, for usually, even with the most active carcinogenic chemicals, cancer development requires the equivalent of one-quarter to one-half the lifespan of the species—six to twenty-four months in rodents, fifteen to thirty years or longer in humans.

Yet, during this long latent period, the change caused by the initiator within the first hours of its contact with the cell remains intact and is passed to all succeeding generations of its progeny during subsequent apparently normal cell divisions. (Cell division is not at all required, however, for "locking in" of the initiated change.) The latent period is characterized by a slow evolution of the initiated cells toward the ultimate malignant cells that are fi-nally recognized as cancer. During the latent period, it is often pos-sible, with appropriate microscopic examination and biochemical measurements, both *in vivo* and *in vitro*, to detect the presence of initiated cells on their way toward full transformation.

The long latent periods typical of cancer raised the question of whether chemicals other than true carcinogens (initiators) might act during the latent period and be responsible for hastening or enhancing the ultimate emergence of the cancer. They do, indeed, and the discovery of these chemicals, known as promotors, has made the entire question of chemical carcinogenesis far more complicated. What promotors do is very different from what initiators do. They must be present for long periods of time in order to stimulate the transformation of initiated cells and, very importantly, their effects, prior to the appearance of the full-blown cancer, are reversible; partially transformed cells may completely disappear or, at the very least, remain in a state of suspended animation, if the promotor is eliminated.

The reversibility of promotion probably accounts for the comforting fact that after fifteen years of not smoking, previously heavy smokers develop lung cancer only to a slightly greater degree than people who have never smoked. Apparently, cigarette smoke provides not only initiators but the promotors required to bring initiated cells to full bloom.

We do not know the molecular events which underlie promotion. There is universal agreement that all promotors act as a stimulus for cell proliferation (i.e., cell division), but it is clear that, by itself, this stimulus is inadequate for promotion since many chemicals which stimulate cell division do not cause any progressive transformation of the dividing cells. Another striking fact about promotors is that there exists a considerable degree of organ specificity for individual promotors; for example, croton oil (the first promotor discovered) is a potent promotor for cancer of the skin, phenobarbital for liver, bile acids (a normally occurring substance!) for the large intestine, and several hormones (again, perfectly normal endogenous substances) for the breast.

To reiterate, most promotors are not, themselves, carcinogens, i.e., they do not cause the initial cell change which makes possible the subsequent events of transformation. Therefore, no amount of most promotors will bring about cancer in the absence of previous initiation by the true carcinogens. But by the same token, most (perhaps all) types of initiated cells require the presence of a promotor, acting over long periods of time, before they will develop into a true cancer. The use of the adjective "most" is necessitated by the fact that some carcinogens can also act as promotors toward cells which they, themselves, or other chemicals, have initiated.

Finally, I should at least mention the term cocarcinogen. These are chemicals which have been observed, empirically, to enhance the development of cancer caused by other chemicals but it is not clear whether they do so via synergistic effects on initiation or by promotion.

The necessity for promotion in the development of most, if not all, cancers has many very important public health implications. For example, imagine for a moment that epidemiologists find that the incidence of pancreatic cancer is rather suddenly beginning to skyrocket all over the country; what should they look for? One possibility is a chemical which came into popular use fifteen to thirty years or more ago and caused a large increase in the rate at which pancreatic cells were initiated; but an equally likely possibility is that no such initiator ever appeared, that the rate of initiation of pancreatic cells hasn't changed for fifty years, and the real villain is a chemical promotor introduced into the environment only within the past few years. Distinguishing between these two possibilities is a crucial public health matter, since if the epidemic is due to an increased initiator, then we are doomed to having the body count rise even further and remain high for another fifteen to thirty years (or longer if we can't figure out what the offending chemical is and eliminate it from the environment). On the other hand, if it is a new promotor that is causing the problem, the epidemic can be stopped rapidly by finding it and eliminating its use (of course, if it persists in the environment for a long time, like DDT and so many other petrochemical products, we are still going to be in deep trouble for a long time to come).

Just as cancer promotors exist, so, apparently, do chemicals which inhibit promotion. Already, several such antipromotors have been discovered, some being normally occurring bodily substances, and their existence holds out the possibility that in an environment loaded with carcinogens, the prophylactic use of an antipromotor might be a powerful weapon in the prevention of cancer.

Immune Defenses Against Cancer

I have already described three types of defenses against cancer. The first line consists of all those responses discussed in chapter 7 which diminish the concentration of free chemical carcinogen reaching the target cells. The second is DNA repair, and the third, one that is presently quite theoretical, is antipromotor chemicals. But perhaps the most important defenses of all are the immune responses, which attack and destroy cancer cells in the same way that transplanted foreign tissues or organs are rejected. (The term "immune" refers simply to those bodily processes which protect against foreign matter.)

This attack is made possible by the fact, mentioned earlier, that virtually all cancer cells have some surface proteins different from those of normal body cells, because they are coded for by altered DNA. The cells can, therefore, be recognized as foreign and be attacked by a particular class of white blood cells known as T lymphocytes (the "T" denotes that these cells, or their precursors, arise within the thymus), the same cells that mediate the rejection of transplants. When an appropriate T lymphocyte encounters the cancer cell, it binds to it, via the abnormal surface protein, and releases a variety of potent chemicals which may either destroy the cancer cell directly or attract to the site another group of cells (phagocytes or "eating cells") which engulf and digest it.

There is presently considerable controversy among experts as to just how important this "immune surveillance" against cancer is. Some believe that we may "get cancer once a day" but that the newly transformed cells are destroyed as fast as they arise. According to this view, only when the T-lymphocyte system is ineffective in either recognizing or destroying cancer cells do they multiply and produce clinical cancer.

In this last regard, there may occur an important interaction between T lymphocytes and another cell type, the B lymphocytes, an interaction which actually protects cancer cells. B lymphocytes are our major defense against bacteria, for they constitute the class of cells which secrete antibodies in response to the presence of these microorganisms; the antibodies attach to the surface of the bacteria and this results, by several means, in their destruction. At one time it was thought that cancer cells, unlike bacteria, did not elicit an antibody response, but now we know that, in many cases, the foreign proteins on the surface of the cancer cell not only activate T lymphocytes but cause specific antibodies to be released by B lymphocytes as well. These antibodies then attach to the surface proteins, the same sites at which T lymphocytes attach. The next events may be quite variable; in some cases, the antibody may facilitate the destruction of the cancer cell whereas in others it may actually protect the cell by preventing T lymphocytes from combining with it. When this occurs, the antibodies are called "blocking antibodies" and the process is called immune enhancement. Whether facilitation or blocking occurs seems to depend upon many poorly understood factors.

Whatever the explanation, it seems clear that the relative amounts of blocking antibody and T lymphocytes elicited by the cancer cell are a major determinant of whether the emergent cancer cell is destroyed or not. Of great potential importance is the finding that dietary protein deficiency greatly decreases the growth of tumors in experimental animals, and much less conclusive data suggests that this may be the case for humans as well. We also know that protein deficiency markedly impairs the production of blocking antibodies and this may account for the anticancer effect. Does our large protein intake favor cancer growth perhaps by enhancing synthesis of blocking antibodies? Can growth of certain cancers be medically controlled by dietary restriction of specific amino acids?

Protein deficiency is not the only nutritional factor to influence our immune defenses against cancer. The possible roles of several vitamins and trace metals are also being investigated at present. The importance of all this is that nutritional factors may influence the development of chemically induced cancers not only by affecting the body's handling of the chemical (the subject matter of the previous chapter) but by altering the body's response to the cancer cells once they are formed.

Animal Tests for Carcinogenicity

There is complete agreement by almost all experts that if a chemical causes cancer in laboratory animals, it is very likely to do so, at some dose, in human beings.[9] This view, endorsed by more than twenty prestigious scientific reports since 1956, is based in part on theoretical considerations of carcinogenetic mechanisms and the "unity of biology" (the similarity of fundamental biological processes such as DNA in all species), but, far more importantly, on experience. In 1978, there were twenty-six specific chemicals (or families of chemicals) known to cause cancer in people, based on overwhelming epidemiological evidence, and twenty-five of these (arsenic compounds being the only exceptions) had also been shown to be carcinogenic for one or more species of laboratory animals. Therefore, knowledgable scientists do not question the qualitative relevance of animal experiments for human beings.

Cancer testing is usually performed on rats and mice. Economy, ease of handling and housing, and the relatively short life spans (two to three years) of these animals (remember that the latency for cancer development is proportional to a species' life span) are considerations dictating these choices. Another important one is that various inbred strains of both species are available; the spontaneous rate of cancer development is much more predictable in these strains than in randomly bred animals as is their relative sensitivity to certain classes of carcinogens. However, the use of a single inbred strain has a disadvantage; it is a poor model for the genetic heterogenicity of human populations. Therefore, more and more cancer tests are utilizing a hybrid of two inbred strains.

The suspected carcinogen is administered by feeding, inhalation, or skin application, the first being by far the most commonly used route, and, ideally, several doses are used, all of them very large compared to the usual human exposure. Indeed, prior to the cancer test, preliminary study is usually made of the largest amount of chemical this species can be given without the animals becoming sick or dying from some noncancerous effect. This so-called maximum tolerated dose is then used as the highest dose in the subsequent cancer tests. In the simplest cancer tests, the chemical is administered during most or all of the animal's life. However, a better test, one used more and more frequently, is the so-called two-generation test. Animals of each sex of the parent generation are fed the chemical from their own weaning on; they are then bred, the mothers continue to be fed the chemical throughout pregnancy and nursing, and the offspring are then started on the chemical following their weaning and for the rest of their lives. The two-generation test thus recognizes the importance of exposure to carcinogens throughout critical periods of development, the usual conditions existing for human beings.

Following the animal's death, its entire body is examined for cancers. This is an extremely laborious procedure as emphasized by Dr. Samuel S. Epstein:

> The process of finding a cancer in the fresh carcass of a mouse or rat is different from the discovery of cancer in a human by a doctor. The rodent cannot complain of painful symptoms before death. Also, since carcinogens may cause cancer in any of a wide range of organs, the entire body must be meticulously searched.[10]

The incredible time, money, space, and trained manpower required to evaluate a single chemical explains why it is simply impossible to use more than 50 to 100 animals in each group (control and different doses in both sexes) of a test. And this limitation in turn explains why such large doses are required to obtain data that can be subjected to meaningful statistical analysis. We must examine this in some detail.

Even in an inbred strain of rats living under controlled laboratory conditions, there exist many interanimal differences in absorption, distribution, metabolism, excretion, end-organ sensitivity, DNA repair mechanisms, and immune responses, so that a range of susceptibility to a particular carcinogen exists. The range is made even wider by the "luck" factor, the sheer chance that the carcinogen will make contact with just the right site on the "cancer gene" in a susceptible cell. Now let us suppose that the amount of saccharin equivalent, on a body weight basis, to that in a single bottle of diet soda is enough to cause bladder cancer in only the most sensitive of rats, 1 in 10,000. I had to say "let us suppose" because, even were this fact true, we would never know it, for we would never use enough rats to detect it. Just think how many would be required. Your first estimate might be 10,000, but that's not really enough. Even though the true incidence is 1 in 10,000, the odds are that that "one" might not appear in the first 10,000 tested. But, even worse, rats have a spontaneous rate of bladder cancer. This means that your control group will also develop some bladder cancers, and so your conclusion that saccharin causes bladder cancer depends not on finding just one case but enough more than the background level for statistical analysis to yield a P value less than 0.05. The numbers of rats actually required would be impossible to handle on a routine basis. This means that, using our usual fifty rats per group, it is impossible to detect a cancer incidence of 1 in 10,000.

Now let us suppose (Watch out! this is another supposition which can never be validated) that humans have precisely the same range of sensitivities to saccharin as our rats, i.e., that the saccharin in one bottle of diet soda ingested every day would cause a bladder cancer in 1 of 10,000 people each year. With a population of 200 million people, this amounts to 20,000 new cases of bladder cancer every year! Yet, the rat tests using fifty animals per group and this "realistic" dose of saccharin would keep telling us, no matter how many times they were repeated, that saccharin is not a carcinogen.

This, of course, is an intolerable situation and, to get out of it, cancer testers use large doses. The logic is very simple. There is no doubt that the likelihood of cancer increases as the dose of the carcinogen is increased (I have said nothing of the shape of this dose-response, which is very much in doubt!), and so, by increasing the dose to maximum tolerated levels, enough of the treated animals will develop cancer to be detected and validated statistically. In the case of saccharin, for example, if (!!) the incidence in rats were really 1 in 10,000 from the equivalent of the saccharin in one bottle and if (!!) the dose-response were such that the magnitude of the response is in direct proportion to the dose, then 800 times the amount in one bottle would produce, on the average, 800 cases in 10,000 animals or 4 cases in our actual group of 50 animals, probably enough (but barely so) cases above the background level in the control group to achieve statistical significance (a good rule of thumb is that a cancer test carried out with 50 animals in each group will give statistically significant results only when the observed incidence is greater than 5 percent).

What are the actual findings for saccharin?[11] There have been eleven single-generation tests of saccharin's carcinogenicity, using doses as high as 2,700 mg/kg/day (the human equivalent of 1,000 bottles of diet soda), and all failed to provide any significant evidence for saccharin causing cancer in any organ. In contrast, the results of the three two-generation studies have been uniformly positive (and have also established that the carcinogenicity is not due to any impurities in saccharin preparations or to the formation of bladder stones). At the highest doses (800 to 1,000 times the human equivalent of one bottle of diet soda) the incidence of bladder cancer in treated second-generation males was always statistically significantly higher than that of controls. In contrast, females were unaffected. The fact that male offspring are the most susceptible group, but only when their parents are also exposed, is a particularly ominous finding in light of the fact, mentioned earlier, that the greatest users of saccharin (on a per weight basis) are women in their childbearing years and males under the age of 10.

Table 9–1 shows the actual data for the second-generation males. Note first that in three of the four control groups one case of bladder cancer occured, emphasizing the point I made earlier about "background" cancers. Second (there is no way you can tell this from the table), these data earn saccharin the title of a "low-potency" carcinogen, that is, the incidence of cancer produced by a certain amount of saccharin in rats is not nearly as great as that produced in this same species by the same amount of most other carcinogens. For example, only 1 μg of aflatoxin ingested daily over a lifetime is adequate to give 50 percent of the test animals cancer, whereas a million times more saccharin (more than 1 g) is required for the same effect. Sometimes, this kind of comparison is used all by itself to argue that saccharin's danger to people is minimal, but this ignores not only the fact, to be emphasized below, that potency in rats and humans cannot be safely equated, but the more obvious fact that a lot of a low-potency carcinogen may be more dangerous than a tiny amount of a high-protency one. In other words, total effect reflects some (unknown) combination of both potency and level of exposure.

But I'm jumping ahead of my story. To continue our perusal of the actual data, note that the WARF and FDA studies tried other lower doses equivalent to from 1.6 to 160 daily bottles of diet soda and the results were uniformly negative. Clearly, had "realistic" doses been used (or even doses only 160 times more than realistic), saccharin would have been pronounced "innocent." Yet, using the assumptions stated above (a directly proportional dose-response for rats and human sensitivity precisely equal to that of rats), a very different picture emerges, as shown by the following calculations. The incidence observed in the Canadian Study at the dose equivalent to 800 bottles per day for a person was 12/45, i.e., 12 out of the 45 rats developed bladder cancer. Presumably, had 45,000 rats been used, 12,000 would have developed cancer (I've simply multiplied

TABLE 9–1   Results of Two-Generation Saccharin Feeding Studies

Study	Saccharin Mfg. Process	Percentage of Diet	Incidence of Bladder Cancer in Male Rats Control	Treated	Statistical Significance P
WARF, 1973 (Wisconsin Alumni Research Foundation)	Remsen-Fahlberg	5	0/14	8/14	0.001
FDA	Remsen-Fahlberg	5	1/25	1/21	N.S.
		7.5	1/25	7/23	0.018
Canadian	Maumee	5	0/42	12/45	0.0002
	Maumee	5	1/36	7/38	0.033

Source: Data from *Saccharin: Technical Assessment of Risks and Benefits. Report #1* (Washington, D.C.: NRC/NAS, 1978).

both the 12 and 45 in the fraction by 1,000). Now comes the first key step: Assuming a directly proportional dose response, we calculate that the *expected* incidence of bladder cancer at a dose equivalent to only 1 bottle per day is (12,000/45,000) ÷ 800, or 15 cancers per 45,000 rats. Now the second key step: Assuming that male humans have the same sensitivity to the cancer-causing action of saccharin as male rats, we conclude that the *expected* incidence in male human is also 15 per 450,000. What does this translate out to be for the entire male population of the United States? There are approximately 100,000,000 males, so the *expected* incidence should be (100,000,000/450,000) × 15, or 33,000 new cases of bladder cancer per year!

To summarize so far: Any chemical shown to be a carcinogen in laboratory animals is likely to be a carcinogen, at some dose, in humans. Animal tests for suspected carcinogens must be performed with the highest doses possible despite the fact that these doses are much greater than those to which humans are ever exposed. This is necessary because we cannot possibly use enough animals to document carcinogenicity, at least for most low-potency carcinogens, at doses to which we are exposed. The use of these large doses is not invalidated by the claim that large amounts of anything will cause cancer, for the claim is false.

The statements of this summary are not controversial. They are accepted by virtually all scientists in this field. Arguments for disregarding the animal tests for saccharin on the grounds that "rat studies have no relevance for people" or "the doses used were idiotically large" are, themselves, utter nonsense, and simply confuse the real scientific issue to which we now turn—the impossibility of making quantitative extrapolations from experimental animals to human beings (I mean "impossible" not "present inability"). The reason I kept emphasizing the "ifs" in the assumptions of dose-response linearity and equality of rat-human sensitivities was to stress that they were only assumptions, unproven and unprovable, as we shall now see.

Quantitative extrapolation to humans of cancer incidences observed in experimental animals consists of two basic steps:[12]

    1. an intraspecies extrapolation of the incidence found at the high doses used to the incidence expected for the same species at doses which correspond to human exposure (I made this extrapolation by assuming a linear dose-response with no threshold).

2. a cross-species extrapolation, from the predicted low-dose incidence in the experimental animals (the first extrapolation, just given above) to that expected for human beings at the same dose (I made this extrapolation by assuming equality of sensitivities).

The extrapolations in both steps are only as valid as the assumptions used in making them. Immediately, in the first step, we encounter two grave problems concerning the shape of the dose-response to be used, the first of which is whether there is a threshold, a minimal level below which the carcinogen exerts absolutely no effect. All of us intuitively feel that thresholds for toxic agents must exist, that one molecule of aspirin or carbon monoxide can't possibly harm us. But, as I have emphasized earlier, based on what we know of carcinogenic initiation, there is a profound difference between carcinogens (as well as noncarcinogenic mutagens) and other kinds of toxic chemicals, since it is possible that one molecule of carcinogen is all that is needed to initiate cancer in the most exquisitely sensitive individual in the population. This is, of course, only theory, but it is all we have. The question of threshold, so crucial for evaluation of carcinogens (not just chemicals but radiation and viruses, as well) is not now and never will be answerable experimentally. How many millions of rats would it take to prove that one molecule of saccharin couldn't cause cancer in some rat under some conditions?

What then do we do? The overwhelming majority of scientists and all governmental agencies opt for assuming no threshold, as evidenced by the committee's report:

Many theoretical dose-response models of carcinogenesis have been proposed. . . . All . . . have one concept in common: that there is no known uniform threshold dose below which any carcinogenic response is impossible for all individuals at risk. Even if thresholds do actually exist, it is scientifically impossible to measure them or prove their existence. In addition, the assumption of one uniform threshold for heterogenous groups is unrealistic. It is much more likely that each member of the population has an individual threshold level which is some complex function of unique biochemical and physiological composition. A further argument against use of threshold models for the estimation of attributable risk is that the environment contains many carcinogenic agents and that the particular chemical in question may be acting additively over and above this background. Therefore, since tumors do appear spontaneously in a control population, the threshold, assuming it does exist, has probably already been exceeded by the environmental background. . . . A review of 151 dose-response curves [for carcinogens] found only one to be inconsistent with the no-threshold hypothesis."[13]

These sentiments only echo the view expressed by a long unbroken series of NAS reports dealing with a variety of carcinogens in food, air, and water; each has concluded that in the evaluation of carcinogenic risk, it must be assumed that thresholds do not exist.

Once we accept the no-threshold assumption, then the first point of the dose-response is established, namely zero-response exists only for zero-dose. But what is the shape of the curve between this zero-zero point and the one actually measured in the animals? Line A in figure 9–1 assumes a linear relationship (as I did in my illustrative calculations for saccharin), based on the assumption that the probability of cancer initiation is directly proportional to the exposure level.

The model of carcinogenesis which predicts a linear dose-response is the "single-event" or "one-hit" hypothesis which as-

Fig. 9–1. **Theoretical dose responses for a carcinogenic chemical.** A = linear, no threshold; B = nonlinear, no threshold; C = linear, threshold. Note that values at the upper (measurable) ends of the curves do not reveal what the lower portions would look like.

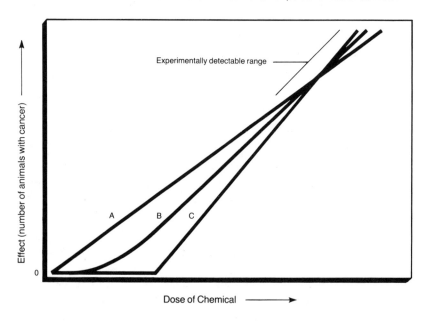

sumes that since only a single event, one molecule of carcinogen hitting one critical site in one DNA molecule in one cell, is required for initiaiton, the probability of cancer initiation is a linear function of the number of carcinogenic molecules around. The evidence usually cited in support of this model is the extensive data existing for radiation-induced cancer; many of these dose-responses are linear down to an incidence of at least 1 in 1,000. However, below this point (and we are almost always interested in such lower incidences), no reliable data exist, again because of the impossibility of testing enough animals. Moreover, radiation-cancer dose-responses are not always linear; indeed, the controversy over the true dose-response for radiation carcinogenesis is every bit as great as for chemical carcinogenesis. Finally, radiation may not be a valid comparison for chemicals, since ionizing radiation encounters none of the restrictions that a chemical does in getting at the critical site, the cell nucleus. A chemical has to be absorbed, be metabolized (for most carcinogens), get into the target organ, and move across multiple membranes to finally get at the cell nucleus. Thus, there are potential roadblocks for the chemical but none for high-energy ionizing radiation.

A second line of evidence favoring the single-event model comes from studies of mutagenesis in a variety of systems (like the bacterial one to be described later) which permit detection of much lower incidences; the dose-responses here are generally linear (with no evidence of threshold), but it can be argued, quite appropriately, that mutagenesis in bacteria is a far different matter from cancer in a rat or person. The fundmental processes might be different and, again, bacteria don't have the roadblocks to carcinogens that mammals do.

Finally, the only carcinogens to which enough "animals" have been exposed are those in cigarette smoking. The data for humans strongly suggest a linear dose-response, but again the data are meaningful only down to an incidence of about 1 percent.

Other models much more sophisticated (this, of course, doesn't mean they are any more likely to be correct) than the single-event one have been hypothesized. These all produce dose-responses which still go through zero-zero (they all presume no threshold) but which are, more or less, upwardly concave (line B on fig. 9–1), i.e., the incidence of cancer is expected to rise very slowly at low doses but then rise steeply at higher doses. For example, this would be

SACCHARIN, CANCER, AND THE DELANEY AMENDMENT

expected if multiple events, not a single hit, were required for the cancer's development. Unhappily, the question of which theory is valid, and therefore which dose-response curve should be used, is not solvable experimentally; the incidences they predict at all doses high enough for the experiment to be meaningful (5 percent or more response rates) are indistinguishable, and it is only at the low doses, those in which we are really interested but cannot experiment with, that the predicted incidences diverge. The differences at these levels are not trivial but may differ from each other by several hundred-fold. For example, applied to the actual saccharin data, extrapolation, using two different theoretical models, from the observed incidence of cancer at the dose actually used in the experiment to that predicted for the rats at 1/800th of the dose yields values which differ from each other by a factor of 200; one model predicts an incidence in rats at this dose of 1 in 5,000, whereas the other predicts 1 in 500 million!

At least one laboratory, the National Center for Toxicological Research, has made a valiant effort to see whether the true dose-response could be determined for at least one carcinogen with the obvious hope of then extrapolating this shape to other carcinogens. They have used seven doses of 2-AFF, a very potent liver and bladder carcinogen, and 24,192 mice! This so-called mega-mouse experiment is failing in its aim, for even with such huge numbers of animals, incidences of less than 1 percent would be missed, and this is still too high to distinguish among the possible models.

It is no wonder then that the committee concluded:

> The fact that . . . [an] animal bioassay that is conducted at dose levels high enough to give observable response rates cannot discriminate among these various models and the fact that these same models are substantially divergent at lower doses provides the major uncertainty for high to low-dose extrapolation.[14]

Most believe that the solution to this problem, if it comes at all, will not be derived from animal carcinogenicity experiments but from a more complete understanding of the actual mechanisms of carcinogenicity. In the meantime, those who favor making educated guesses as to quantitative risk assessments must commit themselves to the use of one of the models; the most conservative one (in the sense that it predicts the highest risk) is the linear single-hit model, and this is the one used by the EPA in making its assessments.

Let me remind you that this terrible uncertainty in extrapolating from high-dose to low-dose is for a single species! When one takes the next step, extrapolating an extremely uncertain prediction of low-dose incidence in the animal to an equivalent dose in a second species—human beings—the situation becomes utterly hopeless. All the factors we dealt with in the previous chapter—absorption, distribution, metabolism, excretion, DNA repair, and immune responses—may differ markedly from species to species and, thereby, influence the carcinogenic potential of the chemical (metabolism, the greatest source of variability, does not apply in the case of saccharin).

As is the case for high-dose to low-dose extrapolation, the best hope for improving interspecies extrapolations in the future lies in an expansion of basic scientific knowledge, in this case in the realm of interspecies differences in chemical metabolism, defenses against emergent cancer cells, and so on. In the meantime, the National Academy of Sciences has expressed an "expect the worst" view in urging that cancer testing be performed in more than one species, or more than one strain of a single species, and that the results obtained from the most sensitive species or strain be used for the extrapolation to people. But, of course, people may still be far more sensitive than any of the species or strains used. If human-rat or human-mouse differences are at least as great as interstrain differences among either rats or mice, we can expect that, in some cases, human beings will be 1,000 times more sensitive (or less sensitive) to carcinogens than the most sensitive rats or mice. This prediction is borne out by beta-naphthylamine, one of the few chemicals for which any comparative carcinogenicity data are available, which is far more carcinogenic in humans than in rats.

There are important scientific reasons for expecting the worst. The lab experiments are carried out in a controlled environment, whereas human beings are exposed not only to the suspected carcinogen but simultaneously to promotors and cocarcinogens, and chemicals which can induce the MES so as to increase the generation of active carcinogens (of course, the optimist might point out that we may also be exposed to antipromotors and agents that inhibit the MES). Diet and stress, too, have been shown to influence the response to carcinogens in experimental animals and almost certainly do so in humans as well. There is simply no way to duplicate this multiplicity of human environments in a laboratory.

Finally, there is another reason that the usual laboratory tests might underestimate the risk of a suspected carcinogen; they do not evaluate the likelihood that the chemical may not only be a carcinogen, itself, but may either promote the action of other carcinogens or synergize with them (as cocarcinogens). This seems to be a fairly common phenomenon, and fortunately it is testable in laboratory animals using special tests. Thus, saccharin in a dose which, by itself, produced no cancers, caused a fivefold to sixfold increase in the number of cancers produced by another carcinogen, FANFT. In a second study, saccharin alone caused a 2 percent incidence of cancer, and a second chemical (NMU) produced none; the incidence was 52 percent for the two together. Thirdly, a combination of saccharin and cyclamate (the banned sweetener previously used with saccharin) yielded a much higher incidence of cancer than did the same dose of either chemical alone. Finally, cholesterol and saccharin, implanted as pellets in the bladder, also have been shown to synergize in causing cancer. In fairness, it must be pointed out that not all studies have revealed a promotor or cocarcinogenic effect of saccharin, and, in one, saccharin actually reduced the incidence of mammary gland and ear duct cancer caused by the chemical AAF (the authors speculate that this was due to a saccharin-induced decrease in food intake and therefore of AAF dose, since the AAF was given in the food.)[15]

In summary, their analysis of the animal studies of saccharin left the committee members only one conclusion:

> The committee accepts the logic that results obtained from valid animal experiments can, in principle, be extrapolated to humans. However, requirements for high doses and long periods of exposure, as well as our current inability to make quantitative extrapolations from animals to humans makes it impossible to estimate with confidence the magnitude of risk to humans from the use of saccharin.[16]

Substitute "almost any carcinogen" for "saccharin" in the last sentence, underline the entire quotation in red pencil and put asterisks all around it. We have spent the better part of two chapters getting there, and like it or not, we must recognize that conclusive *quantitative* extrapolations from animal experiments to the human situation are not "difficult," not "awaiting more data," but "impossible." The value judgments we choose to make about whether the Delaney Amendment is wise or foolish must use this unequivocal fact as a point of departure, but let us hold off on that for the moment until we have described another type of laboratory evaluation for carcinogenesis as well as the contribution of cancer epidemiology.

The Ames Test

Animal tests for cancer are, by all estimates, long (three years), expensive ($200,000 for a thorough test), and require large numbers of highly trained personnel, particularly in the final step of examining the tissues microscopically. For these reasons, many toxicologists believe that, even if it were possible (which they strongly doubt) to test the 700 to 1,000 new chemicals introduced commercially each year, there is no hope whatever of evaluating the backlog of 55,000 untested chemicals already in general use. There is a tremendous need, therefore, for rapid inexpensive techniques to serve, at the very least, as screening techniques for deciding which chemicals should be subjected to animal studies, or ideally, to replace the animal studies altogether.

Several "quick tests" employing *in vitro* techniques have been around for a long time; for example, exposing animal cells in tissue culture to the suspected chemical and examining them for cytoplasmic or biochemical evidence of carcinogenic change. Although these tests were useful adjuncts to the animal studies, it was clear that none of them was really adequate for the job. This situation has changed dramatically in the last few years with the introduction of the Ames test (its developer was Bruce N. Ames, a biochemistry professor at the University of California, Berkeley).[17]

The Ames test, which uses bacteria as its test organism, does not look for cancer at all, for bacteria do not develop expanding masses of malignant cells. Rather it looks for mutations. The Ames test, then, is really a test for mutagenesis, and the theoretical basis for its use is the assumption that since the initiation step of carcinogenesis is probably an alteration of DNA, carcinogens are likely to be mutagens, and vice versa. I'll describe later the evidence Ames and his colleagues have accumulated to document the validity of this theoretical underpinning; suffice it to point out for now that the success of the Ames test in spotting carcinogens has completed the circle by providing a major support for the theory that carcinogenesis really does represent genetic mutation.

The bacteria used in the test are salmonella, more specifically, strains of salmonella which bear a mutation rendering them unable to make a key enzyme required for synthesis of histidine, an amino acid found in most proteins. Therefore, these strains cannot make protein and so cannot grow and multiply in a medium lacking histidine. When these bacteria are exposed to a mutagenic chemical, they undergo additional mutations, some of which restore the previously mutated gene coding for the histidine-synthesizing enzyme. The result of this "back-mutation" is that the bacteria are now able to grow in a histidine-deficient medium. Each of the back-mutated bacteria, over the course of several days, multiples rapidly, forming a single discrete colony which appears on the nutrient plate as a white spot. Counting the white spots tells how many of the bacteria underwent this particular mutation (of course, the test completely ignores all of the other mutations that the chemical may have produced).

This test has some enormous advantages. It is cheap ($200 per chemical) and fast (three days). It permits testing of complex mixtures of chemicals (such as polluted air or cigarette condensate), body fluids (urine, for example), and even solid materials (a slice of sausage, in one case) which are impractical or too "dirty" to be administered to animals. It permits extensive and easy testing of suspected promotors or synergistic reactions between chemicals, and most of all, it is extremely sensitive. Approximately 10 billion bacteria are added to a single plate, and if the mutagenic chemical is so weak that it causes only one of these 10 billion bacteria to develop the appropriate mutation, this will be detected because of the single colony formed (the sensitivity is not quite this good since there is a certain low level of spontaneous mutations in the control plate). Finally, there has been enough experience with it to document that good dose-responses are generated even over the lowest range of sensitivity; interestingly, they are linear and show no threshold, just what many scientists have predicated but cannot prove is the case for cancer in animals.

I hope that somewhere during this description, many of you have cried out: "There's something wrong; this test can't possibly work for carcinogens if what you told us in the last chapter about most carcinogens requiring metabolic conversion to their active forms by the MES is true. Unless, of course, salmonella have an analogous MES." They don't, and you are right, the test won't work as I described it. Indeed, for years, *in vitro* tests employing similar principles had tested chemicals known to be carcinogens in animals and failed to detect mutagenicity for most of them. This had lead to the generalization that most carcinogens are not mutagens. In contrast, it appeared that almost all mutagens (as documented in these *in vitro* tests) were also carcinogenic when tested in animals. Only after the role of the MES in activating carcinogens was appreciated did scientists recognize how they had been misled. The proven mutagens were those chemicals which did not require the MES for activation, and so could act on the bacteria (and also cause cancer when given to animals). In contrast, all those chemicals which required MES activation could cause cancer in animals but couldn't cause mutation *in vitro* because the MES was lacking.

The breakthrough came when Ames thought of adding an extract of liver to the nutrient plate. The enzymes of the MES in this extract went to work metabolizing the originally inactive chemical being tested, and lo and behold, mutated colonies now appeared; the great majority of carcinogens are, indeed, mutagenic as well.

Ames and his colleagues have introduced other tricks to make the test more versatile and sensitive. They developed another mutant form of salmonella which has a defective surrounding membrane rendering it much more penetrable to the test chemicals. With appropriate biochemical techniques, they eliminated the bacteria's DNA repair apparatus so that mutations could not be healed, and they made DNA replication more error-prone than normal. But all these changes are minor compared to the central importance of adding the liver extract. Extracts of other tissues, like lung, are also being experimented with to make the test even more analagous to what occurs throughout the human body.

Ames recognized immediately that despite all its advantages and intellectual beauty, the test would not really be accepted for detecting carcinogens unless its results paralleled those of the animal experiments. After all, bacteria are not mammalian cells, it is impractical to add extracts of all tissues and organs, and a host of other as yet unsuspected circumstances within the mammalian body might render chemicals more or less carcinogenic. Therefore, he set about validating the test with 300 chemicals reported as carcinogens or noncarcinogens in animal experiments. Only 13 of 108 reported noncarcinogens tested out as mutagenic, i.e., gave false positive results, and it is certainly possible, given the limitations of the animal tests, that these are not really false positives, but that the carcinogenicity test was falsely negative; indeed, in at least one case, a food additive used widely in Japan, the extraordinary mutagenicity revealed by the Ames test stimulated yet another attempt to demonstrate the chemical's carcinogenicity in animals (the first two had been negative), and this time the more thorough tests produced positive results in three different species.

Ninety percent (158 of 176) of the known carcinogens were found to be mutagenic in the salmonella test. A similar fraction (16 of 18) of chemicals known as or strongly suspected of being carcinogens in human beings were mutagenic. Nevertheless, there are whole classes of carcinogens (heavily chlorinated chemicals, for example) for which the success rate is much lower, and Ames acknowledges that some chemicals may never be detected by the salmonella test, no matter what improvements may be made in the test, if they cause cancer by some means other than a direct action on DNA.

Ames believes that the problem of these false negatives may be solved through the use of several of the other short-term tests, the development of which has been greatly stimulated by the obvious success of the Ames test. These include the use of animal cells in tissue culture, mutagenicity testing in fruit flies (Drosophila), and a variety of others. His hope is for a standardized battery of short-term tests, each detecting a few carcinogens that the others do not.

Finally, Ames and other scientists are in the process of making a quantitative comparison between carcinogenic potency as revealed by the animal studies and mutagenic potency in the salmonella test. Thus far, the correlation between the two is fairly good, another argument that the salmonella test may be able to serve as a substitute for animal tests.

This substitution is, in fact, the issue being debated at present. Industry has, by and large, adopted the Ames test, and governmental regulatory agencies are also considering placing major reliance on them. This total substitution is a source of concern to some scientists who believe that the practical role of the Ames test has been exaggerated, that the correlation between results from animal tests and the Ames test may diminish as more and more carcinogens are studied, and that there are simply too many false negatives. Moreover, they cite recent estimates that the testing in animals of 700 chemicals per year is quite feasible, that the manpower and facilities are available, and that the $140 million required are trivial compared to the gross sales of the chemical industry and the many billions of dollars which cancer costs this country.

Their criticisms of the Ames test are important, and we must take great care not to place our full faith in the Ames test or any other short-term test until it has been thoroughly validated and its weaknesses understood. Saccharin provides a good example of what those who oppose complete substitution of the Ames test for animal studies fear. The Ames test alone would have declared saccharin a noncarcinogen, for in three separate studies, highly purified saccharin was found to be nonmutagenic. A fourth study reported very weak mutagenic activity of urine collected from mice given saccharin. Other types of short-term tests of mutagenicity have yielded similar results—weakly positive in a few cases but negative in most. Actually, these data are consistent with the relatively weak carcinogenic activity exhibited by saccharin in rats, and the fact that it is not seen at all in one-generation animal studies. Coupled with its unusual feature of not requiring metabolism to bring out carcinogenicity (and its inability to bind to DNA, an experimental finding I haven't mentioned before) these facts suggest that saccharin may cause cancer in a way different from most carcinogens. In any case, it seems clear that if saccharin were to be synthesized tomorrow and its potential carcinogenicity evaluated only by the Ames test, it would probably be given a clean bill of health.

Nevertheless, there are still the untested 50,000 chemicals hanging over our heads. To me, it seems inescapable that at least the initial screening of these chemicals must depend on a "quick test" like the Ames test, or better yet, a battery of them. Based on the carcinogenic potencies revealed by these tests, decisions could then be made as to which should be subjected to subsequent animal testing. Even more important, the continued use of both types of tests, rather than outright substitution of one for the other, should fairly soon reveal the classes of carcinogens that the Ames test consistently misses. Knowing this, we could then submit all such chemicals to animal testing regardless of what the Ames test showed.

Epidemiological Studies of Saccharin

Whenever it is announced that a chemical has been shown to be carcinogenic in animals, there is usually an accompanying disclaimer that "the chemical has not been found harmful to humans." Every time you read this kind of statement in the press, or hear it announced on the radio or television, you should mentally insert the word "yet." You should ask yourself the question, "If the chemical is carcinogenic to humans, how would we know?" We can only know if the appropriate epidemiological study has been done and its results are conclusive beyond doubt—which is rare—or if the chemical induced an extremely rare tumor.[18]

This is not cynicism but plain truth. The failure of the public (as well as scientists and regulatory agencies, who should know better) to understand this ranks with misinterpretation of the use of high doses in animal experiments as the leading causes of confusion concerning our ability (or lack of ability) to detect carcinogens and quantitate their risk for humans. I have previously described (in chap. 2) the limitations inherent in epidemiological studies, and saccharin provides us with an excellent opportunity to review some of them.

Approximately 30,000 new cases of bladder cancer are diagnosed in the United States each year, 75 percent in males. The age-adjusted incidence has been rising steadily for males since at least 1930, particularly for black males (from 3.7 per 100,000 in 1935 to 10 in 1975). In contrast, the incidence has been very slowly declining for all females. This striking sex difference is a beautiful example of (unknown) environmental risk factors at work. The single most important known risk factor is smoking, which has been estimated (based on the correlation coefficient relating smoking and bladder cancer in epidemiological surveys) to account for 39 percent of bladder cancers in men and 29 percent in women. Next comes occupational exposure (especially to dye stuffs and rubber processing), accounting for 18 percent and 6 percent of bladder cancer in men and women, respectively. This leaves 43 percent of male bladder cancers and 65 percent of female unaccounted for—about 15,000 cases per year.

If we can so glibly point the finger (and even assign percentages), based on epidemiological studies, to smoking and occupation, why can't we do the same thing for saccharin? The answer, of course, is given by the guidelines enumerated in chapter 2; the association relating smoking and bladder cancer is very strong, and is consistently observed in each of the many studies on the epidemiology of smoking, studies which involved huge numbers of people in many geographic areas and walks of life. The association with occupation is based on relatively few people but is so strong that no other interpretation is really possible. Indeed, of the twenty-six chemicals known to be carcinogens for humans on the basis of epidemiological studies, the major type of exposure for approximately two-thirds of them is occupational. The remaining one-third is medicinal. In both these types of exposure, a clearly delineated exposed group is identifiable as is a nonexposed control group, and under these circumstances, epidemiology has its best shot at establishing strong clear-cut association. Cigarette smoking is really the only instance of a nonoccupational and nonmedicinal chemical conclusively identified as a cause of human cancer, and this too reflects the facts that exposed and control groups are easily separable and that lung cancer is an extremely uncommon cancer in nonsmokers.

In contrast, for widely dispersed environmental chemicals like DDT (and saccharin, too, when you consider how difficult it is to find persons completely unexposed to this agent or to quantitate total exposure), it is difficult to obtain a really good control group; moreover, most cancers have multiple causes so that the "background" rate due to factors other than the one being investigated may be so high as to obscure any increment caused by the chemical in question. As a general rule of thumb, there is really no hope of establishing an association convincingly unless the specific carcinogen at least doubles the background risk, and then the studies would have to be extremely well designed and include large numbers of people. Small wonder that so few of the hundreds of chemicals known to be carcinogens in animals have been documented for humans by epidemiological studies. As implied by Dr. Epstein, "the chemical has not been found harmful to humans" is generally both meaningless and misleading. What makes it really pernicious is that, given the long latency of cancer, there is not even the slightest chance of an epidemiological study establishing association between a chemical and a cancer if the chemical has been in use just a few years. Only decades later, when the death rate from the chemical starts rising, is epidemiological validation possible.

At the time the FDA included the reassuring statement about human health and saccharin in its announcement of the ban, there existed a fair number of epidemiological saccharin studies which fell into one of two groups.[19] The first group had compared the incidence of bladder cancer in diabetics, who presumably use large amounts of saccharin, with that for nondiabetics. No difference was seen, but the NAS committee dismissed these studies out of hand, emphasizing that diabetics are not useful in epidemiological studies of carcinogens since they differ in so many ways from normal persons (they eat different foods, smoke more, differ metabolically and genetically, and so on).

The second group consisted of three retrospective studies designed to determine whether patients suffering from bladder cancer had consumed more saccharin than matched controls. All these failed to document a difference, but this only proved that saccharin is not the dominant cause of bladder cancer, not that it has no effect. The problem was, as you might have predicted, too few persons. One study used 135 females, a strange choice of sex in light of the animal studies. The male patients in the other two studies numbered 157 and 158. It is easy to show that, because of the high rate of background bladder cancers, i.e., those not caused by saccharin, studies using such small numbers could not possibly yield statistically significant differences were saccharin responsible for only a modest fraction of all bladder cancers, say 5 to 30 percent.

The committee also devoted several pages to specific methodological criticisms of these studies (poor choice of controls, failure to guard against interviewer bias, etc.) but I do not even want to dwell on these at all, for the far more important point, just described, is that even had they been done perfectly, they could not have exonerated saccharin.

The committee's other substantive criticism of these studies (as well as the others to be mentioned below) which is worth stressing is that saccharin just hasn't been around long enough to place much faith in the results of present epidemiological studies. If the latent period extends over two generations, as the rat studies indicate, we may not yet be seeing the full effects of saccharin on our population. An important implication of this possibility is that the present total incidence of bladder cancer, 30,000 per year, does not provide us with a maximal risk that we might use in risk-benefit analysis; twenty years from now, when the latent period is over, the incidence could be far greater than 30,000.

Two more retrospective studies were reported in 1977 and 1978, both of which used larger numbers of male cases, 365 and 480.[20] (Nineteen seventy-nine and 1980 studies are briefly described in the postscript to this chapter. Here I have restricted the discussion to those studies available to the committee.) One found no difference in saccharin use between patients with bladder cancer and controls; the other found a highly significant difference, consistent with saccharin being presently responsible for 7 percent of all bladder cancers found in males. Very importantly, the increased risk remained quantitatively unchanged after factoring out education, high-risk occupations, history of bladder or kidney infections, smoking, and consumption of coffee (which some believe is a major risk factor for bladder cancer). Finally, there was a significant direct relationship of cancer incidence to both amount consumed and duration of use.

I do not mean at all to imply that this one study provides conclusive evidence for a carcinogenic effect of saccharin in humans, for the association, although significant, is certainly not strong, nor have we any idea, in the absence of enough good large-scale studies, of the consistency of the association. I, for one, believe that bladder cancer has so many causes that really conclusive evidence for or against a causal role for saccharin will not be possible from epidemiological studies in the near future, particularly if the latent period extends over two generations. If we ultimately do prove a positive relationship, it will be only because enough time has passed for the body count to mount high enough.

In summary, epidemiological studies have limitations biasing them powerfully toward the yielding of negative results for the relatively weak carcinogens. Epidemiology will not, in the great majority of cases, help us avoid the painful conclusion we drew from analysis of the animal studies: *It is impossible to estimate with confidence the magnitude of risks to humans from chemicals known, from animal studies, to be carcinogens.*

Benefits of Saccharin

The committee has found no studies that permit objective assessment of the asserted health benefits of saccharin use. . . . Data available to the committee do not permit the evaluation of the efficacy of saccharin in the control of diabetes or body weight. Also, . . . it remains unclear whether the use of . . . saccharin has a major effect in decreasing the incidence or severity of [dental caries].[21]

This is a startling piece of news, since the major argument for not banning saccharin was that it is so important in the control of diabetes, life-prolonging weight control, and dental caries. It turns out that these claims were purely assumptions, *never subjected to careful scientific validation.* The italics emphasize that there was no evidence to *disprove* health benefits of saccharin, just no evidence in either direction.

Beyond simply the power that certain intuitively logical assertions wield over us (having full iron stores *must* be healthier; substituting a nonnutrient for sugar *must* help cut down total calories), there is another reason for these questions having been pretty much ignored. The FDA does not require proof of benefit from industry before allowing the marketing of food additives (or cosmetics), in direct contrast to their policy on drugs. The food additive must be shown to be safe under conditions of intended use and capable of accomplishing its intended technical effect (sweetening, preserving, coloring, etc.). Proof that this effect has any value is not required, and so industry makes no attempt to assess it. The committee, in its review, did come up with a few studies, both human and animal, but the limited data, most of it not indicating any benefits of saccharin, precluded definitive conclusions. (Apparently, a number of the committee members felt the data were adequate to state outright that saccharin had no health benefits but ultimately settled for what I also believe to be the more accurate statement quoted above.)

The committee also struggled with the major nonhealth benefit of saccharin, the simple fact that people derive pleasure from sweet things. Predictably, the members were at a complete loss as to how to quantitate this pleasure (or the loss of it resulting from banning saccharin), and it is amusing to see them trying to reduce the issue to more comfortable scientific terms like "psychological dependence" and "acquired preferences." The obvious fact, of course, is that there is no way to quantitate the benefits of either pleasure or the freedom to choose to ingest known carcinogens.

What is Your Decision?

If you are now convinced that animal studies, as presently performed, are relevant for establishing the carcinogenicity of a chemical, that any attempt to quantitate the actual risk of the chemical for people based on either the animal results or epidemiology may be extremely inaccurate, then you are as qualified as the members of the NAS saccharin committee to vote for or against the Delaney Amendment and the saccharin ban. For such a vote reflects one's value system, not any further information. Look back at the pros and cons given earlier for the Delaney Amendment and you will see that this is true.

If you vote for the Delaney Amendment, then you automatically vote for banning saccharin, as well, and your task is completed. If you vote against the Delaney Amendment, then your next job is to decide what to do about saccharin; specifically you must make educated guesses about both the risk and benefits of saccharin.

Most of the committee members did, in fact, vote against the Delaney Amendment.

> The lack of scientific plausibility in the notion of zero risk in any class of compounds raises the question of more feasible goals, taking into account feasibility in a free society, as well as securing for the society the maximum public health benefit. Second, the Delaney clause treats cancer differently from other diseases in safety legislation. Under the clause, it is difficult to avoid focusing scientific and regulatory attention on cancer. In general, the Delaney and the general safety clause represent statutory specification and rigidity. Included are lack of acknowledgment of benefits, whether health or nonhealth, nonacceptance of the reality that nothing is absolutely safe, and lack of a mechanism for adjusting the regulatory process to developments in testing technology, to new findings about unanticipated health risks, and to new approaches for targeting safety regulation to the population groups at greatest risk. The Delaney clause specifically excludes . . . intermediate regulatory measures, such as tolerance levels, warning labels, or restrictions on use.[22]

Their decision seems, in large part, to have reflected a strong desire for a consistent policy toward all potentially toxic chemicals in food, and most of Part II of their report, the section dealing with policy recommendations, dealt with this broad issue. The most succinct summary of these recommendations is to be found in a letter by Philip Handler, president of the National Academy of Sciences, to HEW.

> Part II recommends: (a) that there be a single policy applicable to all foodstuffs, food additives, and food contaminants and that the public official responsible for implementation of that policy be given sufficient flexibility to factor risks, benefits and other considerations into account when making a decision concerning a material that has been called into question; (b) that there be available to that official options other than decisions simply to ban or not ban; and (c) that to facilitate such implementation, materials under consideration first be categorized as exhibiting low, moderate, or high risk.[23]

Seven members of the committee disagreed with these recommendations, and issued a minority report supporting continuation of the Delaney Amendment.

> There is no scientifically defensible way to divide carcinogens or other irreversible toxins into different risk categories. This was the conclusion of Panel I's report on saccharin, and is the predominant scientific opinion for carcinogens in general.[24]

As though to illustrate the truth of this statement in practice, rather than just theory, the majority committee members themselves were unable to agree on which of the three categories to recommend assignation of saccharin, and finally decided to simply leave it up to the FDA.

The minority report also argued that some classes of substances do deserve different degrees of regulatory rigor.

> Irreversible toxicities are deserving of special regulation.... Risks from foods should be lower than other types of risks.... Direct food additives should be regulated differently than other classes of food additives or contaminants.... A safe food policy should involve little agency discretion.... The relative simplicities of our current food safety policy cannot be tampered with because the structure of which it is part can only support regulatory decisions no more complicated than a stop sign on the street corner.[25]

Remember that the Delaney Amendment applies only to one class of toxins—carcinogens—and one category of chemicals—food additives. If you believe the principle of zero tolerance should not apply in this case, then you would surely not be in favor of creating Delaney-type amendments for other situations. On the other hand, if you favor the present Delaney Amendment, then you should force yourself to ask the next question: If zero tolerance is appropriate for carcinogenic food additives, then why not for carcinogenic food contaminants or indirect ingredients, or for carcinogens in air and water, not just food? Why not for other extremely serious nonreversible types of toxicity, notably mutagens (all mutagens are not carcinogenic) and teratogens?

Such expansion has been advocated by many, who point out that the logic which leads one to accept the Delaney Amendment applies equally to all these other situations. Those who disagree, including many who support the Delaney principle for carcinogenic food additives, argue that this view is completely unrealistic, that because our methods of chemical analysis are becoming so powerful and because almost all chemicals inevitably end up in air, food, or water, we would end up banning an incredible number of chemicals. A risk-free existence and complete certainty are impossible, they say, and some risk from toxic chemicals is the price we pay for our standard of living.

Decisions, decisions, decisions....

Postscript

In 1980 and late 1979, three new retrospective epidemiological studies were published; in none of them was a significant correlation observed between bladder cancer and exposure to saccharin. Predictably, newspapers all over the country reported that these studies refuted the rat experiments and proved that saccharin does not cause cancer in people. The *Washington Post* announced "Saccharin Scare Debunked," and the *New York Times* stated, "The evidence contrasts sharply with results from studies that have shown increased risk of cancer from animals."

As R. J. Smith sadly pointed out in *Science* magazine, "Unfortunately, all these reactions are based on an incorrect premise. The three new epidemiological studies do not refute the animal tests, but rather are generally compatible with them."[26] The litany of confusion should be familiar to you. One problem, of course, is that the numbers of subjects studied were too few to detect a relatively weak carcinogenic effect, which is what the rat studies suggest is the case for saccharin. The largest of the three new studies surveyed 3,000 patients with bladder cancer and 6,000 control subjects. The scientists knew in advance that this survey size would be inadequate to detect a saccharin-induced change in cancer incidence of less than 15 percent; they have emphasized that nothing in their study (or the other two) argues against saccharin being a weak carcinogen.

Secondly, as emphasized by the authors of all three papers, their survey populations had not been exposed to large amounts of saccharin *in utero* (the crucial event in the rat studies) and had not been using saccharin long enough to assure completion of a thirty- to fifty-year latent period between exposure and emergence of the cancer. "If this explanation is correct," stated the author of one of the papers, "more consistently positive results may be expected in studies conducted over the next few decades."[27]

Thus, the involved scientists have correctly urged great caution and restraint in the interpretation of their "negative" results, whereas the mass media, because of ignorance or the desire for a story, have presented the public with a one-sided and unjustified interpretation of the results. At least for now, Congress seems to be taking its cue from the media and breathing a collective sigh of relief that the "saccharin scare" is at last behind us.

On September 28, 1979, the heads of the major federal regulatory agencies announced they had reached agreement on a national policy for regulating chemical carcinogens. The policy document strongly supports the validity of animal tests for the prediction of human hazard. As for the Delaney principle of zero tolerance, the language of the document was deliberately left hazy, so that a consensus could be maintained.[28] "In some cases, zero risk will be an appropriate regulatory goal, . . . [but] zero risk will not routinely be considered achievable." Finally, "these principles . . . will not be rigidly and uniformly applied in all cases." As *Science* magazine commented, "Explicit direction, that is not."[29]

Afterword

This book is an unabashed plea for the expansion of research into environment-health issues, and I would like here to make one component of this plea more manifest—the requirement for basic research into *normal* body mechanisms. There is no question that the solutions to environment-health questions ultimately require controlled-exposure experiments and epidemiological studies dealing directly with suspected environmental causes of disease (or health). Research in any field is a slow, expensive, and difficult activity. All these characteristics are greatly magnified when one is dealing with questions of health and disease involving a host of interacting factors often operating over many decades. Frustration and impatience could easily lead us to succumb to the temptation to take shortcuts, to focus all of our efforts on those lines of research—controlled-exposure and epidemiological studies—directly involved in the search for causes. This strategy, while it might be successful on occasion, courts disaster, and one of my aims in this book has been to emphasize how much any real understanding of disease origins depends on a thorough knowledge of basic science—the kidney's handling of vitamin C, amino acid metabolism, iron absorption by the gut, cholesterol carriage in the blood, normal neuroendocrine responses to stress, and biotransformation of lipid-soluble chemicals, to name just a small number of the many basic physiological and biochemical processes we have dealt with.

I firmly believe that, given "a lot of time and patience," biomedical research can provide us with the solutions to many environment-health questions or, as in the case of saccharin and carcinogenesis, it can at least delineate the limits of our knowledge, a crucial antidote against hubris. But in the meantime we scientists must share with the public not just the beauty of our most recent discoveries, but the unsightly depths of our ignorance as well.

Notes

.

Chapter 1

1. S. S. Epstein, *The Politics of Cancer* (San Francisco: Sierra Club Books, 1978), p. 47.
2. Ibid., p. 46.
3. Ibid., p. 47
4. A. B. Hill, "The Environment and Disease: Association or Causation," *Proceedings of the Royal Society of Medicine* 38 (1965):295.
5. Ibid., pp. 295–96.
6. Ibid., p. 297.
7. W. M. Lowrance, *Of Acceptable Risk: Science and the Determination of Safety* (Los Altos, Calif.: William Kaufmann, 1976), pp. 53–54.

Chapter 2

1. P. T. Baker, "Human Biological Variation as an Adaptive Response to the Environment," *Eugenics Quarterly* 13(1966):81.
2. N. Kretchmer, "Lactose and Lactase," *Scientific American*, October, 1972.
3. F. Sargent II, "Environmental Epidemiology: Concepts of Human Adaptability Relevant to Environmental Epidemiology," *American Journal of Public Health* 58(1968):1652.

Chapter 3

1. Cited in W. J. Broad, "Jump in Funding Feeds Research on Nutrition," *Science* 204 (1979):1060–64.
2. Ibid., p. 1060.
3. L. R. Brown and G. W. Finsterbusch, *Man and His Environment: Food* (New York: Harper and Row, 1972), pp. 30–31.

4. R. J. Williams, *Nutrition in a Nutshell* (Garden City N. Y.: Doubleday & Co., 1962), p. 23.

5. N. S. Scrimshaw and V. R. Young, "The Requirements of Human Nutrition," *Scientific American*, October, 1971, p. 54.

6. Ibid, p. 56.

7. R. J. Williams, "Nutritional Individuality," *Human Nature*, June, 1978, p. 46–53.

8. Scrimshaw and Young, p. 64.

9. M. Halberstam, "The A, B-12, C, D, and E of Vitamins," *New York Times Magazine*, March 17, 1974, p. 16.

10. L. Pauling, *Vitamin C, the Common Cold, and Influenza* (San Francisco: W. H. Freeman and Co., 1976).

11. Ibid.

12. Ibid., p. 51.

13. D. W. Cowan, H. S. Diehl, and A. B. Baker, "Vitamins for the Prevention of Colds," *Journal of the American Medical Association* 120(1942):1268–71.

14. M. H. M. Dykes and P. Meier, "Ascorbic Acid and the Common Cold: Evaluation of Its Efficacy and Toxicity," *Journal of the American Medical Association* 231(1975):1073–79.

15. G. Ritzel, "Kritische Beurteilung des Vitamins C als Prophylacticum und Therapeuticum der Erkaltungskrankheiten," *Helvetica Medica Acta* 28(1961):63–68.

16. Dykes and Meier, p. 1073.

17. T. W. Anderson, D. B. W. Reid, and G. H. Beaton, "Vitamin C and the Common Cold: A Double-Blind Trial," *Canadian Medical Association Journal* 107(1972):503–8.

18. Dykes and Meier.

19. T. W. Anderson, "New Horizons for Vitamin C," *Nutrition Today*, January-February, 1977, p. 13.

20. A. Hoffer, "Pellagra and Schizophrenia," *Psychosomatics* 11(1970):8.

21. H. J. Morowitz, "Food for Thought," *Hospital Practice*, November, 1976, p. 179.

Chapter 4

1. N. S. Scrimshaw and V. R. Young, "The Requirements of Human Nutrition," *Scientific American*, October, 1971, p. 59.

2. B. Commoner, "Global Food Supply: A Question of Balance," *Hospital Practice*, December, 1974, p. 120.

3. E. Eckholm, *The Picture of Health; Environmental Sources of Disease* (New York: W. W. Norton, 1977), p. 56.

4. N. S. Scrimshaw, "Through a Glass Darkly," *Nutrition Today*, January-February, 1978, pp. 14–15.

5. N. S. Scrimshaw, "Strengths and Weaknesses of the Committee Approach: An Analysis of Past and Present Recommended Dietary Allowances for Protein in Health and Disease," *New England Journal of Medicine* 294(1976):136.

6. A. E. Harper, P. R. Payne, and J. C. Waterlow "Human Protein Needs," *Lancet*, June 30, 1973, p. 1518.
7. Scrimshaw, "Through a Glass Darkly," p. 15.
8. Scrimshaw, "Strengths and Weaknesses."
9. Scrimshaw, "Through a Glass Darkly."
10. "Strengths and Weakness," pp. 202–3.
11. Harper, Payne, and Waterlow, p. 1518.

Chapter 5

1. A. M. Schmidt, " . . . By Bread Alone," *Nutrition Today*, January-February, 1978, p. 11.
2. Center for Disease Control, *Ten-State Nutrition Survey, 1968–1970, Vol. 4: Biochemical*, DHEW Publication No. (HSM) 72-8132, (Atlanta: Center for Disease Control, 1972).
3. Schmidt, p. 11.
4. W. H. Crosby, "Serum Ferritin and Iron Enrichment," *New England Journal of Medicine* 290(1974):1435–36.
5. Ibid., p. 1435.
6. P. C. Elwood, in "The Experts Debate: A Round-Table Discussion," *Nutrition Today*, March-April, 1972, p. 5.
7. P. C. Elwood, "The Enrichment Debate," *Nutrition Today*, July-August, 1977, p. 19.
8. W. H. Crosby, "The Iron-Enrichment-Now Brouhaha," *Journal of the American Medical Association* 231(1975):1055.
9. Elwood, "Experts Debate" and "Enrichment Debate."
10. G. A. Goldsmith, in "Experts Debate," p. 22.
11. M. M. Wintrobe, "The Proposed Increase in the Iron Fortification of Wheat Products," *Nutrition Today*, November-December, 1973, p. 19.
12. Goldsmith, p. 7.
13. W. H. Crosby, "The Safety of Iron-Fortified Food," *Journal of the American Medical Association* 239(1978):2026.
14. K. S. Olsson, P. A. Heedman, and F. Staugard, "Preclinical Hemochromatosis in a Population on a High-Iron-Fortified Diet," *Journal of the American Medical Association* 239(1978):1999–2000.
15. Crosby, "Safety of Iron-Fortified Food," p. 2027.
16. Elwood, "Enrichment Debate," p. 23.
17. "Anatomy of a Decision," *Nutrition Today*, January-February, 1978, p. 6.
18. W. H. Crosby, "Letter to the Editor," *New England Journal of Medicine* 291(1974):738.
19. "Anatomy of a Decision," p. 7.
20. H. J. Morowitz, "Food for Thought," *Hospital Practice*, November, 1976, p. 179.
21. Elwood, "Enrichment Debate," p. 19.
22. H. A. Pearson, "Experts Debate," p. 8.
23. Goldsmith, p. 13.
24. Schmidt, p. 11.
25. Goldsmith, pp. 16 and 19.

26. Elwood, "Experts Debate," p. 19.
27. Elwood, "Enrichment Debate," p. 24.

Chapter 6

1. J. L. Marx, "Prevention of Heart Disease: Clinical Trials at What Cost?" *Science* 190(1975):764.
2. G. V. Mann, "Diet-Heart: End of an Era," *New England Journal of Medicine* 297(1977):644.
3. J. F. Mueller, "Plain Talk about a Confusing Matter," *Nutrition Today*, May-June, 1974, pp. 19-27.
4. R. I. Levy, "Stroke Decline: Implications and Prospects," *New England Journal of Medicine* 300(1979):490–92.
5. E. P. Benditt, "The Origin of Atherosclerosis," *Scientific American*, February, 1977, pp. 74–85.
6. J. Stamler, "The Primary Prevention of Coronary Heart Disease," *Hospital Practice*, September, 1971, pp. 49–61.
7. Ibid.
8. R. B. McGandy, D. M Hegsted, and F. J. Stare, "Dietary Fats, Carbohydrates, and Atherosclerotic Vascular Disease," *New England Journal of Medicine* 277(1967):417–19.
9. Ibid.
10. J. Brown "Nutritional and Epidemiologic Factors Related to Heart Disease," *World Review of Nutrition and Dietetics* 12(1970):1–42.
11. W. B. Kannel and T. Gordon, *The Framingham Diet Study: Diet and the Regulation of Serum Cholesterol* (Washington, D. C.: Department of Health, Education and Welfare, 1970), Section 24; A. B. Nichols et al., "Daily Nutritional Intake and Serum Lipid Levels: The Tecumseh Study," *American Journal of Clinical Nutrition* 29(1976):1384–92.
12. A. Antonis and I. Bersohn, "Influence of Diet on Serum Lipids in South African White and Bantu Prisoners," *American Journal of Clincial Nutrition* 10(1962):484–99.
13. Mueller, pp. 19–27.
14. N. L. Jacobson, "The Controversy over the Relationship of Animal Fats to Heart Disease," *BioScience* 24(1974):141–48; Mann, pp. 644–50.
15. Mann, p. 645.
16. Mueller, p. 24.
17. F. Ederer et al., "Cancer among Men on Cholesterol-Lowering Diets: Experience from Five Clinical Trials," *Lancet* 2(1972):835–38; M. L. Pearce and S. Dayton, "Incidence of Cancer in Men on a Diet High in Polyunsaturated Fat," *Lancet* 1(1971):464–67.
18. Jacobson, pp. 141–48.
19. Committee of Principal Investigators, "A Cooperative Trial in the Primary Prevention of Ischemic Heart Disease Using Clofibrate," *British Heart Journal* 40(1978):1069–1118.
20. M. F. Oliver, "Cholesterol, Coronaries, Clofibrate and Death," *New England Journal of Medicine* 299(1978):1362.

21. Mann, p. 648.
22. Mueller, pp. 24–25.

Chapter 7

1. L. Levi, *Stress and Distress in Response to Psychosocial Stimuli* (Oxford: Pergamon Press, 1972).
2. H. Selye, *Stress Without Distress* (Philadelphia: J. B. Lippincott, 1974), p. 15.
3. J. Mason and J. Brady, "The Sensitivity of Psychoendocrine Systems to Social and Physical Environment," in *Psychobiological Approaches to Social Behavior*, ed. P. H. Leiderman and D. Shapiro (Stanford: Stanford University Press, 1964), p. 9.
4. J. Mason, "A Review of Psychoendocrine Research on the Pituitary-Adrenal-Cortical System," *Psychosomatic Medicine* 30(1968):596.
5. D. DeWied, "Hormonal Influences on Motivation, Learning, and Memory," *Hospital Practice*, January, 1968.
6. Ibid., p. 89.
7. S. Kiritz and R. H. Moos, "Physiological Effects of Social Environments," *Psychosomatic Medicine* 36(1974):108.
8. Mason, p. 676.
9. S. Levine, "Stress and Behavior," *Scientific American*, January, 1971, p. 136.
10. J. P. Henry and P. M. Stephens, *Stress, Health, and the Social Environment: A Sociobiologic Approach to Medicine* (New York: Springer-Verlag, 1977).
11. J. M. Weiss, "Psychological Factors in Health and Disease," *Scientific American*, June, 1972.
12. Ibid., p. 112.
13. Henry and Stephens.
14. B. Lown and R. L. Verrier, "Neural Activity and Ventricular Fibrillation," *New England Journal of Medicine* 294(1976):1165.
15. Ibid., pp. 1165–70.
16. M. G. Marmot and S. L. Syme, "Acculturation and Coronary Heart Disease in Japanese-Americans," *American Journal of Epidemiology* 104(1976):225–47.
17. C. Stout, J. Morrow, E. N. Brandt, Jr., and S. Wolf. "Unusually Low Incidence of Death from Myocardial Infraction: Study of an Italian-American Community in Pennsylvania," *Journal of the American Medical Association* 188(1964):845–49.
18. C. B. Caffrey, *Behavior Patterns and Personality Characteristics as Related to Prevalence Rates of Coronary Heart Diseases in Trappist and Benedictine Monks*. Ph.D. diss. No. 67-1830, (Ann Arbor: University Microfilms, 1966).
19. Henry and Stephens; J. P. Henry and J. C. Cassel, "Psychosocial Factors in Essential Hypertension: Recent Epidemiologic and Animal Experimental Evidence," *American Journal of Epidemiology* 90(1969):171–200.

20. Henry and Stephens, p. 203.
21. E. D. Freis, "Salt, Volume, and the Prevention of Hypertension," *Circulation* 53(1976):589–94.
22. Ibid.
23. T. H. Holmes and R. H. Rahe, "The Social Readjustment Rating Scale," *Journal of Psychosomatic Research* 11(1967):213–18.
24. R. H. Rahe and R. J. Arthur, "Life Change and Illness Studies: Past History and Future Directions," *Journal of Human Stress*, March, 1978, pp. 3–15.
25. J. G. Rabkin and E. L. Struening, "Life Events, Stress, and Illness," *Science* 194(1976):1015.
26. C. D. Jenkins, "Recent Evidence Supporting Psychologic and Social Risk Factors for Coronary Disease. Pt II," *New England Journal of Medicine* 294(1976):1033.
27. J. Connally, "Life Events Before Myocardial Infarction," *Journal of Human Stress*, December, 1976, p. 8.
28. Jenkins, p. 1034.
29. Ibid.
30. O. R. Galle, W. R. Gove, and J. M. McPherson, "Population Density and Pathology: What Are the Relations for Man?" *Science* 176(1972):23–30.
31. C. Holden, "Cancer and the Mind," *Science* 200(1978):1363–70.
32. M. Friedman and R. H. Rosenman, *Type A Behavior and Your Heart* (New York: Fawcett, 1974).
33. C. D. Jenkins, R. H. Rosenman, and S. J. Zyzanski, "Prediction of Clinical Coronary Heart Disease by a Test for the Coronary-Prone Behavior Pattern," *New England Journal of Medicine* 290(1974):1271.
34. Jenkins, "Recent Evidence."
35. R. S. Lazarus, "A Strategy for Research on Psychological and Social Factors in Hypertension," *Journal of Human Stress*, September, 1979, p. 35.
36. Ibid., p. 38.

Chapter 8
1. B. Commoner, *The Closing Circle* (New York: Knopf, 1971), p. 41.
2. J. McCaull, "Questions for an Old Friend," *Environment* 13(1971):2–9; W. M. Lowrance, *Of Acceptable Risk: Science and the Determination of Safety* (Los Altos, Calif.: William Kaufman, 1976), chap. 6.
3. J. L. Marx, "Drugs during Pregnancy: Do They Affect the Unborn Child?" *Science* 180(1973):174–75.
4. G. Kellermann, C. R. Shaw, and M. Luyten-Kellermann, "Aryl Hydrocarbon Hydroxylase Inducibility and Bronchogenic Carcinoma," *New England Journal of Medicine* 289(1973):934–37.

Chapter 9
1. W. M. Lowrance, *Of Acceptable Risk: Science and the Determination of Safety* (Los Altos, Calif.: William Kaufmann, 1976).
2. Cited in L. J. Carter, "Dispute over Cancer Risk Quantification," *Science* 203(1979):1324–25.

3. W. E. Burrows, "The Cancer Safety Controversy," *New York Times Magazine*, March 25, 1979, p. 56.
4. R. J. Smith, "Toxic Substances: EPA and OSHA Are Reluctant Regulators," *Science* 203(1979):28.
5. Cited in A. Johnson, "The Case Against Poisoning Our Food," *Environment* 21(1979):7.
6. Committee for a Study on Saccharin and Food Safety Policy, *Saccharin: Technical Assessment of Risks and Benefits*, Report No. 1, Assembly of Life Sciences, Institute of Medicine (Washington, D.C.: National Research Council/National Academy of Sciences, 1978); Committee for a Study on Saccharin and Food Safety Policy, *Food Safety Policy: Scientific and Societal Considerations*, Report No. 2, Assembly of Life Sciences, Institute of Medicine (Washington, D.C.: National Research Council/National Academy of Sciences, 1979).
7. S. S. Epstein, "Control of Chemical Pollutants," *Nature* 228(1970):816–19.
8. T. H. Maugh II, "Cancer and Environment: Higginson Speaks Out," *Science* 205(1979):1363–67.
9. See note 6, *Saccharin*.
10. S. S. Epstein, *The Politics of Cancer* (San Francisco: Sierra Club Books, 1978), p. 67.
11. See note 6, *Saccharin*.
12. Ibid., p. 3-61.
13. Ibid., pp. 3-62 and 3-63.
14. Ibid., p. 3-66.
15. Ibid., pp. 3-19 through 3-28.
16. Ibid., p. ES-5.
17. B. N. Ames, "Identifying Environmental Chemicals Causing Mutations and Cancer," *Science* 204(1979):587–93.
18. Epstein, "The Politics of Cancer," p. 54.
19. See note 6, *Saccharin*, pp. 3-75 through 3-103.
20. Ibid.
21. Ibid., p. ES-7.
22. See note 6, *"Food Safety,"* pp. 3-16 and 3-17.
23. Ibid., pp. II and III.
24. Ibid., p. MS-2.
25. Ibid., p. MS-3.
26. R. J. Smith, "Latest Saccharin Tests Kill FDA Proposal," *Science* 208(1980):154.
27. A. S. Morrison and J. E. Buring, "Artificial Sweeteners and Cancer of the Lower Urinary Tract," *New England Journal of Medicine* 302 (1980):541.
28. Cited in R. J. Smith, "Cancer Policy Announced," *Science* 206 (1979): 313.
29. Ibid.

Selected Readings

The following list presents a small fraction of the readings I have used in preparing this book, ones which I feel are most readable by nonscientists desirous of going into greater detail. I have not included primary research articles but have emphasized brief review articles. You will notice that many of them come from the magazine, *Science,* a publication of the American Association for the Advancement of Science (AAAS). This organization has placed great emphasis on public education, and the short reviews published in *Science* (many written by professional science writers) provide accurate and up-to-date summaries not only of research findings but of the politics of science as well. AAAS has recently gone one step further and begun publication of a new magazine, *Science, 80,* aimed specifically at the lay public. The *New York Times* provides the only other vehicle for the detailed objective reporting for the nonscientist of progress in all three of the fields covered by this book—nutrition, stress, and toxicology.

Chapter 1
Bernarde, M. A. *Our Precarious Habitat.* New York: W. W. Norton & Co., 1970.
Eckholm, E. P. *The Picture of Health: Environmental Sources of Disease.* New York: W. W. Norton & Co., 1977.
Epstein, S. S. *The Politics of Cancer.* San Francisco: Sierra Club Books, 1978.

Fisher, R. A. *Statistical Methods and Scientific Inference*. New York: Hafner, 1973.

Fox, J. P; Hall, C. E.; and Elvaback, L. A. *Epidemiology and Disease*. New York: Macmillan, 1970.

Higgenson, J. "Environment and Cancer." In *Fundamental Cancer Research*. pp. 69–92. Baltimore: Williams & Wilkins, 1972.

Hill, A. B. "The Environment and Disease: Association or Causation." *Proceedings of the Royal Society of Medicine* 38(1965):295.

Lowrance, W. W. *Of Acceptable Risk: Science and the Determination of Safety*. Los Altos, Calif.: William Kaufmann, 1976.

World Health Organization. *Health Hazards of the Human Environment*. Geneva: World Health Organization, 1972.

Chapter 2

Dill, D. B., ed. *Handbook of Physiology. Section 4: Adaptation to the Environment*. Washington, D. C.: American Physiological Society, 1964.

Dubos, R. *Man Adapting*. New Haven: Yale University Press, 1965.

Eckholm, E. P. *The Picture of Health: Environmental Sources of Disease*. New York: W. W. Norton, & Co., 1977.

Lee, D. H. K., and Minard, D., eds. *Physiology, Environment, and Man*. New York: Academic Press, 1970.

Slonim, N. B., ed. *Environmental Physiology*. St. Louis: C. V. Mosby Co., 1974.

Vander, A. J.; Sherman, J. H.; and Luciano, D. S. *Human Physiology: The Mechanisms of Body Function*. 3d ed. New York: McGraw-Hill, 1980.

Vander, A. J., ed. *Human Physiology and the Environment in Health and Disease: Readings from Scientific American*. San Francisco; W. H. Freeman and Co., 1976.

Chapter 3

Anderson, T. W. "New Horizons for Vitamin C." *Nutrition Today*, January-February, 1977, p. 6.

Brown, L. R., and Finsterbusch, G. W. *Man and His Environment: Food*. New York: Harper and Row, 1972.

Burkett, D. P. "Economic Development—Not All Bonus." *Nutrition Today*, January-February, 1976, p. 6.

Dykes, M. H. M., and Meier, P. "Ascorbic Acid and the Common Cold: Evaluation of Its Efficacy and Toxicity." *Journal of the American Medical Association* 231(1975):1073.

Halberstam, M. "The A, B-12, C, D, and E of Vitamins." *New York Times Magazine*, March 17, 1974, p. 16.

Harper, A. E. "Those Pesky RDAs." *Nutrition Today*, March-April, 1974, p. 15.

Morowitz, J. P. "Food for Thought." *Hospital Practice*, November, 1976, p. 179.

Passmore, R. "How Vitamin C Deficiency Injures the Body." *Nutrition Today*, March-April, 1977, p. 6.

Pauling, L. "The New Medicine?" *Nutrition Today*, September-October, 1972, p. 18.

————. *Vitamin C, the Common Cold, and Influenza*. San Francisco: W. H. Freeman and Co., 1976.

Scrimshaw, N. S., and Young, V. R. "The Requirements of Human Nutrition." *Scientific American*, October, 1971, p. 51.

Shneour, E. A. *The Malnourished Mind*. Garden City, N. Y.: Anchor Press/Doubleday, 1975.

Task Force on Vitamin Therapy in Psychiatry. "Megavitamin and Orthomolecular Therapy in Psychiatry." *Nutrition Reviews*, Supplement, July, 1974, p. 44.

Vander, A. J.; Sherman, J. H.; and Luciano, D. S. *Human Physiology: The Mechanisms of Body Function*. 3d ed. New York: McGraw-Hill, 1980.

Williams, R. J. "Nutritional Individuality." *Human Nature*, June, 1978, p. 46.

Winikoff, B. "Nutrition, Population, and Health: Some Implications for Policy." *Science* 200(1978):895.

Wohl, M. G., and Goodhart, R. S. *Modern Nutrition in Health and Disease*. 5th ed. Philadelphia: Lea & Febiger, 1975.

Young, V. R., and Scrimshaw, N. S. "The Physiology of Starvation." *Scientific American*, October, 1971, p. 51.

Chapter 4

Berg, A. "Nutrition, Development, and Population Growth." *Population Bulletin* 29, no. 1(1973).

Harper, A. E. "Adaptability and Amino Acid Requirements." In *Metabolic Adaptation and Nutrition*. Pan-American Health Organization. Vol. 222. 1971.

————."Those Pesky RDAs." *Nutrition Today*, March-April, 1974, p. 15.

Harper, A. E.; Payne, P. R.; and Waterlow, J. C. "Human Protein Needs." *Lancet*, June 30, 1973, p. 1518.

"Human Energy and Protein Requirements." *Lancet*, August 18, 1973, p. 363.

Lappe, F. M. *Diet for a Small Planet*. New York: Ballantine Books, 1971.

Scrimshaw, N. S. "Strengths and Weaknesses of the Committee Approach: An Analysis of Past and Present Recommended Dietary Allowances for Protein in Health and Disease." *New England Journal of Medicine*. 294(1976):136 and 198.

————. "Through a Glass Darkly." *Nutrition Today*, January-February, 1978, p. 14.

Young, R. "Protein Requirements of Man." *Journal of Nutrition* 103 (1973):1164.

Chapter 5

"Anatomy of a Decision." *Nutrition Today*, January-February, 1978, p. 6.

Crosby, W. H. "The Safety of Iron-Fortified Food." *Journal of the American Medical Association* 239(1978):2026.

————. "Serum Ferritin and Iron Enrichment." *New England Journal of Medicine.* 290(1974):1435.

————. "Who Needs Iron?" *New England Journal of Medicine* 297(1977):543.

Crosby, W. H., et al. "The Dietary Iron Controversy." *Nutrition Today,* March-April, 1972.

Elwood, P. C. "The Enrichment Debate." *Nutrition Today,* July-August, 1977, p. 18.

Norman, C. "Iron Enrichment." *Nutrition Today,* November-December, 1973.

Chapter 6

Benditt, E. P. "The Origin of Atherosclerosis." *Scientific American,* February, 1977, p. 74.

Biss, K., et al. "Some Unique Biological Characteristics of the Masai of East Africa." *New England Journal of Medicine* 284(1971):694.

Blackburn, H.; Chapman, J. M.; Dawber, T. R.; Doyle, J. T.; Epstein, F. H.; Kannel, W. B.; Keys, A.; Moore, F. E.; Paul, O.; Stamler, J.; Taylor, H. L. "Revised Data for 1970 ICHD Report: Letter to the Editor." *American Heart Journal* 94(1977):539–40.

Broad, W. J. "Jump in Funding Feeds Research on Nutrition." *Science* 204(1979):1060.

————. "NIH Deals Gingerly with Diet-Disease Link." *Science* 204(1979):1175.

Garraway, W. M., et al. "The Declining Incidence of Stroke." *New England Journal of Medicine* 300(1979):449.

Epstein, F. H. "Coronary Heart Disease Epidemiology Revisited." *Circulation* 48(1973):185.

Inter-Society Commission for Heart Disease Resources, Atherosclerosis Study Group and Epidemiology Study Group. "Primary Prevention of the Atherosclerotic Diseases." *Circulation* 42(1970):A55–A95.

Jacobson, N. L. "The Controversy over the Relationship of Animal Fats to Heart Disease." *BioScience* 24(1974):141.

Keys, A. "Bias and Misrepresentation Revisited: Perspective on Saturated Fat." *American Journal of Clinical Nutrition* 27(1974):188.

Kolata, G. B. "Atherosclerotic Plaques: Competing Theories Guide Research." *Science* 194(1976):592.

Kolata, G. B., and Marx, J. L. "Epidemiology of Heart Disease: Search for Causes." *Science* 194(1976):509.

Mann, G. V. "Diet-Heart: End of an Era." *New England Journal of Medicine* 297(1977):644.

Marx, J. L. "Atherosclerosis: The Cholesterol Connection." *Science* 194 (1976):711.

————. "The HDL: The Good Cholesterol Carriers?" *Science* 205(1979):677.

McGandy, R. B.; Hegsted, D. M.; and Stare, F. J. "Dietary Fate, Carbohydrates, and Atherosclerotic Vascular Disease." *New England Journal of Medicine.* 277(1971):417 and 469.

Mueller, J. F. "Plain Talk about a Confusing Matter." *Nutrition Today*, May-June, 1974, p. 19.

Pooling Project Cooperative Group. "Relationship of Blood Pressure, Serum Cholesterol, Smoking Habit, Relative Weight and ECG Abnormalities to Incidence of Major Coronary Events: Final Report of the National Cooperative Pooling Project." *Journal of Chronic Diseases* 31(1978):201–306.

Reiser, R. "Oversimplification of Diet: Coronary Heart Disease Relationships and Exaggerated Diet Recommendations." *American Journal of Clinical Nutrition* 31(1978):865.

Ross, R., and Glomsett, J. A. "Atherosclerosis and the Arterial Smooth Muscle Cell." *Science* 180(1973):1332.

Stamler, J. "The Primary Prevention of Coronary Heart Disease." *Hospital Practice*, September, 1971, p. 49.

Wissler, R. W. "Development of the Atherosclerotic Plaque." *Hospital Practice*, March, 1973.

Chapter 7

Benson, H. *The Relaxation Response.* New York: William Morrow & Co., 1975.

Calhoun, J. B. "Population Density and Social Pathology." *Scientific American*, February, 1962, p. 139.

Friedman, M., and Rosenman, R. H. *Type A Behavior and Your Heart.* New York; Fawcett, 1974.

Henry, J. P., and Stephens, P. M. *Stress, Health, and the Social Environment: A Sociobiologic Approach to Medicine.* New York: Springer-Verlag, 1977.

Holden, C. "Cancer and the Mind." *Science* 200(1978):1363.

Jenkins, C. D. "Recent Evidence Supporting Psychologic and Social Risk Factors for Coronary Disease. Pt. II. *New England Journal of Medicine* 294(1976):987 and 1033.

Kaplan, N. M. "Stress, the Sympathetic Nervous System and Hypertension." *Journal of Human Stress*, September, 1978, p. 29.

Kiritz, S., and Moos, R. H. "Physiological Effects of Social Environments." *Psychosomatic Medicine* 36(1974):96.

Lazarus, R. S. "A Strategy for Research on Psychological and Social Factors in Hypertension." *Journal of Human Stress*, September, 1978, p. 35.

Levi, L. *Stress and Distress in Response to Psychological Stimuli.* Oxford: Pergamon Press, 1972.

Levine, S. "Stress and Behavior." *Scientific American*, January, 1971, p. 136.

Lynch, J. J. *The Broken Heart: The Medical Consequences of Loneliness.* New York: Basic Books, 1977.

Marx, J. L. "Stress: Role in Hypertension Debated." *Science*, 198(1977):905.

Rabkin, J. G., and Struening, E. L. "Life Events, Stress, and Illness." *Science* 194(1976):1013.

Rahe, R. H., and Arthur, R. J. "Life Change and Illness Studies: Past History and Future Directions." *Journal of Human Stress*, March, 1978, p. 3.

Rahe, R. H.; Rubin, R. T.; and Arthur, R. J. "The Three Investigators Study: Serum Uric Acid, Cholesterol, and Cortisol Variability During Stresses of Everyday Life." *Psychosomatic Medicine* 36(1974):258.

Selye, H. *Stress Without Distress*. New York: J. B. Lippincott, 1974.

Vander, A. J.; Sherman, J. H.; and Luciano, D. S. *Human Physiology: The Mechanisms of Body Function*. 3d. ed. New York; McGraw-Hill, 1980.

Weiss, J. M. "Psychological Factors in Health and Disease." *Scientific American*, June, 1972.

Chapter 8

Arena, J. M. "Contamination of the Ideal Food." *Nutrition Today*, Winter, 1970, p. 2.

Commoner, B. *The Closing Circle: Man, Nature, and Technology*. New York; Knopf, 1971.

Conney, A. H., and Burns, J. J. "Metabolic Interactions Among Environmental Chemicals and Drugs." *Science* 178(1972):576.

Horning, M. G.; Butler, C. M.; Nowlin, J.; and Hill, R. M. "Drug Metabolism in the Human Neonate." *Life Sciences* 16(1977):651.

Kappas, A., and Alvares, A. P. "How the Liver Metabolizes Foreign Substances." *Scientific American*, June, 1975.

Koch-Weser, J. "Bioavailability of Drugs." *New England Journal of Medicine* 291(1974):233 and 503.

Lee, D. H. K., ed. *Handbook of Physiology. Section 9: Reactions to Environmental Agents*. Bethesda, Md.: American Physiological Society, 1977.

Lieber, C. S. "The Metabolism of Alcohol." *Scientific American*, March, 1976.

Loomis, T. A. *Essentials of Toxicology*. Philadelphia: Lea & Febiger, 1968.

Lowrance, W. W. *Of Acceptable Risk: Science and the Determination of Safety*. Los Altos, Calif.: William Kaufmann, 1976.

McCaull, J. "Questions for an Old Friend." *Evnironment* 13(1971):6.

Peakall, D. B. "Pesticides and the Reproduction of Birds." *Scientific American*, April, 1970.

Schroeder, H. A. *The Poisons Around Us*. Bloomington: Indiana University Press, 1974.

Shakman, R. A. "Nutritional Influences on the Toxicity of Environmental Pollutants." *Archives Environmental Health* 28(1974):105.

Strauss, B. S. "Repair of DNA in Mammalian Cells." *Life Sciences* 15 (1976):1685.

Vander, A. J.; Sherman, J. H.; and Luciano, D. S. *Human Physiology: The Mechanisms of Body Function*. 3d ed. New York: McGraw-Hill, 1980.

Chapter 9

Ames, B. N. "Identifying Environmental Chemicals Causing Mutation and Cancer." *Science* 204(1979):587.

Cairns, J. "The Cancer Problem." *Scientific American*, November, 1975.

Committee for a Study on Saccharin and Food Safety Policy. *Saccharin: Technical Assessment of Risks and Benefits*. Report No 1. Assembly of Life

Sciences, Institute of Medicine. Washington, D.C.: National Research Council/National Academy of Sciences, 1978.

————. *Food Safety Policy: Scientific and Societal Considerations.* Report No. 2. Assembly of Life Sciences, Institute of Medicine. Washington, D.C.: National Research Council/National Academy of Sciences, 1979.

Coon, J. M. "The Delaney Clause." *Preventive Medicine* 2(1973):150.

Cornfield, J. "Carcinogenic Risk Assessment." *Science* 198(1977):693.

Devoret, R. "Bacterial Tests for Potential Carcinogens." *Scientific American,* August, 1979.

Epstein, S. S. "The Delaney Amendment." *Preventive Medicine* 2(1973):140.

————. *The Politics of Cancer.* San Francisco: Sierra Club Books, 1978.

Kennedy, D. "What Animal Research Says About Cancer." *Human Nature,* May, 1978.

Marx, J. L. "Tumor Promoters: Carcinogenesis Acts More Complicated." *Science* 201(1978):515.

Maugh, T. H. II. "Chemical Carcinogenesis: A Long-Neglected Field Blooms." *Science* 183(1974):940.

————. "Chemical Carcinogenesis: How Dangerous Are Low Doses?" *Science* 202(1978):37.

Smith, R. J. "Latest Saccharin Tests Kill FDA Proposal." *Science* 208 (1980):154.

Weinberg, A. M. "Science and Trans-Science." *Minerva* 10(1972):209.

Index

and crowding, 228
and DDT, 295
disease-producing effects of, 218–
21
effects of, 202–3
Cortisone, 200
Cost-benefit analysis, 302
CRH, 201
Critical periods, 52
Crosby, William H., 139, 140, 141,
145, 148, 149
Crowding, 227–29
and human disease, 244–45
Cycasin, 255, 297
Cyclamates, 257, 310
Cytochrome P-450, 284

DDT, 259–61
effects on reproduction of, 294–95
in fat, 273–74
in fetal blood, 271
and the MES, 285–86
in milk, 268
and protein deficiency, 289
renal excretion of, 280
Deamination, 113
in protein homeostasis, 115–16
Delaney amendment, 305–9, 340–
42
Denial, 212
DES, 53
Detoxification, 282
Developmental acclimatizations,
61–62
Diabetes, 218–19
Dietary changes in industrialized
countries, 77
Dietary Goals for the United States,
154
Dietary lipid
and coronary heart disease, 181–
84
and plasma cholesterol, 185–86
Diet-heart hypothesis, 154–56
animal experiments, 175–76
epidemiological data, 176–84
Diethylstilbestrol. *See* DES

Disease patterns, 3–11
DNA
and cancer, 314
structure of, 47
DNA repair, 56–57
and cancer, 314
Dose-response for carcinogens, 321–
22
Double-blind study, 28
Drug metabolizing enzymes, 283
Dykes, M. H. M., 106, 107

Eckholm, Erick, 122
E. coli, 49, 50
Egg cholesterol. *See* Cholesterol, egg
Elwood, P. C., 140, 142, 143, 146,
149, 150, 151
End-product inhibition, 51
Environmental chemicals
biotransformation of, 281–97
excretion of, 275–81
internal distribution of, 271
storage of, 271–75
Enzyme activity, alteration of, 50–
51
Enzyme induction, 49
Enzyme repression, 49–50
Enzymes defined, 46
EPA, 301, 304
Epidemiological data
for coronary heart disease, 176–
84
for psychosocial stress, 233–48
for saccharin, 343–44
Epidemiology, 12–22, 335–40
Epinephrine, 198
Epoxide, 290
Epstein, Samuel S., 15, 320, 336,
337
Error-signal, 43
Eskimos, 63
Essential fatty acids, 80–81
Essential nutrients
defined, 80
homeostasis of, 79–89
Estrogen, 204, 294
Ethanol, 286, 288

for coronary heart disease, 177–
84
Rosenman, Ray H., 246, 247
Roseto, Pennsylvania, 181, 234

Saccharin
    Ames test for, 335
    benefits of, 339–40
    dose-response extrapolation, 328
    epidemiology of, 335–40, 343–44
    lab animal data on, 322–24
    metabolism of, 309–12
    NAS committee decisions on,
        341–42
    as a promotor, 330
    use of, 310–11
Safe allowances for protein, 127–
    31
Salmonella tests, 331
Salt. See Sodium
Sargent, Frederick, 67
Saturated fatty acids
    and cancer, 190
    defined, 158
    effects on plasma cholesterol, 173
Saturation, nutrient, 93
Schmidt, Alexander M., 134, 135,
    136, 150
Scrimshaw, Nevin S., 121, 124, 126,
    127, 130, 131
Selye, Hans, 196, 197, 207, 221
Sickle-cell anemia, 54–56
Significance, statistical, 33
Silent Spring, 259
Single-hit model, 315, 326
Skin, foreign chemicals and, 268
Skin cancer, 314
Smith, R. J., 343
Sodium
    homeostasis of, 44
    and hypertension, 236
Species differences, 299
Specific hungers, 84–85
Stamler, Jeremiah, 154
Standard deviation, 32
Statistical methods, 31–37
Status incongruity, 244

Steroids, 156
Sterols, 156
Stone, Irwin, 101
Storage depots, 87–88
Stress. See also Psychosocial stress
    defined, 195–96
    in infancy, 213–14
    and learning, 205–10
Stroke, 159
Struening, Elmer L., 240
Sympathetic nervous system
    and coronary heart disease, 215–
        18
    effects of, 199
    and fight-or-flight, 198–200
Synthetic chemicals, 256–57

Temperature regulation, 40–42
Ten-State Nutrition Survey, 135,
    139
Testosterone, 204
Thalidomide, 21, 53
Thiamine, 88
Thomas, Lewis, 21, 142, 251
Threshold, 325–26
Thyroxin, 88
T lymphocytes, 318
Tolerance levels, 306
Total calories, 89
    distribution of, 75
    and protein homeostasis, 116–17
Toxic chemicals, classification of,
    255–56
Trace elements defined, 81
Transcendental meditation, 249–50
Transcription, 49
Transport mechanisms, 262–68
Triglycerides, 157
2-AFF, 328
Two-generation tests, 320
    for saccharin, 322–23
Type A behavior, 246–48

Unsaturated fatty acids, 157. See
    also Polyunsaturated fatty
    acids
Urea, 114

Vasopressin, 203
  and learning, 210
Ventricular fibrillation, 159
  and psychosocial stress, 231–33
Vernix caseosa, 272
Verrier, Richard L., 231, 232
Very low density lipoproteins. *See*
  VLDL
Virchow, Rudolf, 164
Vitamin B$_{12}$, 83, 97–98
Vitamin C, 100–108
Vitamin C and the Common Cold,
  105
Vitamin D, plasma cholesterol and,
  175
Vitamin K, 83

Vitamins, function of, 81
VLDL, 158

Weak acids, 265
Weak bases, 265
Weiss, Jay, 225, 226
White, Paul Dudley, 154
White House Conference on Food,
  Nutrition, and Health, 135
Williams, Roger J., 96
Wintrobe, Maxwell M., 144
Wolfe, Sidney, 304
Work-pressure, disease and, 243–44

Xeroderma pigmentosa, 314

Young, Vernon R., 121